CLINICAL MANAGEMENT OF COMPLICATED URINARY TRACT INFECTION

Edited by **Ahmad Ali Nikibakhsh**

Clinical Management of Complicated Urinary Tract Infection
Edited by Ahmad Ali Nikibakhsh

Published by InTech
Janeza Trdine 9, 51000 Rijeka, Croatia

Publishing Process Manager Dragana Manestar

Technical Editor Teodora Smiljanic

Cover Designer InTech Design Team

Additional hard copies can be obtained from orders@intechopen.com

Clinical Management of Complicated Urinary Tract Infection,
Edited by Ahmad Ali Nikibakhsh
p. cm.
ISBN 978-953-307-393-4

For EU product safety concerns:
IN TECH d.o.o., Prolaz Marije Krucifikse Kozulić 3, 51000 Rijeka, Croatia,
info@intechopen.com or visit our website at intechopen.com.

Meet the editor

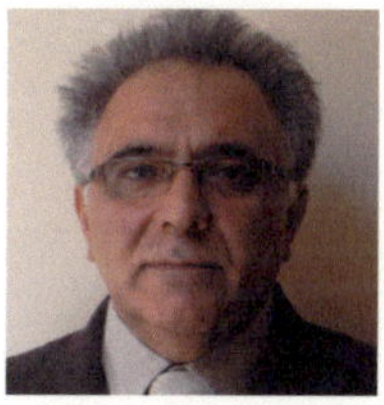

Ahmad Ali Nikibakhsh is an associated professor in pediatric nephrology, head of The Department of Pediatrics as well as a member of education council and esearch council at Urmia University of Medical Sciences. He is also a member of urology-nephrology and transplantation research center and a member of Iranian society of nephrology. He has been involved in training medical students and pediatric residents in Urmia University of Medical Science, Mothahry and Imam Khomainy Hospital for more than 20 years . He has dedicated the period of his sabbatical leave to improving his clinical and research experiences in nephrology, dialysis and transplantation in Regina Margherita Children Hospital and Nephrology, Dialysis and Transplantation center in Turin, Italy. He has authored more than 25 papers in urology and nephrology journals and 50 Congress presentations in international congresses - most of them on complicated urinary tract infection in children.

Contents

Preface

Complicated urinary tract infections (cUTIs) are a major cause of hospital admissions and are associated with significant morbidity and health care costs. Knowledge of baseline risk of urinary tract infection can help clinicians to make informed diagnostic and therapeutic decisions. Prevalence rates of UTI vary by age, gender, race, and other predisposing risk factors. In this regard, this book provides comprehensive information on etiology, epidemiology, immunology, pathology, pathogenic mechanisms, symptomatology, investigation and management of urinary tract infection. The chapters cover common problems in urinary tract infection and put emphasis on making the correct clinical decision and choosing the appropriate therapeutic approach.

Topics of Chapters are organized to address all of the major complicated conditions frequently seen in urinary tract infection. The authors have paid particular attention to urological problem like the outcome of patients with vesicoureteric reflux, the factors affecting renal scarring, obstructive uropathy, voiding dysfunction and catheter associated problems.

This book will be indispensable for all professionals involved in the medical care of patients with urinary tract infection.

My sincere thanks to all expert contributors from different countries because of the recommended therapeutic approachs which will be gauged at an international standard applicable to most regional referral centers.

Ahmad Ali Nikibakhsh
Health Science Center Motahari Hospital
Pediatric Department Urmia,
IRAN

Part 1

Epidemiology of Urinary Tract Infection

1

Epidemiology and Control of Urinary Tract Infections in Intensive Care Patients

Antonella Agodi and Martina Barchitta
Department GF Ingrassia,
University of Catania
Italy

1. Introduction

Healthcare-associated infections (HAIs) are one of the most common complications in hospitalized patients, leading to increased hospitalization, morbidity and mortality and associated with additional costs (Geffers and Gastmeier, 2011).

Urinary tract infection (UTI) is common in hospitalized patients. It has been reported that in U.S. hospitals, among adults and children outside of the intensive care units (ICUs), the urinary tract is the most common site of HAI, accounting for 36% of infections, followed by surgical site infections (20%), bloodstream infections and pneumonia (11%, each) and other infection types (all 22%) (Klevens et al., 2007).

Almost all healthcare-associated UTIs are caused by instrumental urinary tract procedures. In fact, the presence of a foreign body in the urinary tract predisposes the patient to UTI and alters the body's ability to eradicate bacteria (Gray et al., 2010). It has been estimated that more than 80% of UTIs are associated with an indwelling catheter (Anderson et al., 2007) and notably, catheter-associated UTI (CAUTI) has been related with such complications that prolonged hospital stay, and increased cost, morbidity and mortality (Gould et al., 2009).

Urologic patients should be considered at high risk for a healthcare-associated UTI, because they are usually exposed both to urethral catheterization and instrumentation of the urinary tract. In a surveillance study conducted in an urologic clinic of an Italian university hospital the incidence of symptomatic UTIs was 1.4 per 1000 patient-days (Agodi et al., 2007).

1.1 Epidemiology of UTI in intensive care units

Since of intrinsic (such as, severity of illness or impaired immunity) and extrinsic (such as, devise exposure: mechanical ventilation, urinary and central line catheterization) risk factors, patients admitted in ICUs are at high risk of HAIs (Lambert et al., 2011). Particularly, in Europe, the *Annual Epidemiological Report on Communicable Diseases in Europe* of the European Centre for Disease Prevention and Control (ECDC, 2009), show that 3% of patients staying more than two days in ICUs, acquire bloodstream infections, and 6.2% of patients acquire pneumonia.

UTI is one of the most common infection in ICU. The mean incidence density of UTI in patients admitted in European ICUs is 5.4 UTI episodes per 1000 patient-days. The majority of UTI (96.2%) are associated with the use of a urinary catheter (HELICS, 2005), that is the most important risk factor for development of UTI (Meddings et al., 2010). It has been reported that about 15% - 25% of patients may be exposed to short-term indwelling urinary catheters (Warren JW, 2001) and in several cases, catheters are placed for inappropriate indications. Urinary catheters are used frequently in ICUs for correct monitoring of urinary output, but, once inserted, catheters tend to remain in place until appropriate indications for their use end and thus CAUTI incidence increases as the duration of catheter use increases. Use of urinary catheters in the ICU causes breaches in the mucosa or may provide a surface for colonization, thus, increasing the incidence of CAUTI. The risk for infection is at least 5% per day of catheterization (Tissot et al., 2001; Elpern et al., 2009).

Other factors have been reported as potential risk factors for CAUTI including constitutional factors such as female gender, pregnancy and older age and potential modifiable factors such as poor nutrition, fecal incontinence, use of systemic antibiotics, severity of illness, impaired immune system function, and elevated creatinine level (Gray, 2010).

A recent multicenter study was conducted in a cohort of patients from 10 countries (Argentina, Brazil, Colombia, Greece, India, Lebanon, Mexico, Morocco, Peru, and Turkey) to estimate the excess length of stay (LOS) and mortality in ICU due to CAUTI. Results show that CAUTI lead to a small increase LOS in ICU, particularly, prolonging length of ICU stay by an average of 1.59 days, but CAUTI increase the risk of death by 15% (Rosenthal et al., 2011).

Thus, it is necessary to implement every possible preventive measure that have proven useful in the prevention of CAUTI.

Furthermore, UTIs are often underdiagnosed due the lack of physician requesting systematic laboratory tests and urine cultures (Agodi et al., 2007). Diagnosis, particularly in the ICU setting, is very difficult, as asymptomatic bacteriuria may be hard to be differentiated from symptomatic UTI (Shuman and Chenoweth, 2010).

The National Healthcare Safety Network (NHSN) is a system for the surveillance of HAI that aggregates data of surveillance, reported by hospitals participating in the network, into a single national database (Edwards et al., 2007). In the framework of the "Patient Safety component" of the NHSN, data are collected using standardized methods and definitions and are grouped into specific module protocols. Particularly, in the device-associated module infection control professionals collect data on CAUTIs that occur in patients staying in a patient care location such as an ICU, specialty care area, or ward. Indicators are calculated in terms of urinary catheter associated infection rate and urinary catheter utilization ratio (Table 1).

Indicator	
Urinary catheter associated infection rate	$\frac{\text{Number of urinary catheter-associated UTI}}{\text{Number of urinary catheter-days}} \times 1000$
Urinary catheter utilization ratio	$\frac{\text{Number of urinary catheter-days}}{\text{Number of patient-days}}$

Table 1. Calculation of urinary catheter-associated infection rate and urinary catheter utilization ratio.

The NHSN reports that in 2006 pooled mean urinary catheter utilization ratios in ICU and non-ICU wards ranged from 0.23 in inpatient medical/surgical ward to 0.91 in trauma ICU. The pooled mean of CAUTI rates ranged from 3.1 infections per 1000 catheter-days in medical/surgical ICU to 7.5 infections per 1000 catheter-days in burn ICUs.

In Europe, the German National Reference Centre for surveillance of nosocomial infections was started in 1997 creating a nationwide surveillance system: the Krankenhaus Infektions Surveillance System (KISS) (Gastmeier et al., 2008). The surveillance methods of the National Nosocomial Infections Surveillance (NNIS) System (Garner et al. 1988; Emori et al., 1991) were used and for diagnosing HAIs the definitions of the CDC were adopted. Surveillance data obtained from January 2005 to December 2009 in German ICUs, report an urinary catheter utilization ratio of 0.81 and a CAUTI rate of 1.97 per 1000 device-days (Geffers and Gastmeier, 2011).

1.2 Case definitions of UTI

Major challenges in appraising the quality of evidence in the CAUTI literature are represented by the limitations due to heterogeneity of definitions of UTI used in various published studies. Researchers have often used numerous different definitions for UTI, ranging from simple bacteriuria to symptomatic infection defined by combinations of bacteriuria and various signs and symptoms. Furthermore, the heterogeneity of definitions may reduce the quality of evidence for a given intervention and often precludes meta-analyses (Gould et al., 2009).

Case definition of UTI proposed by the Hospitals in Europe Link for Infection Control through Surveillance (HELICS) system is reported in Table 2 (HELICS-ICU, 2004). Particularly, in the HELICS protocol three different types of UTIs are identified and defined: microbiologically confirmed symptomatic UTI (UTI-A), not microbiologically confirmed symptomatic UTI (UTI-B) and asymptomatic bacteriuria (UTI-C) (HELICS-ICU, 2004). Of note is that UTIs may be added or not, optionally, in the HELICS protocol surveillance.

The case definitions of UTI by the HELICS are similar to the case definition by the Centers for Disease Control and Prevention/National Healthcare Safety Network (CDC/NHSN) (NHSN Manual; Horan et al., 2008), where CAUTIs are classified into two groups with specific sets of criteria for each: symptomatic urinary tract infections (SUTI) and asymptomatic bacteriuria (ASB). The only difference is that, in the HELICS, asymptomatic bacteriuria is defined as the subcategory UTI-C, and not as a separate category. Otherwise, the subcategories UTI-A and UTI-B are the same as respectively criterion 1 and 2 of the CDC/NHSN definition of symptomatic urinary tract infection. NHSN in January 2009 has revised the UTI definition criteria. Among the changes are removal of the ASB criterion and refinement of the criteria for defining symptomatic SUTI. The time period for follow-up surveillance after catheter removal also has been shortened from 7 days to 48 hours to align with other device-associated infections (NHSN Manual).

1.3 Pathogenesis of UTIs

Microorganisms causing CAUTI can be acquired by an endogenous source (such as, via meatal, rectal, or vaginal colonization) or an exogenous one (such as, via contaminated hands of healthcare personnel or devices).

UTI-A: microbiologically confirmed symptomatic UTI	Patient has at least one of the following signs of symptoms with no other recognized cause: - Fever (>38°C) - Urgency - Frequency - Dysuria - Suprapubic tenderness and Patient has a positive urine culture ($\geq 10^5$ microorganisms per ml of urine) with no more than two species of microorganisms
UTI-B: not microbiologically confirmed symptomatic UTI	Patient has at least two of the following with no other recognized cause: - Fever (>38°C) - Urgency - Frequency - Dysuria - Suprapubic tenderness and, at least one of the following: - Positive dipstick for leukocyte esterase and/or nitrate - Pyuria urine specimen with ≥10 WBC/ml or ≥ 3 WBC/high-power field of unspun urine - Organisms seen on Gram stain of unspun urine - At least two urine cultures with repeated isolation of the same uropathogen (gram-negative bacteria or *S. saprophyticus*) with $\geq 10^2$ colonies/ml urine in nonvoided specimens $\leq 10^5$ colonies/ml of a single uropathogen (gram-negative bacteria or *S. saprophyticus*) in a patient being treated with effective antimicrobial agent for a urinary infection - Physician diagnosis of a urinary tract infection - Physician institutes appropriate therapy for a urinary - infection
UTI-C: asymptomatic bacteriuria	Patient has no fever (>38°C), urgency, frequency, dysuria, or suprapubic tenderness and either of the following criteria: 1. Patient has had an indwelling urinary catheter within 7 days before urine is cultured and Patient has a urine culture, that is, $\geq 10^5$ microorganisms per ml of urine with no more than two species of microorganisms. 2. Patient has not had an indwelling urinary catheter within 7 days before the first positive culture and Patient has had at least two positive urine cultures $\geq 10^5$ microorganisms per mm^3 of urine with repeated isolation of the same microorganism and no more than two species of microorganisms

Table 2. Case definition of Urinary Tract Infection (HELICS-ICU, 2004).

The NHSN reported that between 2006-2007, the most frequent pathogens associated with CAUTI were *Escherichia coli* (21.4%) and *Candida* spp. (21.0%), followed by *Enterococcus* spp. (14.9%), *Pseudomonas aeruginosa* (10.0%), *Klebsiella pneumoniae* (7.7%), and *Enterobacter* spp. (4.1%). A smaller proportion of CAUTI was caused by other gram-negative bacteria or by *Staphylococcus* spp. (Hidron et al., 2008).

Finally, it is important to underline that bacteriuria associated to CAUTI commonly leads to antimicrobial use, that would have been avoidable, as well as to urinary drainage systems that are often reservoirs for multidrug-resistant bacteria and a potential source of transmission to other patients (Gould et al., 2009).

As reported in the *Annual Epidemiological Report on Communicable Diseases in Europe* (ECDC, 2010), the antimicrobial resistance of microorganisms is to be considered the most important disease threat. In 2008 a Europe-wide increase of resistance to all antibiotic classes under surveillance was observed for the most common Gram-negative bacteria - *E. coli* - responsible for bacteraemia and UTIs.

1.4 Prevention of CAUTI

CAUTIs are generally considered an avoidable complication. It has been estimated that between 17% and 69% of all observed CAUTIs may be prevented by implementation of an evidence based prevention program that is particularly important in the ICU setting with a high prevalence of urinary catheterization and a high percentage of patients with comorbidities (Gould et al., 2009).

The CDC/Healthcare Infection Control Practices Advisory Committee (HICPAC) published a specific document - *Guideline for Prevention of Catheter-associated Urinary Tract Infections* – that addresses the prevention of CAUTI for patients with short- or long-term urinary catheterization admitted in any type of healthcare facility and evaluates the evidence for several options of methods of urinary drainage, including intermittent catheterization, external catheters, and suprapubic catheters (Gould et al., 2009). The guideline is based on a specific systematic review of the best available evidence on CAUTI prevention; it uses the Grading of Recommendations Assessment, Development and Evaluation (GRADE) approach (Atkins et al., 2004; Guyatt et al., 2008a; Guyatt et al. 2008b) in order to provide clear links between the available evidence and the resulting recommendations.

Particularly, in this document, recommendations include: i) appropriate urinary catheter use; ii) proper techniques for urinary catheter insertion; iii) proper techniques for urinary catheter maintenance; iv) quality improvement programs; v) administrative infrastructure; and vi) surveillance.

As suggested by the Authors of this guideline further research in order to prevent CAUTIs should focuse on catheter materials (antimicrobial and antiseptic-impregnated catheters and standard catheters), appropriate urinary catheter use (in incontinent patients and appropriate indications for continued use in postoperative patients), use of antiseptics (for periurethral cleaning prior to catheter insertion and to prevent CAUTI), alternatives to indwelling urethral catheters and bag drainage (suprapubic catheters, urethral catheters, use of catheter valves and other alternative methods of urinary drainage), optimal methods for preventing encrustation in long-term catheterized patients, other prevention measures and prevention of transmission of pathogens colonizing urinary drainage systems.

A specific recommendation for the appropriate urinary catheter use (category IB) is: "Minimize urinary catheter use and duration of use in all patients, particularly those at higher risk for CAUTI or mortality from catheterization such as women, the elderly, and patients with impaired immunity" (Gould et al., 2009).

In this contest, a recent study (Elpern et al., 2009) has been conducted in a medical ICU in order to implement and evaluate the efficacy of an intervention, based on the decreasing use of urinary catheters, to reduce CAUTI. Results of this study report that the implementation of an intervention targeting the appropriate use of indwelling urinary catheters may result in a significant reduction in the duration of catheterization as well as in the occurrences of CAUTIs.

A systematic literature review and meta-analysis was performed to evaluate the effect of interventions that remind clinicians of the presence of urinary catheters to prompt the timely removal of catheters during hospitalization. Results of the meta-analysis report that the rate of CAUTI was significantly reduced by 52% with the use of a reminder or stop order. Furthermore, the mean duration of catheterization decreased by 37%. Thus, interventions to routinely prompt physicians or nurses to remove unnecessary urinary catheters appear to reduce the rate of CAUTI and should be strongly considered to enhance the safety of hospitalized patients (Medding et al., 2010).

The Institute for Health Care Improvement (IHI) developed the model of "bundles" to help health care workers more consistently deliver the best possible care for patients undergoing particular treatments (Institute for Health Care Improvement, 2006). "A bundle is a structured way of improving the processes of care and patient outcomes: a small, straightforward set of evidence-based practices — generally three to five — that, when performed collectively and reliably, have been proven to improve patient outcomes" (Resar et al., 2005).

A recent observational study (Venkatram et al., 2010) was conducted in order to study the effect of bundle strategies on the device use adjusted rate of HAI in adult medical ICU, to prevent HAIs associated with endovascular catheters, mechanical ventilation, and urinary tract catheters. Particularly, the UTI bundle regards the use of antimicrobial catheters, closed drainage systems, and daily assessment for removal. During the study period, HAIs declined from 47 in 2004 to 3 in 2007. Particularly, CAUTI decreased from 6.23 to 0.63 per 1000 device-days. However, the decline in infection rates cannot be accounted by the decline in device use by itself, in fact, when adjusted to device use, the decrease in HAI rates still showed statistical significance. Therefore, it is not easy to attribute this decline to any one component of the bundle. Results of this study demonstrate that best practices using a multidisciplinary bundle strategy including device use can lead to optimal outcomes with respect to HCAI rates.

2. Surveillance of urinary tract infections in ICUs

Epidemiologic surveillance of HAI in ICUs is an important tool of internal quality management in the hospital setting (Zuschneid et al., 2010), and together with appropriate infection control activities, can decrease infection rates significantly (Haley et al., 1985).

A specific recommendation, of category II, included in the CDC/HICPAC *Guideline for Prevention of Catheter-associated Urinary Tract Infections* is: "Consider surveillance for CAUTI when indicated by facility-based risk assessment". Particularly, it is recommended to identify the patient groups or units on which to conduct surveillance based on frequency of catheter use and potential risk of CAUTI and to use standardized methodology for

performing CAUTI surveillance (Category IB). Furthermore, providing regular feedback of CAUTI rates to the staff should be also considered (Gould et al., 2009).
In order to explore the epidemiologic *scenario* and control of UTIs in intensive care patients, surveillance of HAI was performed on three Sicilian ICUs participating in the first two edition of the SPIN-UTI (Sorveglianza Prospettica delle Infezioni Nosocomiali nelle Unità di Terapia Intensiva) project.

2.1 Methods of surveillance

The Italian Nosocomial Infections Surveillance in ICUs, SPIN-UTI project, established in Italy by the Italian Study Group of Hospital Hygiene (GISIO) of the Italian Society of Hygiene, Preventive Medicine and Public Health (SItI) (Agodi et al., 2010), started the first edition in 2006 - 2007, the second edition of the project was implemented in 2008 – 2009, and the third, in 2010 – 2011 is in progress.
The methodology of surveillance are describes in great details elsewhere (Agodi et al., 2010) and is based on the HELICS-ICU protocol, in order to participate in the European benchmark (HELICS-ICU, 2004; Suetens et al., 2007). The enrollment of patients was prospective, and data regarding ICU stay, patient's risk factors including exposure to invasive devices (such as intubation, central venous catheter and urinary catheter), were collected using a web-based data collection procedure for each patient staying longer than two days in the ICU (Figure 1).
The definitions of HAI used in the SPIN-UTI project are the same proposed by the HELICS-ICU protocol for pneumonia, bloodstream infections (BSIs), central venous catheter-related bloodstream infections (CRIs) and UTIs (HELICS-ICU, 2004; Suetens et al., 2007). UTI data collection was mandatory.
The indicators included cumulative incidence and, to adjust for length of stay, incidence density. Furthermore, device-associated infection rates and device utilization ratios were also calculated as the number of infections per 1000 device-days and the number of days with the device divided for the number of patient-days.

2.2 Web-based data collection and statistical analysis

Surveillance data collection was performed from all patients enrolled in the project using four electronic data forms - designed using SPSS "Data Entry Enterprise Server" - as instruments for data collection. Particularly, the following data forms were used: 1) 'Characteristics of hospital and of ICU', 2) 'Patient', 3) 'Infection' and 4) 'Microorganism' (Figure 1). The electronic forms were characterized by functional instruments. Using these electronic forms data are entered via Web and each record is sent to the server, where it is automatically routed to the appropriate database. Cleaning and analyses were performed using SPSS for Windows (version 14.0): univariate analyses and the above reported indicators were calculated. Furthermore, categorical variables were compared using the chi-square-test, and continuous variables by Student's t-test; $p < 0.05$ was considered statistical significant.

3. Results of surveillance

3.1 ICU setting

The study was conducted at three Sicilian ICUs participating in the first two edition of the SPIN-UTI Project. The ICU identified as ICU 1 is a 12-bed interdisciplinary ICU, from a 700-bed acute care hospital; the ICU identified as ICU 2 is a 7-bed interdisciplinary ICU, from a

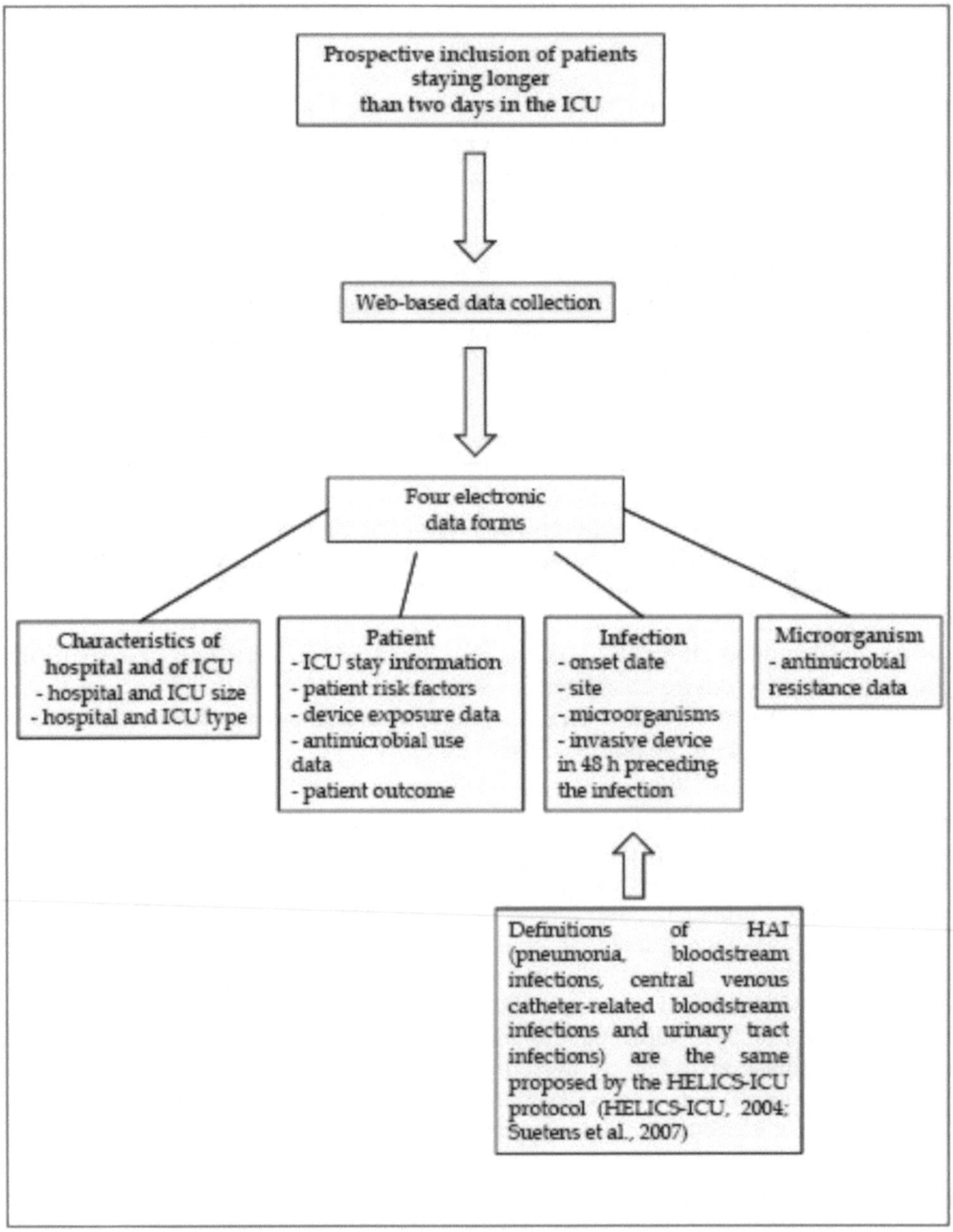

Fig. 1. Methods of Surveillance and web-based data collection.

830-bed tertiary care hospital; the ICU identified as ICU 3 is a 6-bed interdisciplinary ICU, from a 200-bed tertiary care hospital.

3.2 Patient's characteristics and device usage

A total of 501 patients with length of stay >2 days, for a total of 9681 patient-days, were admitted in the three ICUs during the two edition of the SPIN-UTI project and thus were enrolled in the study. A summary of patient characteristics and urinary catheter use is shown in Table 3.

Characteristic	ICU 1		ICU 2		ICU 3		Total	
	(2006-07)	(2008-09)	(2006-07)	(2008-09)	(2006-07)	(2008-09)	(2006-07)	(2008-09)
Number of patients	133	80	103	91	44	50	280	221
Mean age in years (range)	54.4 (5-94)	59,3 (22-92)	65.8 (2-94)	62,6 (1-97)	64.7 (19-87)	62,9 (13-87)	60.2 (2-94)	61.5 (1-97)
Male (%)	59.8	53,8	53.5	56	43.2	46	54.9	52.9
Mean SAPS II score (range)	41.85 (6-98)	51,58 (16-87)	31.38 (5-64)	27,41 (6-62)	34.06 (9-68)	43,80 (7-114)	37.37 (5-98)	40.84 (6-114)
Mean length of stay in days (range)	12.92 (3-65)	30,23 (6-106)	13.86 (3-79)	26,71 (3-120)	10.55 (3-57)	24,42 (3-84)	12.9 (3-79)	27.47 (3-120)
Total length of stay in ICU (in days)	1719	1598	1428	1335	464	736	3611	3669
Urinary catheter (%)	127 (95.5)	60 (75.0)	102 (99.0)	75 (82.4)	41 (93.2)	36 (72.0)	270 (96.4)	171 (77.4)
Total length of urinary catheterization (in days)	1576	1565	1269	1297	412	713	3257	3575
Mean length of urinary catheter in days (range)	12.5 (1-65)	19.8 (3-106)	12.6 (1-79)	14.3 (3-87)	10.1 (1-58)	14.9 (3-78)	12.2 (1-79)	16.4 (3-106)
Urinary catheter utilization ratios	0.92	0.97	0.89	0.97	0.89	0.97	0.90	0.97

Table 3. Main characteristics of patients included in the study.

Particularly, in the first edition of the project a total of 280 patients for a total of 3611 patient-days and a total of 221 patients for a total of 3669 patient-days in the second edition, were admitted. During the two edition of the project, a significant reduction of the proportion of patients with urinary catheter was observed (chi-square test, p <0.05). Particularly, in the first edition the overall proportion of patients with urinary catheter was 96.4% (range: 93.2%

- 99.0%) and in the second edition was 77.4% (range: 72.0 – 82.4%). Furthermore, in the first edition the total length of urinary catheterization was 3257 days (mean: 12.2 days; range: 1-79) and increased significantly (comparison between means, Student's t test, $p < 0.05$), in the second edition where was 3575 days (mean 16.4 days; range: 3-106 days).
Considering all three ICUs, an increase of urinary catheter utilization ratio, from 0.90 to 0.97, was observed in the second edition of the project.

3.3 Infection's indicators

Table 4 reports infection's indicators. Considering all ICUs, in the first edition of the SPIN-UTI project, the most frequently reported ICU-acquired infection type was pneumonia (38.2%) followed by bloodstream infections (30.9%), urinary tract infections (20.9%) and central venous catheter-related bloodstream infections (10.0%). In the second edition, the most frequently reported ICU-acquired infection type was bloodstream infections (43.7%) followed by urinary tract infections (29.1%), pneumonia (23.2%) and central venous catheter-related bloodstream infections (4.0%). Thus, in the last edition of the SPIN-UTI project an increase of the proportion of infections due to bloodstream infections and to urinary tract infections were registered, both considering all ICUs and each ICU separately. Instead, a decrease of the proportion of infections due to pneumonia infections and to central venous catheter-related bloodstream infections were registered, both considering all ICUs and each ICU separately.
The risk of ICU-acquired infections for all sites was estimated by computing the cumulative incidence: 39.3 per 100 patients in the first edition and 68.3 per 100 patients in the second one; and the incidence density: 30.5 per 1000 patient-days in the first edition and 41.2 per 1000 patient-days in the second one. Particularly, the cumulative incidence and the incidence density of UTI were increased in the second edition compared with the first one (Table 4).
Notably, in the two edition of the project, all UTIs were related to the presence of urinary catheter.
Urinary catheter-associated UTI rates (i.e. the number of urinary catheter-associated UTI per 1000 urinary catheter-days) was 7.1 per 1000 urinary catheter-days in the first edition and 12.3 per 1000 urinary catheter-days in the second edition.

3.4 Microorganisms associated to HAI

Considering all infection sites, relative frequencies of the five most common isolated microorganisms in ICU-acquired infections are reported in Table 5.
Despite difference among ICUs (data not shown), in the first edition of the SPIN-UTI project, the most frequently reported microorganism associated with ICU-acquired infections overall was *P. aeruginosa* (18.1%), followed by *Acinetobacter baumannii* (15.5%), *S. epidermidis* (14.7%), *K. pneumoniae* (7.8%) and *E. coli* (6.9%). In the second edition *A. baumannii* became the most frequently reported microorganism (20.3%), followed by *K. pneumoniae* (15.8%), *P. aeruginosa* (12.4%), *S. epidermidis* (6.8%) and *E. coli* (4.5%).
Considering only UTIs, in the first edition of the SPIN-UTI project, the reported microorganism overall were *P. aeruginosa* (30.8%), followed by *A. baumannii* and *Escherichia coli* (15.4%, each), *K. pneumoniae* (11.5%), *Candida albicans, Candida tropicalis* and *Enterobacter cloacae* (11.5%, each) and *Enterococcus* spp. (3.8%). In the second edition *K. pneumoniae* became the most frequently reported microorganism (22.2%), followed by *E. coli* and *P. aeruginosa* (13.3%), *Enterococcus faecalis* (11.1%), *A. baumannii* and *Candida glabrata* (8.9%, each) and *C. albicans* (6.7%) (Table 6).

	ICU 1		ICU 2		ICU 3		Total	
	(2006-07)	(2008-09)	(2006-07)	(2008-09)	(2006-07)	(2008-09)	(2006-07)	(2008-09)
Total number of infections	54	86	52	52	4	13	110	151
Total number of UTI (%)	10 (18.5)	18 (20.9)	13 (25.0)	22 (42.3)	0	4 (30.8)	23 (20.9)	44 (29.1)
Total number of Pneumonia (%)	24 (44.4)	29 (33.7)	16 (30.8)	5 (9.6)	2 (50.0)	1 (7.7)	42 (38.2)	35 (23.2)
Total number of CRI (%)	11 (20.4)	6 (7.0)	0	0	0	0	11 (10.0)	6 (4.0)
Total number of BSI (%)	9 (16.7)	33 (38.4)	23 (44.2)	25 (48.1)	2 (50.0)	8 (61.5)	34 (30.9)	66 (43.7)
Total length of stay in ICU (in days)	1719	1598	1428	1335	464	736	3611	3669
Cumulative incidence of infection (all sites) (/100 patients)	40.6	107.5	50.5	57.1	9.1	26.0	39.3	68.3
Incidence density of infection (all sites) (/1000 patient-days)	31.4	53.8	36.4	39.0	8.6	17.7	30.5	41.2
Cumulative incidence of UTI (/100 patients)	7.5	22.5	12.6	24.2	0	8.0	8.2	19.9
Incidence density of UTI (/1000 patient-days)	5.8	11.3	9.1	16.5	0	5.4	6.4	12.0
Cumulative incidence of Pneumonia (/100 patients)	18.0	36.3	15.5	5.5	4.5	2	15.0	15.8
Incidence density of Pneumonia (/1000 patient-days)	14.0	18.1	11.2	3.7	4.3	1.4	11.6	9.5
Cumulative incidence of CRI (/100 patients)	8.3	7.5	0	0	0	0	3.9	2.7
Incidence density of CRI (/1000 patient-days)	6.4	3.8	0	0	0	0	3.0	1.6
Cumulative incidence of BSI (/100 patients)	6.8	41.2	22.3	27.5	4.5	16.0	12.1	29.9
Incidence density of BSI (/1000 patient-days)	5.2	20.7	16.1	18.7	4.3	10.9	9.4	18.0

Table 4. Infection's indicators in the three ICUs.

	All ICUs (all infection types)	
	(2006-07)	**(2008-09)**
1st microorganism (n; %)	*P. aeruginosa* (21; 18.1)	*A. baumannii* (36; 20.3)
2nd microorganism (n; %)	*A. baumannii* (18; 15.5)	*K. pneumoniae* (28; 15.8)
3rd microorganism (n; %)	*S. epidermidis* (17; 14.7)	*P. aeruginosa* (22; 12.4)
4th microorganism (n; %)	*K. pneumoniae* (9; 7.8)	*S. epidermidis* (12; 6.8)
5th microorganism (n; %)	*E. coli* (8; 6.9)	*E. coli* (8; 4.5)

Table 5. Relative frequencies of the five most common isolated microorganisms in ICU-acquired infections.

All ICUs (only UTIs: n; %)	
(2006-07)	**(2008-09)**
P. aeruginosa (8; 30.8)	*K. pneumoniae* (10; 22.2)
E. coli and *A. baumannii* (4; 15.4, each)	*E. coli* and *P. aeruginosa* (6; 13.3, each)
K. pneumoniae (3; 11.5)	*E. faecalis* (5; 11.1)
C. albicans, C. tropicalis, E. cloacae (2; 7.7, each)	*A. baumannii* and *C. glabrata* (4; 8.9, each)
Enterococcus spp. (1; 3.8)	*C. albicans* (8; 6.7)

Table 6. Relative frequencies of the isolated microorganisms in UTIs.

4. Discussion

In several high-income countries, device-associated HAI surveillance in the ICU plays a considerable role in hospital infection control and quality assurance (Edwards et al., 2009).
A recent study was performed in the framework of the German KISS with the aim of investigating whether surveillance of CAUTI in ICUs leads to reduced infection rates. When comparing the symptomatic CAUTI rates in the third and first years of the surveillance, a significant reduction in CAUTI was shown. However, before-and-after studies are limited by confounding variables such as the difficulties of ICU patients in recognizing and reporting UTI symptoms, that leads to the availability of microbiological reports as a major criterion for diagnosing symptomatic UTI. Thus, in the case of CAUTI diagnosis, microbiological reports may have decreased over time and have influenced reduction of CAUTI rates (Gastmeier et al., 2011).

In the same study, it has been reported that the overall surveillance effect was highest for ventilator-associated pneumonia and central venous catheter bloodstream infection. This could be explained by the perception of the clinicians that ventilator-associated pneumonia and central venous catheter bloodstream infection are more serious infections demanding more effective responses rather than CAUTI. However, CAUTI may also lead to sepsis, and changes in CAUTI rate over time, with consistent microbiology diagnostic procedures, may lead to the introduction of appropriate infection control measures (Gastmeier et al., 2011).

The SPIN-UTI project was implemented to create a HAI surveillance network of Italian ICUs (Agodi et al., 2010). The validation study of the SPIN-UTI project has showed a high sensitivity, specificity, and positive and negative predictive values of surveillance data (Masia et al., 2010).

Comparison of results of the two editions of the SPIN-UTI project revealed that, the risk of ICU-acquired infections for all sites, estimated by computing the cumulative incidence and the incidence density, increased in the second edition compared to the first one.

Differences were presented considering infection by site. In the second edition of the project a decrease of the proportion of infections due to pneumonia and to CRIs were registered. On the contrary, an increase of the proportion of infections due to BSIs and to UTIs were observed, either considering all ICUs or each ICU separately. Particularly, after comparing results of the two studies, in the second edition a higher proportion of the patients acquired a UTI in ICU than in the first edition. The cumulative incidence of UTI increased from 8.2 per 100 patients to 19.9 per 100 patients. The incidence density also increased from 6.4 per 1000 patient-days to 12.0 per 1000 patient-days.

Hospital wide prevalence rates for indwelling catheterization vary from 25% to 35% (Haley et al., 1981; Junkin & Selekof, 2007). Prevalence rates in ICU are substantially higher at 67% to 76% (Huang et al., 2004; Gray, 2010). In our study, a high proportion of patients were with urinary catheter (range: 72.0%- 99.0%), and although a significant reduction of the proportion of exposed patients was observed in the second edition of the project an increase of the mean length of urinary catheterization from 12.2 days to 16.4 days was observed. Furthermore, urinary catheter utilization ratio was significantly higher in the second edition compared with the first edition (from 0.90 to 0.97).

Notably, in the two edition of the project, all UTIs were related to the presence of urinary catheter. Urinary catheter-associated UTI rates increased from 7.1 per 1000 urinary catheter days in the first edition and 12.3 per 1000 urinary catheter days in the second edition.

It is advised that device-associated infection rates and device utilization ratios should be examined together so that preventive measures may be appropriately targeted. Since urinary catheter use is a significant risk factor for UTI, efforts must be redirected to reducing their use or limiting the duration with which they are used and to addressing the best consensus guidelines and recommendations in their insertion and maintenance (Edwards et al., 2007). In fact, it has been reported that targeted strategies for prevention of UTI include limiting the use and duration of urinary catheterization, using aseptic technique for catheter insertion, and adhering to proper catheter care (Shuman and Chenoweth, 2010).

The most frequently isolated microorganisms causing CAUTI in the ICU setting are enteric Gram-negative bacilli, enterococci, *Candida* species, and *P. aeruginosa* (Shuman and Chenoweth, 2010). Microorganisms are often multidrug resistant probably following the increasing use of broad-spectrum antibiotics in hospitals and this is a considerable problem in ICU.

In our surveillance survey, despite difference among ICUs, in the first edition of the project, the most frequently reported microorganism associated to UTI was *P. aeruginosa*, in the second one, *K. pneumoniae* (22.2%) was the first species isolated. Notably, in the second edition an increase of *K. pneumoniae* isolation and a decrease of *P. aeruginosa* isolation were observed.

5. Conclusion

Our study represents a contribution to improve the quality of care in the ICU setting. A major item was identified for planning future intervention: focusing on the appropriate urinary catheter use. HAIs can be prevented by constant use of "bundles" of simple and effective measures, including the monitoring of device use, recommended by CDC and IHI (Institute for Health Care Improvement, 2006; Gould et al., 2009). To improve patient safety, an integrated, multimodal and comprehensive "bundles" approach is the means to reducing the impact of HAI.

6. Acknowledgements

This work was supported in part by grants from the University of Catania (Progetti di Ricerca di Ateneo to A.A.).
The authors wish to thank all physicians and nurses in the participating ICUs for providing surveillance data and for their co-operation during the development of this surveillance system.

7. References

Agodi, A., Barchitta, M., Anzaldi, A., Marchese, F., Bonaccorsi, A., & Motta M. (2007). Active surveillance of nosocomial infections in urologic patients. *Eur Urol*, vol.51, pp. 247-253.

Agodi, A., Auxilia, F., Barchitta, M., Brusaferro, S., D'Alessandro, D., Montagna, M.T., Orsi, G.B., Pasquarella, C., Torregrossa, V., Suetens, C., Mura, I., & GISIO. (2010). Building a benchmark through active surveillance of ICU-acquired infections: the Italian network SPIN-UTI. *J Hosp Infect*, Vol.74, pp. 258-265.

Anderson, D.J., Kirkland, K.B., Kaye, K.S., et al. (2007). Underresourced hospital infection control and prevention programs: penny wise, pound foolish? *Infect Control Hosp Epidemiol*, Vol.28(7), pp. 767–773.

Atkins, D., Best, D., Briss, P.A., et al. (2004). Grading quality of evidence and strength of recommendations. *BMJ*, Vol.328(7454), p. 1490.

Edwards, J.R., Peterson, K.D., Andrus, M.L., et al. (2007). National healthcare safety network (NHSN) report, data summary for 2006, issued June 2007. *Am J Infect Control*, Vol.35(5), pp. 290-301.

Edwards, J.R., Peterson, K.D., Mu, Y., Banerjee, S., Allen-Bridson, K., Morrell, G., et al. (2009). National Healthcare Safety Network (NHSN) report: data summary for 2006 through 2008, issued December 2009. *Am J Infect Control*, Vol. 37, pp. 783–805.

Elpern, E.H., Killeen, K., Ketchem, A., Wiley, A., Patel, G., & Omar. (2009). Reducing use of indwelling urinary catheters and associated urinary tract infections. *Am J Crit Care*, Vol.18, pp. 535-541

Emori, T.G., Culver, D.H., Horan, T.C., et al. (1991). National Nosocomial Infection Surveillance System (NNIS): description of surveillance methodology. *Am J Infect Control*, Vol. 19, pp. 19-35.

European Centre for Disease Prevention and Control. (2009). Annual epidemiological report on communicable diseases in Europe 2009. Stockholm, Sweden: European Centre for Disease Prevention and Control.

European Centre for Disease Prevention and Control. (2010). Annual Epidemiological Report on Communicable Diseases in Europe 2010. Stockholm Sweden: European Centre for Disease Prevention and Control.

Garner, J.S., Emori, W.R., Horan, T.C., & Hughes, J.M. (1988). CDC definitions for nosocomial infections. *Am J Infect Control*, Vol.16, pp.128-140.

Gastmeier, P., Sohr, D., Schwab, F., et al. (2008). Ten years of KISS: the most important requirements for success. *J Hosp Infect*, Vol.70(Suppl. 1), pp.11-16.

Gastmeier, P., Behnke, M., Schwab, F., & Geffers, C. (2011). Benchmarking of urinary tract infection rates: experiences from the intensive care unit component of the German national nosocomial infections surveillance system. *Journal of Hospital Infection*, Vol.78, pp. 41-44.

Geffers, C., Gastmeier, P. (2011). Nosocomial infections and multidrug resistance organisms - epidemiological data from KISS. *Dtsch Arztebl Int*. Vol.108(6), pp. 87–93.

Gould, C.V. Umscheid, G.A., Agarwal, R.K. Kuntz, G., Pegues, D.A. & Healthcare Infection Control Practices Advisory Committee (HICPAC). (2009). Guideline For Prevention Of Catheter-Associated Urinary Tract Infections 2009.

Gray, M. (2010). Reducing Catheter-Associated Urinary Tract Infection in the Critical Care Unit. *AACN Advanced Critical Care*, Vol.21, Number 3, pp.247–257.

Guyatt, G.H., Oxman, A.D., Kunz, R., et al. (2008). What is "quality of evidence" and why is it important to clinicians? *BMJ*, Vol.336(7651), pp. 995-998.

Guyatt, G.H., Oxman, A.D., Kunz, R., et al. (2008). Going from evidence to recommendations. *BMJ*, Vol.336(7652), pp. 1049-1051.

Junkin, J., & Selekof, J.L. (2007). Prevalence of incontinence and associated skin injury in the acute care inpatient. *J Wound Ostomy Continence Nurs*, Vol.34(3), pp.260–269.

Haley, R.W., Hooton, T.M., Culver, D.H., et al. (1981). Nosocomial infections in US hospitals, 1975–76: estimated frequency by selected characteristics of patients. *Am J Med*, Vol.70(4), pp. 947–959.

Haley, R.W., Culver, D.H., White, J.W., et al. (1985). The efficacy of infection control programs in preventing nosocomial infections in U.S. hospitals. *Am J Epidemiol*, Vol.212, pp. 182-205.

HELICS-ICU working group. (2004). Surveillance of nosocomial infections in intensive care units. Protocol, version 6.1. IPH/EPI reports D/2004/2505/48. Brussels: Scientific Institute of Public Health.

HELICS-ICU working group. (2005). Surveillance of nosocomial infections in intensive care units. HELICS implementation phase II. HELICS-ICU Statistical Report 2000-2004. Brussels: Scientific Institute of Public Health.

Hidron, A.I., Edwards, J.R., Patel, J., et al. (2008). NHSN annual update: Antimicrobial-resistant pathogens associated with healthcare-associated infections: Annual summary of data reported to the national healthcare safety network at the centers for disease control and prevention, 2006-2007. *Infect Control Hosp Epidemiol*, Vol.29(11), pp. 996-1011.

Horan, T.C., Andrus, M., & Dudeck, M.A. (2008). CDC/NHSN surveillance definition of health care–associated infection and criteria for specific types of infections in the acute care setting. *Am J Infect Control*, Vol.36, pp. 309-332.

Huang, W.C., Wann, S.R., Lin, S.L., et al. (2004). Catheter-associated urinary tract infections in intensive care units can be reduced by prompting physicians to remove unnecessary catheters. *Infect Control Hosp Epidemiol,* Vol.25(11), pp.974–978.

Institute for Healthcare Improvement (IHI) (2006). Critical Care: What is a Bundle? Available from http://www.ihi.org/ IHI/ Topics/ CriticalCare/ IntensiveCare/ ImprovementStories/WhatIsaBundle.htm.

Klevens R.M., Edward J.R., et al. (2007). Estimating health care-associated infections and deaths in U.S. hospitals, 2002. *Public Health Reports,* Vol.122, pp. 160-166.

Lambert, M.L., Suetens, C., Savey, A., Palomar, M., Hiesmayr, M., Morales, I., Agodi, A., Frank, U., Mertens, K., Schumacher, M., & Wolkewitz, M. (2011). Clinical outcomes of health-care-associated infections and antimicrobial resistance in patients admitted to European intensive-care units: a cohort study. *Lancet Infect Dis,* Vol.11, pp. 30-38.

Masia, M.D., Barchitta, M., Liperi, G., Cantù, A.P., Alliata, E., Auxilia F., Torregrossa, V., Mura, I., Agodi, A., & Italian Study Group of Hospital Hygiene (GISIO). (2010). Validation of intensive care unit-acquired infection surveillance in the Italian SPIN-UTI network. *J of Hosp Infect,* Vol.76, pp. 139-142.

Meddings, J., Rogers, M.A.M., Macy, M, & Saint, S. (2010). Systematic Review and Meta-Analysis: Reminder Systems to Reduce Catheter-Associated Urinary Tract Infections and Urinary Catheter Use in Hospitalized Patients. *Clin Infect Dis,* Vol.51, pp. 550–560.

NHSN Manual: Patient Safety Component Protocol. Available from www.cdc.gov/ncidod/dhqp/nhsn.html.

Resar R, Pronovost P, Haraden C, Simmonds T, et al. Using a bundle approach to improve ventilator care processes and reduce ventilator-associated pneumonia. (2005). Joint Commission Journal on Quality and Patient Safety, Vol.31(5), pp. 243-248.

Rosenthal, V.D., Dwivedy, A., Rodrıguez Calder, M.E., Esen, S., Hernandez, H.T., Abouqal, R., Medeiros, E.A., Espinoza, T.A., Kanj, S.S., Gikas, A., Barnett, A.G., Graves, N., & International Nosocomial Infection Control Consortium (INICC) Membersl. (2011). Time-dependent analysis of length of stay and mortality due to urinary tract infections in ten developing countries: INICC findings. *Journal of Infection,* Vol.62, pp. 136-141.

Shuman, E.K., Chenoweth, C.E. (2010). Recognition and prevention of healthcare-associated urinary tract infections in the intensive care unit. *Crit Care Med.* Vol. 38, pp. 373-379.

Suetens, C., Morales, I., Savey, A., et al. (2007). European surveillance of ICU-acquired infections (HELICS-ICU): methods and main results. *J Hosp Infect,* Vol. 65, pp. 171-173.

Tissot, E., Limat, S., Cornette, C., & Capellier, G. (2001). Risk factors for catheter-associated bacteriuria in a medical intensive care unit. *Eur J Clin Microbiol Infect Dis,* Vol. 20(4), pp. 260-262.

Venkatram, S., Rachmale, S., & Kanna, B. (2010) Study of device use adjusted rates in health care–associated infections after implementation of "bundles" in a closed-model medical intensive care unit. *J of Crit Care.* Vol.25, pp. 174.e11–174.e18

Warren, J.W. (2001). Catheter-associated urinary tract infections. *Int J Antimicrob Agents,* Vol.17(4), pp.299-303.

Zuschneid, I., Rucker, G., Schoop, R., Beyersmann, J., Schumacher, M., Geffers, C., Ruden, H., & Gastmeier, P. (2010). Representativeness of the Surveillance Data in the Intensive Care Unit Component of the German Nosocomial Infections Surveillance System. *Infect Control Hosp Epidemiol,* Vol.31, pp. 934-938.

2

The Changing Epidemiology of Extended Spectrum Beta-Lactamases (ESBL) Infections of the Urinary Tract Focusing on Clinical Resistance and Therapeutic Options

Suresh J. Antony
Texas Tech University Medical Center/Paul Foster School of Medicine and The Center for Infectious Diseases and Travel Medicine
El Paso, Texas
USA

1. Introduction

The first beta- lactamases were identified in a species of *E.coli* in 1940 (1). However, the ability of bacteria to produce enzymes that destroy the b-lactam ring was noted even before penicillin was developed. In fact, many of the gram-negative bacteria possess chromosomally mediated b- lactamases, which help the bacteria find a niche when faced with competition from other bacteria that naturally produce b-lactams.

In 1965, the first plasmid mediated beta- lactamases was discovered. This occurred in a strain of *E.coli* isolated from the blood culture of a patient from Greece whose name was Temoniera. The beta -lactamases was named TEM-1 after the patient's name from whom it was isolated. (2) This strain soon spread to other members of the Enterobacteriaceae species, *Hemophilus influenza, Neisseria gonorrhoeae* and *Pseudomonas aeruginosa* due to the plasmid mediated transfer.

Around the same time a second plasmid mediated beta-lactamases was found in *Klebsiella pneumonaie* and *E.coli*. This was called SHV-1 (sulfhydryl variable) (3). The advent of the b-lactam class of antibiotics was influenced largely by the discovery of these enzymes. An example of this was the development of oxyimino-cephalosporin, which showed good stability against the TEM-1 and SHV-1 b-lactamases (4). This class of antibiotics soon became the workhorse for these types of serious infections.

Unfortunately, resistance to this class soon became evident in 1985 with beta-lactamases showing the ability to hydrolyze these compounds in *K.pneumoniae* (5). Because this enzyme was noted to be active against expanded spectrum b-lactams these enzymes were labeled as "extended spectrum beta-lactamases" –ESBL.

Several b-lactamases have continued to be with over 130 TEMS types and over 50 SHV types known to date. These are mainly found in *E.coli, K.pneumoniae* and *P.mirabilis,* but have also been found in other species of the Enterobacteriacae family and even in some nonenteric bacteria such as *Acinetobacter* species.

Shortly after the introduction of new broad-spectrum cephalosporins such as cefotaxime and ceftazidime, non-TEM and non SHV ESBL's were discovered. This new class of ESBL's has been called CTX-M in reference to the potent hydrolytic activity of these enzymes against cefotaxime(6). There are over 40 of these enzymes reported. CTX-M producing ESBL pathogens usually have cefotaxime in the resistant range (MIC>64).

More recently, and of greater concern is the occurrence of carbapenemases which show activity against oxyimino-cephalosporins and cephamycins but also against carbapenems (7). There are two major groups in this class called metallo-b-lactamases (Verona integron encoded metallo b lactamases) (VIM) and carbapenemases. Structural studies of ESBL indicate that active site expansion and remodeling are responsible for the extended hydrolytic activity (8).These enzymes are globally present and appear to cause clinically significant disease such as urinary tract infections, abscesses and bacteremia.

With the advent of the ESBL pathogens, there has been a significant increase in the morbidity and mortality related to these infections. If the number of carbapenemase-producing organisms continues to increase, the treatment options will be seriously compromised.

In addition, ESBL producing pathogens are not only resistant to penicillin and cephalosporins but also to trimethoprim-sulphamethoxazole and fluroquinolones which can compromise the treatment of both nosocomial and community acquired infections caused by *Enterobacteriaceae* and other species (9).

One of the major clinical problems has been the recognition of both nosocomial and community acquired urinary tract infections resulting from ESBL pathogens. The treatment options for these infections are limited, especially in the out patient setting.

This chapter will review the epidemiology, risk factors, clinical features and therapeutics options for ESBL-induced infections of the urinary tract.

2. Recent epidemiological data

ESBL producing organisms have been implicated in nosocomial infections. Over the last decade, there has been a steady increase of these infections in the community.

In fact, a recent study from Spain suggest there was been an increase in ESBL *E.coli* producers from 0.3% to 4.8% between 1995 and 2002. (10) Interestingly, during this same period there was a drop in the rate of ESBL producing *K.pneumoniae* following the control of nosocomial transmission of this pathogen. These *K. pneumoniaie* were mostly clonally related and produced SHV and TEM.

In contrast, the ESBL *E.coli* strains were not clonally related and the predominant strain was a CTX-M. In addition, half of these strains were isolated from outpatients (10,11).

France was one of the first countries to report an outbreak of ESBL infections in 1986. In this study, 30% of *Enterobacter aerogenes* isolates in 2000 were ESBL producers (12). Since that time, virtually every country in Europe has reported ESBL producers with considerable geographical variability in the occurrence of ESBL's. Examples of this include a prevalence rate of ESBLs

K. pneumoniaie in Sweden of 3% to 34% in Portugal (13). In one study done in France, it was noted that intestinal carriage prevalence of ESBL-*E.coli* was 8.0%, mainly the CTX-M type. At the same time, it was noted that there was an increase in antibiotic usage, especially the beta-lactams. This variability probably occurred because of the repeated introduction of new strains and plasmids and from inter-individual dissemination (14)

In Central and South America ESBL, rates in *Klebsiella* varied from 30 to 60% in countries such as Brazil, Columbia and Venezuela (15). The ESBL strains included SHV-2, 5, CTX-M and even non-TEM and non-SHV with no geographical predilection. (16, 17)

In Africa and the Middle East there has been a number of outbreaks of ESBL producing infections from South Africa to northern Africa. The rates of ESBL were variable depending on the country (18 19) .

In North America the first case of an ESBL producer was in 1988and since then a variety of infections produced by TEM strains, SHV type and CTM-X have been reported. In fact, in a recent survey it was noted that non-susceptibility to third generation cephalosporin's may be as high as 13 %.(20,21). In the outpatient, setting 1.8% of *k.pneumoniae* and 0.4% were ceftazidime resistant (22)

In Asia, there seems to be a larger proportion of ESBL pathogens. Studies from several countries, including China, India, Japan, Korea, and Malaysia showed ranges from 30% to 40 % (23,24). Reports of a possible predominant CTM-X ESBL in countries like India, China Korea, Japan and Taiwan indicate that there may be a dominant ESBL type in Asia (25,26). More recently, there have been studies showing increasing numbers of carbapenemase producing pathogens, which is of increasing clinical importance due to the lack of effective antimicrobial therapy. (27-31).

Current data suggest that the incidence of ESBL producing infections is on the rise globally resulting in increasing difficulty in the diagnosis and treatment of these infections.

3. *In vitro* resistance studies for ESBL

In- vitro susceptibility testing of cephalosporins for ESBL producing enterobacteriacae can be misleading. Testing may suggest that an isolated strain is susceptible to a given cephalosporin, but the drug may not be effective when used to treat a serious infection caused by the organism. Thus, CLSI guidelines recommend that laboratories report ESBL producing isolates as resistant to all penicillin's, cephalosporins and aztreonam irrespective of in vitro results. (32).

In vitro studies performed in Turkey found that *E.coli* isolated from CA-UTI infections had simultaneous resistance to trimethoprim-sulphamethaxazole, ciprofloxacin, and gentamicin in 4.6% of an ESBL negative group and 39.2% in the ESBL positive group. 90% of these ESBL isolates were found to have CTX-M 15. (33). This data is worrisome as therapeutic options are limited when oral antibiotics are used.

In Taiwan, Lau and colleagues looked at 201 patients with and without bacteremia in CA-ESBL UTI. They found that *e.coli* was the most common pathogen and was more frequent in the bacteremic than non-bacteremic group. Non-*E.coli* isolates such as *K.pneumoniae, Morganella morganii* etc were more common in the non-bacteremic group. E.*coli* isolates had a high rate of resistance to ampicillin (80%), gentamicin (29%) trimethoprim-sulphamethaxazole (56%). (34). Similar findings have been documented from other parts of the world such as Saudi Arabia (35).

Detection of ESBL's is based on the fact that ESBL producers should be reported as resistant to all penicillin's, cephalosporins (except cephamycins) and aztreonam irrespective of routine antimicrobial susceptibility testing. (32)

Both broth dilution and disk diffusion can be used for the screening of ESBL producers. Specific phenotypic confirmatory tests should be done if the E.coli, K.pneumoniae, show MIC's>8ug/ml for cefpodoxime or MIC's >2 ug/ml against ceftazidime, cefotaxime or aztreonam. (36,37)

The E-test can also be used in the detection of ESBL. Automated methods for bacterial identification and susceptibility testing are also used in the detection of ESBL producing organisms. These include the BD Phoenix system, Vitek 2 system and the Micoscan Walkway -96 system.

4. Risk factors for colonization /infection with ESBL

There have been several case controlled studies looking at the risk factors for colonization with or without infection due to ESBL producers. However, the results are conflicting due to study populations, geographical areas, selection of cases and controls and sample size. (38-48).

Despite these statistical differences, some generalizations can be made. (Table 1)

Diabetes mellitus
Previous antimicrobial exposure (quinolones, third generation cephalosporins, penicillin)
Previous hospital admissions
Older age
Male patients

Table 1. Risk factors for the Development of Community ESBL Infections.

Some of these risk factors include seriously ill patients with prolonged hospital stays (11-67 days) who have usually had multiple invasive devices and co-morbidities such as urinary catheters, central lines, nasogastric tubes, jejunostomy tubes, arterial lines, total parental administration, recent surgery, decubitus ulcers, hemodialysis catheters and poor nutritional status.

The use of previous antibiotics such as third generation cephalosporins, quinolones, trimethoprim-sulphamethoxazole, aminoglycosides and metronidazole have also been implicated in several studies. (38,42,45,49,44,50,47, 48,51).

5. Community –acquired infections involving ESBL pathogens

In a large French study in 1993, looking at *E.coli, K.pneumoniae and P .mirabilis* (2500 isolates) from non-hospitalized patients, there was no evidence of community acquired ESBL infections (52). Since then, there have been several studies of true community acquired ESBL infections. These involved patients with diarrheal diseases such as *Shigella, Salmonella, Vibrio cholerae and E. coli*. (53-56)

The prevalence of colonization with enterobacteria is unknown. The percentage of ESBL producing *Enterobacteria* faecal carriers in Spain increased from 2.1% to 7.5% IN 2002. (57) . The most frequent types of ESBL were CTX-M, followed by SHV. In India, the rate of fecal carriage was 7% in a sample of healthy adults (60). In Canada, Pitout found 5.5 cases per 100,000 populations with 69% being community acquired. (59)

Three case controlled studies looking at risk factors for ESBL *E.coli* outpatient infections found that diabetes mellitus, previous use of antibiotics such as quinolones and cephalosporins, recurrent urinary tract infections, prior hospital admissions and older age were independent risk factors (59,60). However, infections due to ESBL producing *E.coli* in patients can occur without obvious risk factors. This may be related to the increase in healthy carriers colonized with this pathogen.

Colodoner et al evaluated 128 cases of UTI caused by ESBL *E.coli* and *K. pneumoniae* and found that age >60 years, male sex, previous use of quinolones or cephalosporins, previous hospitalization, and previous infections caused by *K. pneumoniae* were independent risk factors.(61)

In community- acquired urinary tract infection (CA-UTI), the rate of ESBL associated UTI's varied from 1.4% in Spain up to 3.3% in the Gaza strip (60,62,63).

In the last 7 years, there have been an increasing number of publications from several countries showing and increase of community acquired ESBL infections, mainly in urinary tract. (64,65,61,57,30,59,60,31) Most of these patients had urinary tract infections (UTI's) with genes encoding for CTM-X type of ESBL's (60). Recently, there has been an increase in the diagnosis of infections caused by ESBL *E.coli* producers diagnosed in the outpatient's setting.(59,60,30)

Romero et al showed an increase from 0.3% in 1995 to 4.8% in 2002 in community acquired ESBL *E.coli* producers. (10). These ESBL *E.coli* producing strains were not clonally related with the majority belonging to the CTX-M family and more than 50% were isolated in the outpatient setting. (10, 11)

In one study in Spain up to 6.5% of community, acquired bacteremia was associated with ESBL *E.coli* UTI (60).

In summary, ESBL infections can range from colonization to carriage to true infections involving sepsis syndromes and bacteremia.

6. Clinical features of CA-UTI infections caused by ESBL pathogens

Several studies have described the microbiological features of ESBL producing organisms in the outpatient setting. However, very few studies have correlated the microbiological findings with that of the clinical features and prognosis of these CA-UTI ESBL infections. Therefore, one may only draw some tentative conclusions from these studies.

In urinary tract infections, the majority of ESBL's isolated, not surprisingly, have been ESBL *E.coli.* This organism has also been isolated from other sources such as wounds, sputum, and occasionally blood. (59,60,11,)

In the United States, Chao Qi et al evaluated 193 single patient ESBL isolates in outpatient urine cultures during a 5-year period. 3% of *E.coli* had ESBL and this was noted to have increased 14 times from 2003 to 2008. This increase may have been in part due to the dissemination of CTX-M type of ESBL. (66) This was also noted in another study from nursing homes and out patient clinics. (67) . Resistance to ciprofloxacin and trimethoprim-sulphamethaxazole was much higher as well.

In another study of 49 patients with ESBL *E.coli* infections, ESBL *E.coli* was isolated from urine in 47 of the cases and from blood in 6 of the patients. Thirty-seven (76%) of these patients were considered to have symptomatic infections and 11 (22%) asymptomatic bactiuria. 1 patient also had cholangitis and 6 (13.5%) of these patients were bacteremic. In this same study, 10 of the 28 patients who received antibiotics actually received an appropriate agent to which the organism was susceptible in vitro. 13% of these patients had a UTI relapse. There were no deaths in this study (60). It appears that the complication rate with CA-ESBL UTI's may not be higher than that associated with routine non-ESBL pathogens, although further studies are still needed. The main predictor of mortality caused by ESBL *E.coli* is probably inadequate initial antimicrobial therapy. In comparison, ESBL-EC associated mortality for hospitalized patients with serous infections such as bacteremia and sepsis was about 25%-31%. This was also associated with inadequate empiric antibiotic therapy. (68,69).

The most frequent cause of community-acquired bacteremia is *E.coli* (70,71) and currently available antibiotics such as quinolones, beta-lactams and third generation cephalosporins are commonly used to treat them. This may need to change with the advent of increasing antimicrobial resistance and increasing mortality associated with these CA-ESBL infections (44,59). Rodriguez-Bano examined CA-ESBL associated bacteremia and its features and found that in 95 patients with blood stream infections 7.3% were due to *E.coli.* The majority belonged to the CTX-M family of ESBL and was clonally unrelated. The risk factors associated with these patients included urinary foley catheter use and previous antimicrobial exposure (60). The sources of bacteremia were the urinary tract, intra-abdominal sites and respiratory tract. Interestingly, mortality associated with blood stream infections due to ESBL-*E.coli* was lower among patients who received empirical therapy with beta-lactam or it combinations or carbapenems than among those that received quinolones. In addition, higher mortality was associated with inappropriate empirical therapy in patients with bacteremia due to *E.coli.* (72)

In patients with solid organ transplants and renal transplants, the major site of infection was the urinary tract in 72% of the cases, with ESBL .*K. pneumoniae* being more common in renal transplant patients (73).

Geriatric patients with ESBL UTI's pose an unusual clinical problem. These patients may be chronically colonized in either the gastrointestinal tract or the skin and reinfection is a possibility. In addition, many of these patients are asymptomatic and do not present with the classic symptoms of dysuria, frequency of urination, fever or leukocytosis. In general, one may not need to treat asymptomatic ESBL infections. If there is a change in the clinical status such as fever, leukocytosis or altered mental status then treatment options should be considered. Numerous outbreaks have been reported of patients with ESBL infections. Much of the spread is plasmid mediated and is therefore through direct and indirect transmission. Contact isolation should be instituted in patients with ESBL infections.

In summary, ESBL infections can present from simple colonization to active UTI's and to serious bacteremia associated with sepsis syndrome.

7. Treatment options for ESBL UTI infections

Treatment options for ESBL infections are the same for both nosocomial and community acquired infections. The major problem at this time is the lack of effective oral antibiotics for the treatment of outpatient ESBL infections.

7.1 Overview of available antibiotics

ESBL's hydrolyze aztreonam, penicillin and cephalosporins (with the exception of cephamycins) with varying degrees of hydrolytic activity. Usually the TEM and SHV type ESBL's have greater hydrolytic activity for ceftazidime than for cefotaxime (74). Therefore, ESBL producing organisms may appear susceptible to some of the above-mentioned antibiotics in vitro. In addition, there is frequent co –expression of resistance by these organisms to classes of antimicrobial agents other than those hydrolyzed by the ESBL's. This has been documented for quinolones, aminoglycosides, tetracycline's (excluding glycylcycline) and trimethoprim-sulphamethoxazole (59)

Some of the other antibiotic classes used to treat ESBL infections include beta lactam/beta-lactamases inhibitors. The level of activity for these agents varies by the type of inhibitor and by the class of ESBL. For example, tazobactam appears to be more effective than clavulanic acid against certain types of CTX-M type ESBL's and both of these agents are more effective than sulbactam in inhibiting TEM and SHV type ESBL. (75,76). This data is mainly from in-vitro studies. Clinical information is sparse in regards to beta-lactam and inhibitor combinations, but some favorable outcomes have been reported with pipercillin/tazobactam. However, it is important to note that favorable results have not been consistently reported (74,77). One possible oral option may be amoxicillin/clavulanate, which has shown some activity in CA-ESBL Enterobacteriaceae UTI infections (60,78)

Few studies have evaluated cephalosporins in the treatment of both bacteremic and non-bacteremic ESBL infections. The results have been equivocal when ceftazidime or cefepeme were compared to Imipenem in *e. coli* bacteremia and in ICU patients with Enterobacteriaceae infections. (79,80). In vitro data also suggests suboptimal outcomes when the cephalosporins were used to treat ESBL infections. Thus, most experts' advise against using cephalosporins in the treatment of ESBL associated infections.(79,80)

Cephamycins have not been well studied in the treatment of ESBL associated infections. In one small retrospective study, there was no obvious difference in the mortality rates between the cephamycins and carbapenems. Recent studies have documented resistance to the cephamycins (49,74).

The glycylcycline class of antibiotics, specifically tigecycline, thus far evaded the common mechanisms of resistance in both gram positive and gram-negative pathogens. It has excellent in vitro activity against ESBL-*E.coli* and *K. pneumoniae*. However, clinical data is sparse in the treatment of ESBL UTI's and bacteremia. In addition, only a fraction of the drug is excreted in the urine as unchanged drug. In addition, tigecycline does not achieve high concentrations in the blood, casting doubts on its potential effectiveness in the treatment of bacteremia.(81)

Fosfomycin has been used in Europe but is not available in most parts of the world. It is a phosphor derivative of streptomycin and inhibits cell wall synthesis and impairs adherence to urogenital mucosa. A study in Spain found that the resistance rate to fosfomycin of ESBL-EC was 0.3%. (82). It has been used in cystitis and asymptomatic UTI in pregnancy. (82,83). In the United States 90% of the isolates in one study were susceptible to fosfomycin and to a combination of cefdinir plus amoxicillin-clavulanate. (84,85)

Pivmecillinam is a beta lactam antibiotic, which binds penicillin-binding protein 2 (PBP-2) and inhibits cell wall synthesis. This drug has been used in the treatment of cystitis due to Enterobacteriaceae. (86).

Nitrofurantoin is a bactericidal drug, which acts by altering bacterial ribosome's proteins and can be used for UTI as well.

Finally, carbapenems are considered the drug of choice for ESBL infections. All the drugs in the class appear to have the same efficiency in the treatment of ESBL. Ertapenem, is the only drug in this class that can be administered once a day. It can be used in the outpatient setting as long as the in vitro activity is similar to imipenem, doripenem or meropenem.(87,88). However, recent reports of carbapenem resistance have emerged and the spread of resistance is of concern. One possible option might be to add amikacin to the empiric regimen in community-acquired sepsis originating in the urinary tract since amikacin resistance among CTX-M isolates is relatively low.

The treatment for upper UTI's may have to be limited to the intravenous antibiotics mentioned above especially as the patients tend to be sicker and may present with systemic

inflammatory response syndrome and occasionally bacteremia. These should include carbapenems. Occasionally, ampicillan-sulbactam and tigecycline may be alternate therapies although data on these drugs in the treatment of ESBL UTI infections is sparse.
In lower UTI's, some of the oral antibiotics such as nitrofurantoin, fosphomycin, amoxicillin-clavulanate and trimethoprim-sulphamethaxazole may be used if the pathogen is susceptible to them.

8. Conclusion

Antimicrobial resistance has become a global problem of increasing importance. It is now essential that laboratories be able to rapidly identify and characterize resistant organisms. This is, of even more importance, in ESBL producing organisms that clearly have a higher morbidity and mortality associated with their infections. There is also increasing evidence, that ESBL organisms frequently possess resistance factors to other classes of other antimicrobials, like the aminoglycosides and quinolones. ESBL producing bacteria are being found both in the hospital and in the community, especially the CTX-M beta –lactamases.
The increasing number of community isolates, especially E. coli producing CTX-M-15 have become global and now are being seen in the hospital as well. It is thought that the CTX-M -15 producing *E.coli* is mostly due to a single clone named ST131, which appears to have originated in the Indian sub-continent. In addition, the increasing number of carbapenemases could also seriously compromise our treatment options. Therefore, empiric antimicrobial coverage may need to be modified in patients who present with serious sepsis syndromes, especially, after travel to countries that are high risk for this clone.
Treatment of ESBL infections requires the use of carbapenems in seriously ill patients. Imipenem, meropenem, doripenem are all viable alternatives. Ertapenem can be used in the out patient setting, in the absence of *Pseudomonas aeruginosa.* Agents such as fosfomycin, nitrofurantoin, amoxicillin/clavulanic acid, pivemecillinam, temocillin can be alternate drugs in uncomplicated UTI's and in patients with drug allergies to the carbapenems. Salvage therapy using tigecycline and colistin can be used in seriously ill patients who are CTX-M producers and Amp-C producing isolates.
In addition to understanding the complex mechanisms involved in ESBL infections, strict antimicrobial stewardship, appropriate infection control measures and aggressive treatment of seriously ill patients is necessary in reducing the mortality and morbidity associated with these infections.

9. References

[1] Abraham EP, Chain E(1940): An enzyme from bacteria able to destroy penicillin (letter). Nature ;146:837
[2] Datta N, Kontomichalau P(1965): Penicillinase synthesis controlled by infectious R factors in Enterobacteriaceae. Nature ;208:239-44
[3] Pitton JS (1972): Mechanism of bacterial resistance to antibiotics. Rev. Physiol Biochem Pharmacol.;65:15-93
[4] Neu HC (1982). The new beta-lactamase stable cephalosporins. Ann Intern Med ;97:408-19
[5] Kiebe C et al (1985): Evolution of plasmid coded resistance to broad-spectrum cephalosporins. Antimicrobial Agents chemotherar .28:302-7

[6] Bonnet R (2004). Growing extended spectrum of beta lactamases: the CTX-M enzymes.Antimicrob Agents Chemother;48:1-14

[7] Nordmann P, Poirel L (2002): Emerging carbapenemases in gram-negative aerobes. Clin Microbiol Infect;8:321-31

[8] Perez F et al (2007): The continuing challenges of ESBL'S. Curr Opin Pharmacol oct 7(5):459-469.

[9] Paterson DL et al (2001). Outcome of cephalosporins treatment for serious infections due to apparently susceptibility organism producing extended spectrum beta lactamases: implications for the clinical microbiology laboratory. J Clin Microbiol;39:2206-12

[10] Romero L et al (2005) A: long-term study of the frequency of ESBL producing e.coli and Klebsiella pneumonia isolates. Clin Microbiol Infect. 11;625-631

[11] Hernandez JR et al (2005) A. Spanish Group for nosocomial infections . Nationwide study of Escheria coli and Klebsiella pneumoniae producing extended spectrum beta lactamases in Spain. Antimicrobial Agents Chemother. ;49;2122-2125

[12] Albertini Mt et al (2002). Surveillance of methicillin resistant staphylococcus aureus and enterobacteriacae producing extended spectrum beta lactamases (ESBL) in Northern France. A 5-year multicentre study. . J hosp Infec;52:107-113.

[13] Handberger H et al(1999): Antibiotic susceptibility among gram negative bacilli in intensive care units in 5 European countries. French and Portuguese ICU study groups. .JAMA 281:67-71

[14] Woerther PL et al (2010). Emergence and dissemination of extended spectrum beta lactamases producing Escherichia coli in the community: lessons from the study of a remote and controlled population. J Infect Dis. Aug 15;(4):515-23

[15] Mendes C et al (2000): evaluation of the in vitro activity of 9 antimicrobials against bacterial strains isolated from patients in the intensive care units in Brazil. MYSTIC antimicrobial surveillance Program.2000. Braz J Infect Dis. 4:236-244

[16] Casellas JM, Quinteros MG . A Latin American point de vu on the epidemiology, control and treatment options of infections caused by extended spectrum beta-lactamase producers. In Anabile-cuevas CF. editor. Antimicrobial resistance in bacteria. Wymondham Horizon bioscience. 99-122

[17] Bauernfeind A et al (1992). A new plasmidic cefotaximase from patients infected with salmonella typhimurium . Infection .20:158-163

[18] Aitmhand R et al (2002). Plasmid mediated TEM 3 extended spectrum beta lactamase production in salmonella typhimurium in Casablanca. J Antimicrobial Chemother.49;169-179

[19] Barguellil F et al (1995). In vitro acquisition of extended spectrum beta lactamases in salmonella enteritis during antimicrobial therapy. Eur j Clin Microbiol Infect Dis. 14:703-706

[20] Neuwirth CS et al (2001). TEM 89 beta lactamase produced by a Proteus mirabilis clinical isolate. New complex mutant with mutations in both TEM 59 and TEM 3. . Antimicrobial Agents Chemother 45:3591-3594

[21] Myers KS et al (1993): Nosocomial outbreak of Klebsiella infection resistant late generation cephalosporin's. . Ann Intern Med. 119:353-358

[22] National Nosocomial Infections Surveillance, 2002 nation nosocomial Infections Surveillance system report, data summary from January 1992 to June 2002, issued august 2002. Am J Infect Control.30:458-475
[23] Bell JM et al (2007). Prevalence and significance of a negative extended spectrum beta lactamase confirmation test result after a positive ESBL screening test result for isolates of Escherichia coli and Klebsiella pneumonaie : result form the Sentry Asia pacific surveillance program. J Antimicrobial Chemother.;45:1478-82
[24] Yu WLet al (2002). Molecular epidemiology of extended spectrum beta lactamase producing fluroquinolones resistant isolates of Klebsiella pneumoniae in Taiwan. J Clin Microbiol.;40:4666-9
[25] Chanawong A et al (2002). Three cefotaximases, CTX-M-9, CTX-M-13 and CTX-M-14 among enterobacteriacae in the People Republic of China. Antimicrobial Agents Chemither.;46;630-637
[26] Karim A, Poirel S, Nagarajan S, Nordmann P (2001): Plasmid mediated extended spectrum beta lactamase (CTX-M like)from India and gene association with insertion sequence ISEcpL. .FEMS Microbiol Lett.201:237-241
[27] Koh TH et al (2001). Carbapenem resistant Klebsiella pneumoniae in Singapore producing IMP-1 beta lactamases and lacking an outer membrane protein. Antimicrobial agents Chemother. ;45:1939-40
[28] Miriagou V, Tassos PT, Legakis NJ, Tzouvelckis LS (2004). Extended spectrum cephalosporin resistance in non-typhoid salmonella. Int. J Antimicrobial Agents;23:547-55
[29] Lincopan NJ et al (2005). First isolation of metallo beta lactamase producing multi-resistent Klebsiella pneumoniae from a patient in Brazil. J clin Microbiol. 25:516-519
[30] Munday CJ et al(2004). Predominance and genetic diversity of community and hospital acquired CTX-M extended spectrum beta –lactamases in York, UK. J Antimicrobial Chemother.;54:628-33
[31] Woodford N et al (2007). Molecular epidemiology of multi resistant Escherichia coli isolates from community onset urinary tract infections in Cornwall, England. J Antimicrob Chemother.59(1)106-109
[32] Clinical and laboratories Standards Institute. Performance standards for antimicrobial susceptibility testing. fifteen Informational supplement. M100-S15, CSI, Wayne PA, USA 2005
[33] Azap OK et al (2010).Risk factors for extended spectrum beta lactamases positivity in uropathogenic Escherichia coli isolated from community acquired urinary tract infections. Clin Microbiol Infect Feb;16 (2): 147-51.
[34] Lau SM, Peng MY, Chang FY (2004). Resistance rates to community used antimicrobials among pathogens of both bacteremic and non-bacteremic community acquired urinary tract infections. J Microbiol Immunol Infect.. Jun ;37(3):185-91
[35] Khanfar H et al (2009). Extended spectrum beta lactamases in Escheria coli and Klebsiella pneumoniae: trends in hospital and community settings. J Infect Dev Ctries. 3(4) 295-299
[36] Carter MW et al (2000): Detection of extended spectrum beta lactamases in Klebsiella with the oxford combination disk method. J Clin Microbiol .38:4228-4232

[37] Weigand I et al (2007). Detection of extended spectrum beta lactamases in Enterobacteriaceae by use of semi automated microbiology systems and manuel detection procedures. . j clin Microbiol .45;1167-1174

[38] Canton R, Coque TM (2006): The CTX-M beta lactamases pandemic. Curr opion Microbiol..9:466-476

[39] Arsenio A et al (2000). Outbreak of a multidrug resistant Klebsiella pneumonaie strain in an intensive care unit: antibiotic use as a risk factor for colonization and infection. . Clin Infect Dis. 30> 55-60

[40] Bisson G et al (2002). Extended spectrum beta lactamase producing E. coli and klebsiella species : risk factors for colonization's and impact of antimicrobial formulary interventions on colonization's prevalence. Infect Control Hosp Epidemiol. 23:254-260

[41] DAgata E et al (1998). The molecular and clinical epidemiology of enterobacteriacae producing extended spectrum beta lactamases in a tertiary care hospital. 36. 279-285.

[42] Lautenbach E et al (2001), Strom BL, Bilker WB, Patel JB, Edelstein PH, Fishman NO. epidemiological investigation of fluroquinolones resistance in infections due to extended spectrum beta lactamase producing Escherichia coli and klebsiella pneumoniae . Clin Infect Dis.;33:1288-94

[43] Mangeney N et al ( ) G. A 5-year epidemiological study of extended spectrum beta lactamases producing klebsiella pneumoniae isolates

[44] Peterson LP (2008). Antimicrobial policy and prescribing strategies for therapy of extended spectrum beta lactamases producing enterobacteriacae: the role of pipercillin tazobactam . Clin Microbiol Infect.14(suppl)181-184

[45] Pena c et al (2008). Infections due to Escherichia coli producing extended spectrum beta lactamase among hospitalized patients: factors influencing mortality. J Hosp Infect. Feb ;68(2):116-22.

[46] Helfand MS, Bonomo RA (2006): Extended spectrum beta lactamases in multidrug resistant Escherichia coli . Changing the therapy for hospital acquired and community acquired infections. Clin Infect Dis.;43:1415-1416

[47] Schiappa D et al (1996), Hayden MK, Matushek MG, Hasemi FM, Sullivan J, Smith KY, Miyashiro D, Quinn JP, Weinstein RA, Trenholme GM. Ceftazidime resistant klebsiella pneumonaie and Escheria coli blood stream infection . a case control and epidemiological investigation. J Infect Dis. 174:529-536

[48] Weiner J et al (1999). Multiple antibiotic resistant Klebsiella and E coli in nursing homes.. JAMA 281:517-523

[49] Lee CH, Su LH, Tang YF, Liu JW (2006). Treatment of ESBL producing Klebsiella pneumoniae bacteremia with carbapenems or flomofef: a retrospective study and laboratory analysis of the isolates. J Antimicrob Chemother.;58:1074-1077.

[50] Silva J, Aguillar C, Becerra Z et al (1999), Lopez Antunano F, Garcia R: extended spectrum beta lactamases in clinical isolated of enterobactericae in Mexico.. Microb drug Resist. 5:189-193

[51] DeChamps C et al (1991), Rouby D, Guelon D, Sirot J, Sirot D, Beytout D, Gourgand JM. A case controlled study of an infections caused by Klebsiella pneumoniae strains producing CTX-M (TEM-3) beta lactamases. . J Hosp Infect. 18:5-13

[52] Goldstein FW, Pean Y, Gartner J (1995): Resistance to ceftriaxone and other beta lactam in bacteria isolated in the community. The Vigil Roc study group. 1995. Antimicrob Agents Chemother.. 39:2516-2519

[53] Baranniak A et al (2002), Sadowy E, Hryniewicz W, Gniadkowski M: Two different extended spectrum beta lactamase(ESBL) in one of the first ESBL producing salmonella isolates in Poland.. J Clin Microbiol.. 40:1095-1097

[54] Fortineau N, Naas T, Gaillot O, Nordmann P (2001). SHV type extended spectrum beta lactamase in a Shigella flexerni clinical isolates. J Antimicrob Chemother.. 47:685-688

[55] Kim S et al (2004). Occurrence of extended spectrum beta lactamases in members of the genus Shigella in the republic of Korea.. J clin Microbiol. 42:5264-5269

[56] Ishil Y et al(1995). Cloning and sequence of the gene encoding a cefotaxime hydrolyzing class A beta lactamase isolated from E coli.. Antimicrob Agents Chemother. 39;2269-2275

[57] Mirelis B et al(2003), Navarro F, Miro E, Mesa RJ, Coll P, Prats G. Community transmission of extended spectrum beta lactamases. Emerg Infect Dis 9;1024-1025

[58] Rodriguez Bano J, Navarro MD (2008). Extended spectrum beta lactamases in ambulatory care: a clinical perspective. Clin Microbiol Infect.. Jan ;14 Suppl 1:104-10

[59] Pitout J et al (2004), Hanson N, Church DL, Laupland KB. Population based laboratory surveillance for Escheria coli producing extended spectrum beta lactamases: importance of community isolates with the bla CtX-m genes. Clin Infec Dis. 38;1736-1741.

[60] Rodriguez Bano J, Alcala JC, Cisneros JM et al (2008). Community infections caused by extended spectrum beta lactamases producing Escheria coli. Arch intern med..168:1897-1902.

[61] Colodner R, Rock W, Chazan B (2004). Risk factors for the development of extended spectrum beta lactamase producing bacteremia in hospitalized patients. Eur J Clin Microbiol Infect Dis..23:163-7

[62] Calbo E et al (2006 J. risk factors for community onset urinary tract infections due to Escheria coli harboring extended spectrum beta lactamases. J Antimicrob. Chemother.. 57; 780-783.

[63] Astal Z, Sharif SA, Abdallah SA et al (2004). Extended spectrum beta lactamases in escheria Coli isolated from community acquired urinary tract infections in the Gaza Strip.. Ann Saudi Med. 24:55-57

[64] Bloomberg B et al (2005). High rate of pediatric septicemia caused by gram-negative bacteremia with extended spectrum beta lactamases in Dar-es- Salam, Tanzania. J Clin Microbiol. 43:745-749fatal cases

[65] Brigante GF et al ( ). Evolution of CTX-M type beta lactamases in isolates of escheria coli infecting hospital and

[66] Chao Qi et al (2010),. Changing prevalence of Escherichia coli with CTX-M type extended spectrum beta lactamases in out patient urinary e.coli between 2003-2008. Diag Microbiol and Infect Dis.. 67:87-91

[67] Hanson ND (2003). Amp C beta lactamases: what do we need to know for the future.?. J Antimicrob Chemother. 52.2-4

[68] Ramphal R, Ambrose P (2006): Extended spectrum beta lactamases and clinical outcomes. Clin Infect Dis;42:S164-72

[69] Kang CL et al (2008), Cheong HS, Chung DR, Peck KP, Song JH, Oh MD, Choe KW. Clinical features and outcome of community onset bloodstream infections caused by extended spectrum beta lactamase producing Escherichia coli. . Eur J Clin Microbiol Infect Dis. Jan; 27(1)85-8

[70] Wisplinghoff H et al (2003). Nosocomial blood stream infections in US Hospitals: analysis of 24,179 cases from a prospective nationwide study. Clin Infect Dis.;39:309-317

[71] Friedman R, Raveh R, Zartzer E, et al (2009).Prospective evaluation of colonization with extended spectrum beta lactamase producing enterobacteriacae among patients at hospital admission and of subsequent colonization with ESBL producing enterobactericae among patients during hospitalization.. Infect Control Hosp Epidemiol. 30:534-542

[72] Kim Y et al (2002), Pai H, Lee HJ, Park SE, Choi EH, Kim J, Kim JH, Kim EC. Blood stream infections by extended spectrum beta lactamases producing escheria coli and klebsiella pneumoniae in children. Epidemiology and clinical outcomes.. Antmicrob Agents Chemother.46:1481-1491.

[73] Cervera C et al (2010), linares L, Hoyo G, Sanclemente G, Marco F, Cofan F, Coftan F, Ricart MJ, Navasa M, Moreno A: Klebsiella pneumoniae infection in solid organ transplant: Epidemiology and antibiotic resistance. Transplantation Proceeding, 42, 2941-2943.

[74] Paterson DL. Bonomo RA (2005). Extended spectrum beta lactamases. C clinical update. Clin Microbiol rev.18;657-686

[75] Bush K et al (1993), Macanthil C, Rasmussen BA, Lee VJ et al.Kinetic interactions of tazobactam with beta lactamases from all major structural classes. Antimicrob Agents Chemother.;37:851-858

[76] Payne DJ et al(1994): comparative activities of clavulanic acid, sulbactam and tazobactam against clinically important beta lactamases. Antimicrob Agents Chemother.;38:767-772

[77] Burgess DS et al (2003). Clinical and microbiologic analysis of a hospitals extended spectrum beta lactamases producing isolates over a two-year period. Pharmacotherapy. ;23:1232-1237

[78] Falagas ME, Polemis M, Alexiou VG et al (2008). Antimicrobial resistance of escheria e.coli isolates from primary care patients in Greece. Med sci Monit;14:CR75-CR79.

[79] Bin C, Hui W, Renyuan Z et al (2006): outcome of cephalosporin treatment of bacteremia due to CTX-M type extended spectrum beta lactamases producing Escherichia coli. Diag Microbiol Infec Dis.;56:351-357.

[80] Goethaert K, Van Looveran M, Lammens C et al: High does cefepeme as an alternative treatment for infections caused by TEM-24 ESBL producing Enterobacter aerogenes in severely ill patients. Clin Microbiol Infect 2006;12:56-62

[81] Morosini MI et al(2006): Antibiotic co resistance in extended spectrum beta lactamases producing enterobacteriacae and in vitro activity of tigecycline. Antimicrob Agents Chemother:50:2695-2699

[82] Garau J (2008). other antimicrobials of interest in the era of extended spectrum beta lactamases: fosfomycin, nitrofurantoin, and tigecycline. Clin Microbiol Infect.14(suppl). P198-202

[83] Auer S, Wojna A, Hell M (2010): Oral treatment options for ambulatory patients with urinary tract infections caused by extended spectrum beta lactamases producing e.coli. Antimicrobial Agents Chemother. Sept .p4006-4008

[84] Prakash V et al (2009), Lewis JS, Herrara ML, Wickes BL, Jorgenson JH: oral and parental therapeutic options for out patient urinary infections caused by enterobacteriacae producing CTX-M extended spectrum beta-lactamase. Antimicrob Agents Chemotherar. March;53(3):1278-80

[85] Depersio JR et al (2005): Evolution and dissemination of extended spectrum beta lactamases producing Klebsiella pneumoniae: Epidemiology and molecular report from the Sentry Antimicrobial surveillance program. (1997-2003).Diag Microbiol infec Dis . 51(1):1-7

[86] Zahar JR, Lortholary O, Martin C et al: Addressing the challenge of extended spectrum beta lactamases. Curr Opion Investig.Drugs 2009;Feb 10.(2):172-80

[87] Hernandez JR et al (2006), Velasco C, Romero C, Martinez,-Martinez L, Pascual A. A comparative in-vitro activity of ertapenem against extended spectrum beta lactamase producing escheria coli and klebsiella pneumoniae isolated in Spain.. Int Antimicrob Agents. 28:457-9.2006

[88] Livermore DM, Oakton KJ carter Mw et al (2001), Warner M: Activity of ertapenem (MK-0826) versus Enterobacteriaceae with potent beta lactamases. Antimicrobial. Agents Chemother 45(10): 2831-2837

Part 2

Uropathogens and Host Characteristics

3

Extended Characterization of Human Uropathogenic *Escherichia coli* Isolates from Slovenia

Marjanca Starčič Erjavec and Darja Žgur-Bertok
University of Ljubljana, Biotechnical Faculty,
Department of Biology
Slovenia

1. Introduction

Escherichia coli (*E. coli*) is a very diverse bacterial species found naturally in the intestinal tract of humans and many other animal species. Even though *E. coli* is known to be part of the normal gut microbiota, some strains - that are pathogenic - cause a wide variety of different intestinal and extraintestinal diseases (Marrs et al., 2005). Typical extraintestinal infections due to *E. coli* include urinary tract infections (UTI), diverse intra-abdominal infections, pneumonia, surgical-site infection, meningitis, osteomyelitis, soft-tissue infections, bacteremia (Russo & Johnson, 2006).

UTIs are one of the most frequently acquired bacterial infections and *E. coli* accounts for as many as 90% of all community-acquired UTIs. Approximately 50% of all women have had a UTI by their late 20s. About 20–30% of women with first UTI will have two or more infections; while 5%, will develop chronic recurring infections which greatly disrupt a woman's life (Marrs et al., 2005). In Slovenia *E. coli* is the causative agent of approximately 80% of uncomplicated UTIs (Lindič, 2005).

E. coli isolates that cause UTI exhibit a number of specific characteristics and are classified, as uropathogenic *E. coli* (UPEC), a subgroup of extraintestinal pathogenic *E. coli* (ExPEC) (Russo & Johnson, 2000). UPEC strains mainly belong to the B2 phylogenetic group and to a lesser extent to the D group, while commensal strains belong to groups A and B1 (Picard et al., 1999). Further, some O-antigens (O1, O2, O4, O6, O7, O18 and O83) are more prevalent among uropathogenic *E. coli* strains and are therefore associated with UTI (Moreno et al. 2006). In comparison to commensal *E. coli* strains, UPEC possess an array of virulence factors namely, adhesins, toxins, polysaccharide coatings, invasins, iron uptake systems and systems to evade host immune responses (Oelschlaeger et al., 2002).

Of serious concern and an increasing health problem, on a global scale, is the appearance and spread of antimicrobial resistance. One of the major health care concerns is emergence of multidrug resistant bacteria and clinical microbiologists increasingly agree that multidrug resistant Gram-negative bacteria pose the greatest risk to public health (Kumarasamy et al., 2010). Therefore, it is essential to determine susceptibility of pathogenic strains for antimicrobial agents and association of antimicrobial resistance with virulence genes.

One of the means for acquiring specific virulence factor genes and antimicrobial resistance genes, is via mobile DNA (*e. g.* conjugal plasmids, transposons/integrons) (Alekshun &

Levy, 2007; Boerlin & Reid-Smith, 2008; Dobrindt et al., 2010). Hence, determining the prevalence of mobile elements and examining the correlation of antimicrobial resistance/virulence factor genes with mobile elements among UPEC is of great significance.

The search for alternative antibacterial agents is of great importance and colicins, toxic, narrow killing spectrum exhibiting proteins produced by colicinogenic *E. coli*, exhibit great potential as an alternative approach in the battle against microbes. It has been reported that colicins are effective against intestinal and UPEC strains (Rijavec et al., 2007; Schamberger et al., 2004; Stahl et al., 2004), and that they prevent colonization of urinary catheters (Trautner et al., 2005). To evaluate the potential of colicins as antimicrobial agents, studies on the prevalence of colicins and colicin resistance are needed.

In summary, to diminish the burden of UPEC, using effective preventive measures, data on phylogenetic groups, serogroups, virulence factor prevalence, antimicrobial resistance, presence of mobile DNA, colicin production and colicin resistance among *E. coli* isolates from different geographic regions must be assessed.

In Slovenia in 2002, we collected 110 *E. coli* isolates from humans with community-acquired urinary tract infections at the Institute of Microbiology and Immunology, Medical Faculty, Ljubljana, Slovenia. Isolation was performed according to standard laboratory protocols and UPEC were isolates from > 10^5 colony-forming units (CFU) (Rijavec et al., 2006). These isolates were studied in order to obtain an extended characterisation, including phylogenetic groups, serogroups, virulence factor prevalence, antimicrobial resistance, presence of mobile DNA and colicinogeny and colicin resistance (Rijavec et al., 2006; Starčič Erjavec et al., 2006; Starčič Erjavec et al., 2007; Starčič Erjavec & Žgur-Bertok, 2008; Starčič Erjavec et al., 2008; Starčič Erjavec et al., 2009; Starčič Erjavec et al., 2010).

2. Phylogenetic groups and subgroups

E. coli strains can be assigned to one of four main phylogenetic groups: A, B1, B2, and D. The four groups were identified on the basis of allelic variation at enzyme-encoding genes detected by multilocus enzyme electrophoresis (Ochman et al., 1983, Whittam et al., 1983). Clermont et al. (2000) established the method of rapid and simple determination of the *E. coli* phylogenetic groups by a triplex PCR. This genotyping method is based on the amplification of a 279 bp fragment of the *chuA* gene; a 211 bp fragment of the *yjaA* gene; and a 152 bp fragment of TSPE4.C2, a noncoding region of the genome. The presence or absence of combinations of these three amplicons is used to assign *E. coli* to one of the four phylogenetic groups. However, to increase the discriminative power of phylogenetic group analysis, Escobar-Paramo et al. (2004) proposed the introduction of phylogenetic subgroups. They defined (Figure 1), apart from the phylogenetic group B1 (lacking *chuA* and *yjaA* and having Tspe4.C2), the following six subgroups: in the phylogenetic group A, subgroupA_0 (lacking *chuA*, *yjaA*, and Tspe4.C2) and subgroup A_1 (lacking *chuA*, having *yjaA*, and lacking Tspe4.C2); in the phylogenetic group B2, subgroup $B2_2$ (having *chuA* and *yjaA* and lacking Tspe4.C2) and subgroup $B2_3$ (having *chuA*, *yjaA*, and Tspe4.C2); in the phylogenetic group D, subgroup D_1 (having *chuA* and lacking *yjaA* and Tspe4.C2) and subgroup D_2 (having *chuA*, lacking *yjaA*, and having Tspe4.C2), Fig. 1.

Analysis of our collection of 110 UPEC isolates showed that 55 (50%) belonged to group B2, 28 (25%) to A, 21 (19%) to D, and 6 (5%) to the B1 group (Rijavec et al., 2006). When subgroups were considered the distribution of the isolates was: 4 (4%) of the studied isolates belonged to the subgroup A_0, 24 (22%) to A_1, 6 (5%) to $B2_2$, 49 (45%) to $B2_3$, 16 (15%) to D_1 and 5 (5%) to D_2 (our unpublished data).

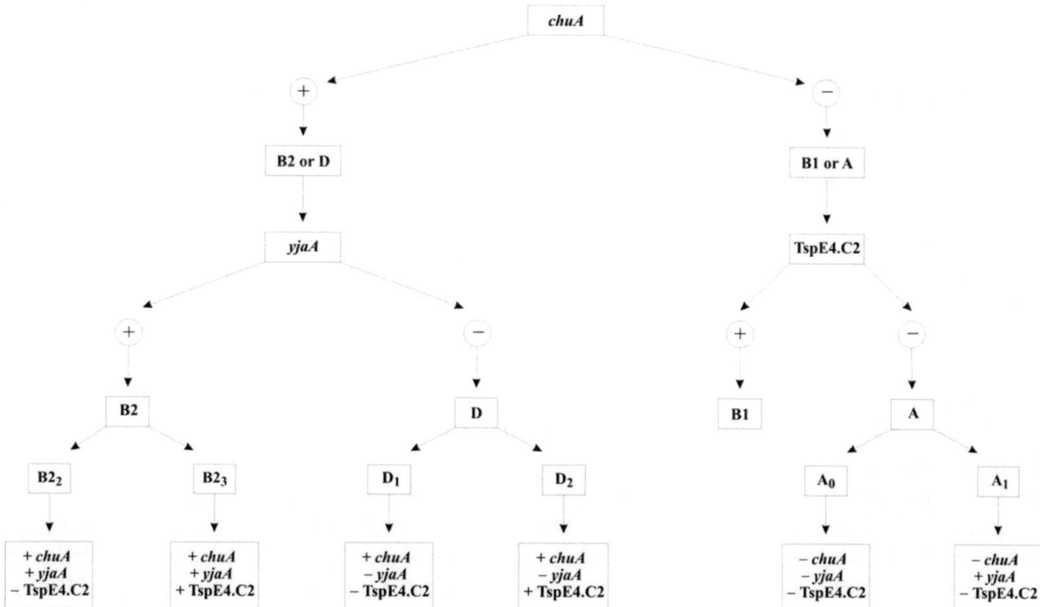

Fig. 1. Diagram of phylogenetic (sub)group determination.

The obtained distribution of the studied isolates into the phylogenetic groups, with the large majority classifying to the B2 group was expected since, it is known that ExPEC isolates mainly belong to the B2 phylogenetic group (Picard et al., 1999) however, the disproportionate distribution into the $B2_2$ (5%) and $B2_3$ (45%), and A_0 (4%) and A_1 (22%) subgroups was surprising.

3. Serogroups

Serotyping of *E. coli* isolates is an often used method for distinguishing possible pathogenic *E. coli* from commensal *E. coli*. It is complex since among *E. coli* 173 O-antigens, 80 K-antigens, and 56 H-antigens can be found. The O-, K-, and H-antigens can occur in many possible combinations therefore, the final number of *E. coli* serotypes is very high, 50,000-100,000 or more. However, the number of frequent pathogenic serotypes is limited. Two main groups of frequent serotypes are: (i) serotypes from diarrhoeal disease and (ii) serotypes from extraintestinal disease (Orskov & Orskov, 1992).

Serotyping of the 110 uropathogenic strains revealed that 77 (70%) were O-antigen typable, 19 (17%) were O-nontypable, and 14 (12.7%) were rough. Sixty-three (57%) of the examined strains were H-antigen typable, 41 (37%) were H-antigen negative, and 6 (5%) were H-antigen nontypable. The O-typable strains were distributed into 31 serogroups. Nevertheless, the most frequent were O2 (9 isolates) and serotype O6:H1 (10 isolates). Five common serotypes were identified in three or more strains: O2:HNT (n = 3), O2:H6 (n = 3), O6:H1 (n = 10), O7:HNT (n = 3), and O74:H39 (n = 4) accounting for 30% of the serotypable isolates. A number of other serotypes were detected in one or two strains (Rijavec et al., 2006).

Serotype analysis of the studied strains revealed that they belonged to diverse serogroups. However, the most frequent were O2 and O6, which are well established as associated with urinary tract infections. The large majority, 96%, of the O2 and O6 isolates were assigned to the B2 phylogenetic group (Rijavec et al., 2006).

4. Virulence factors

Any component of a microbe that is required for, or potentiates its ability to cause disease is designated as a virulence factor. Many different virulence factors exist however, they can all be placed in one of the four major groups of virulence factors: adhesins, toxins, iron uptake systems and host immunity evading systems. Hence, virulence factors facilitate colonization and invasion of the host, avoidance or disruption of host defence mechanisms, injury to host tissue, and/or stimulation of a noxious host inflammatory response (Johnson and Steel, 2000).

4.1 Adhesins

Among the first virulence factors that come into play during establishment of an infection are adhesins. Besides their primary role as adhesin molecules, they can also function as invasins, promoters of biofilm formation and transmitors of signals to epithelial cells resulting in inflammation. Various adhesins have been identified and studied (Zhang & Foxman, 2003). In our analysis we focused on the four mostly studied: type 1 fimbriae, P fimbriae, S fimbriae and the Afa/Dr family of adhesins (Starčič Erjavec & Žgur-Bertok, 2008).

Type 1 fimbriae are the most common adhesive organelles of *E. coli* strains. They are encoded by the vast majority of uropathogenic *E. coli* (UPEC) isolates and many other pathogenic and commensal isolates (Bower et al., 2005). Receptors for type 1 fimbriae are present on erythrocytes, buccal epithelial cells, intestinal cells, vaginal cells and uroepithelial cells (Johnson, 1991). The *fimH* gene that was tested in our study (Starčič Erjavec & Žgur-Bertok, 2008), encodes the minor subunit protein FimH that mediates binding to the receptor. FimH has several variants: UPEC strains have a FimH that binds both monomannose and trimannose containing glycoprotein receptors, while commensal *E. coli* isolates typically show high affinity binding to only trimannose residues (Bower et al., 2005). Type 1 fimbriae function not just as adhesins, but also as invasins for bladder epithelial cells (Martinez et al., 2000).

P fimbriae are among the best studied fimbrial adhesive fibres of UPEC strains. The P fimbrial adhesin molecule (PapG) recognizes globoseries of glycolipids as receptors (Zhang & Foxman, 2003). In our study the *papC, papGII* and *papGIII* genes were included (Starčič Erjavec & Žgur-Bertok, 2008). The *papC* gene encodes the outer membrane usher protein that is required for ordered P fimbriae assembly (Thanassi et al., 1998). Many studies showed that P fimbriae occur more frequently among UPEC than fecal isolates. Based on binding specificities, P fimbriae are grouped into three major classes: I, II and III (Zhang & Foxman, 2003).

S fimbriae bind to sialyl galactosides. Studies showed that *E. coli* UTI isolates were at least two times more likely to carry S fimbriae genes (*sfa* operon) than fecal strains (Zhang & Foxman, 2003). In our study the fimbriae typical gene sequence *sfa/foc* was investigated (Starčič Erjavec & Žgur-Bertok, 2008).

The Afa/Dr family consists of 13 known adhesins that all bind to the Dra blood group antigen present on the complement regulatory molecule CD55, also known as decay-accelerating factor (DAF) (Bower et al., 2005). The *E. coli* strains harbouring these adhesins have been found to be associated with UTIs and also with various enteric infections (Servin, 2005).

Among the tested adhesin genes in the studied UPEC isolates (Table 1), the type 1 fimbriae were the most prevalent - the *fimH* gene nucleotide sequences were detected in 107 strains (97%). The P fimbriae were also abundant, the *papC* encoding gene sequence was found in 54 strains (49%), 37 strains (34%) harboured the class II *papG* adhesin sequence and 14 strains (13%) harboured the class III *papG* adhesin. Twenty-six (24%) possessed the S fimbriae typical gene sequence *sfa/foc*. Only 2 strains (2%) harbored *afa/dra* sequences (Starčič Erjavec & Žgur-Bertok, 2008).

Analysis of the distribution of adhesin gene sequences among phylogenetic groups revealed that adhesin gene sequences were differently distributed (Table 1): *fimH* sequences were found with similar prevalence in strains of all four phylogenetic groups, *papC* sequences were found in all phylogenetic groups, but they were most prevalent (65%) among B2 group strains. The association of *papC* with the B2 group was statistically significant. Nevertheless, *papGII* sequences were found in all phylogenetic groups, in contrast, *papGIII* adhesin sequences were exclusively found among strains of the B2 group.

Further, a very high, statistically significant, prevalence of S fimbriae in the B2 group was detected, 45% of the strains belonging to the B2 group harboured *sfa/foc* sequences (Starčič Erjavec & Žgur-Bertok, 2008).

4.2 Toxins

Toxins affect an astonishing variety of fundamental eukaryotic processes and thereby harm the host (Kaper, 2004) and are important virulence factors in a variety of *E. coli* mediated diseases - in UTI the production of toxins by colonized *E. coli* may cause an inflammatory response that leads to the UTI symptoms (Zhang & Foxman, 2003).

In pathogenic *E. coli* strains several important toxins have been identified, the best known, associated with UPEC strains, are alpha hemolysin (HlyA) and cytotoxic necrotizing factor 1 (CNF1) (Zhang & Foxman, 2003).

Well known toxins are also invasins, the Ibe proteins that help *E. coli* strains to invade the human brain microvascular endothelial cells (Xie et al., 2004). The presence of IbeA protein is statistically significantly higher in strains causing cystitis and/or pyelonephritis (Johnson et al., 2005). The gene for the uropathogenic specific protein (USP) that was found as a homologue of the *Vibrio cholerae* zonula occludens toxin encoding gene (Kurazono et al., 2000), has been significantly more often detected in UPEC strains than in fecal strains from healthy individuals (Bauer et al., 2002).

Among the screened toxin encoding genes in the studied UPEC isolates (Table 1), the *usp* gene had the highest prevalence as *usp* specific nucleotide sequences were detected in 48 strains (44%). The prevalence of *hlyA* and *cnf1* was similar, 28 (25%) and 25 strains (23%), respectively, possessed the tested nucleotide sequences. Only 10 strains (9%) harboured *ibeA* sequences (Starčič Erjavec et al., 2008).

Analysis of the distribution of toxin encoding genes among the determined phylogenetic groups of studied strains (Table 1) revealed that the tested toxin encoding genes *hlyA*, *cnf1*, *ibeA* and *usp* were mostly harboured by UPEC strains belonging to the B2 phylogenetic group, as 26 (93%) of the strains harbouring *hlyA* belonged to the B2 group, 25 (100%) harbouring *cnf1*, 9 (90%) harbouring *ibeA* and 42 (88%) harbouring *usp* belonged to the B2 phylogenetic group (Starčič Erjavec et al., 2008).

Trait	Prevalence (N, [%])				
		Phylogenetic group			
	Total (N=110)	A (N=28)	B1 (N=6)	B2 (N=55)	D (N=21)
Virulence factors					
Adhesins					
fimH	107 (97)	28 (26)	5 (5)	53 (50)	21 (20)
papC	54 (49)	8 (15)	1 (2)	35 (65)	10 (19)
papGII	37 (34)	5 (14)	1 (3)	21 (57)	10 (27)
papGIII	14 (13)	0 (0)	0 (0)	14 (100)	0 (0)
sfa/foc	26 (24)	1 (4)	0 (0)	25 (96)	0 (0)
afa/dra	2 (2)	1 (50)	0 (0)	1 (50)	0 (0)
Toxins					
hlyA	28 (25)	1 (4)	0 (0)	26 (93)	1 (4)
cnf	25 (23)	0 (0)	0 (0)	25 (100)	0 (0)
ibeA	10 (9)	0 (0)	0 (0)	9 (90)	1 (10)
usp	48 (44)	1 (2)	0 (0)	42 (88)	5 (10)
Iron uptake systems					
iucD	46 (42)	8 (17)	0 (0)	27 (59)	11 (24)
iroCD (=*iroN*)	51 (46)	9 (18)	0 (0)	41 (80)	1 (2)
ireA	22 (20)	4 (18)	0 (0)	12 (55)	6 (27)
fyuA	84 (76)	17 (20)	3 (4)	49 (58)	15 (18)
Host immunity evading systems					
K1	6 (5)	1 (17)	1 (17)	4 (67)	0 (0)
K5	11 (10)	2 (18)	1 (9)	8 (73)	0 (0)
traT	63 (57)	20 (32)	4 (6)	29 (46)	10 (16)
tcpC	23 (21)	0 (0)	0 (0)	23 (100)	0 (0)
Antimicrobial susceptibility					
Ampicillin	57 (52)	12 (21)	5 (9)	32 (56)	18 (32)
Ciprofloxacin	99 (90)	23 (23)	5 (5)	52 (53)	19 (19)
Chloramphenicol	50 (45)	7 (14)	3 (6)	32 (64)	8 (16)
Kanamycin	95 (86)	20 (21)	5 (5)	51 (54)	19 (20)
Mezlocillin	59 (54)	12 (20)	5 (8)	34 (58)	8 (14)
Nalidixic acid	64 (58)	12 (19)	3 (5)	38 (59)	11 (17)
Norfloxacin	99 (90)	23 (23)	5 (5)	52 (52)	19 (19)
Streptomycin	69 (63)	15 (22)	5 (7)	40 (60)	9 (13)
Sulfamethoxazole-Trimethoprim	87 (79)	18 (21)	6 (7)	49 (56)	14 (16)
Tetracycline	47 (43)	6 (13)	4 (9)	33 (70)	4 (9)
Trimethoprim	72 (65)	14 (19)	6 (8)	41 (57)	11 (15)
Mobile genetic elements					
RepFIA	20 (18)	7 (35)	0 (0)	10 (50)	3 (15)
RepFIB	57 (52)	18 (32)	2 (4)	26 (46)	11 (19)
RepFIIA	24 (22)	7 (29)	0 (0)	15 (63)	2 (8)
Integron	34 (31)	12 (35)	1 (3)	12 (35)	9 (26)
Colicinogenity	42 (38)	12 (29)	3 (7)	20 (48)	7 (17)

Table 1. Characterized traits in studied UPEC isolates – prevalence and distribution among phylogenetic groups.

4.3 Iron uptake systems

Iron is an essential cofactor for many basic metabolic pathways and bacteria have developed specialized iron uptake systems to capture iron. The most prominent are the siderophores, iron-binding molecules that are taken up by special siderophore receptors and ATP-consuming porin-like transporters in the bacterial outer membrane (Schaible & Kaufmann, 2004). Siderophores can be classified into three groups: (i) the catecholate type (enterobactin, salmochelin = enterochelin), (ii) hydroxamate type (aerobactin) and (iii) a mixed type - a combination of both (yersiniabactin) (Grass, 2006; Schaible & Kaufmann, 2004). In addition to siderophore synthesis strains can use siderophores produced and released into the extracellular medium by other bacteria and even fungi. In the host, bacteria may use iron sources such as heme, hemoglobin, hemopexin, and iron bound to transferrin and lactoferrin (Braun & Braun, 2002). Apart from the siderophores and their receptors, autotransporters, virulence-associated proteins in gram-negative bacteria, can also play a role in obtaining iron for example, the hemoglobin protease Hbp (Otto et al., 2002). All autotransporter proteins are energy-independent secreted via a type 5 secretion system and possess an overall unifying structure, comprising (i) an amino-terminal leader peptide (for secretion across the inner membrane), (ii) the secreted mature protein (or passenger domain), and (iii) a dedicated C-terminal domain, which forms a pore in the outer membrane through which the passenger domain passes to the cell surface (Henderson & Nataro, 2001).

In our study the following iron uptake systems genes were investigated (Table 1): *iucD* for aerobactin, *iroCD* and *iroN* for salmochelin, *fyuA* for yersiniabactin and *ireA* of a putative TonB-dependent siderophore receptor. The iron uptake system with the highest prevalence was yersiniabactin, the *fyuA* gene coding for the ferric yersiniabactin receptor was found in 84 strains (76%). The salmochelin uptake system genes *iroN*, coding for the catecholate siderophore receptor, and *iroCD* coding for proteins needed in salmochelin transport, were found in 51 (46%) of studied strains. The aerobactin iron uptake system gene *iucD*, coding for lysine:N6-hydroxylase needed in aerobactin biosynthesis, was detected in 46 strains (42%) and the *ireA* gene was harboured by 22 studied strains (20%) (our unpublished data).

Analysis of the distribution of iron uptake systems encoding genes among the determined phylogenetic groups of studied strains (Table 1) revealed that all of the studied iron uptake systems were mostly harboured by UPEC strains belonging to the B2 phylogenetic group, as 41 (80%) of the strains harbouring *iroCD* and *iroN* belonged to the B2 group, 49 (58%) harbouring *fyuA*, 27 (59%) harbouring *iucD* and 12 (55%) harbouring *ireA* belonged to the B2 phylogenetic group (our unpublished data).

4.4 Host immunity evading systems

Pathogenic microbes avoid host defences using a wide array of virulence factors, ranging from polysaccharide capsules, serum resistance proteins to immune system modulating agents (Kaper et al., 2004).

Capsules are the discrete structural layers of extracellular polysaccharides that envelope the cell and allow the bacteria to evade or counteract the host immune system (Roberts, 1996). Capsules protect pathogens from assaults such as opsonophagocytosis and complement-mediated killing (Roberts, 1995); and in case of acidic capsules they can act as "sponges" to sequester and neutralize antimicrobial peptides (Llobet et al., 2008). Virtually all UPEC have a K-type polysaccharide capsule. Most UPEC express Group 2 or 3 capsules on their surfaces (Goller and Seed, 2010) and the K-antigens K1, K5, K30 and K92 are the most prevalent among UPEC (Johnson, 1991).

TraT, the surface exclusion protein of the plasmid transfer system, has been implicated in increased serum resistance (Binns et al., 1979). TraT is one of the most prevalent virulence factors in pathogenic *E. coli* isolates, as *traT* sequences have been found in 50% of *E. coli* isolates from sepsis (Ananias & Yano, 2008), in 68% of uroseptic *E. coli* (Johnson & Stell, 2000), and in 65% of UPEC isolates from cystitis, pyelonephritis, prostatitis (Johnsons et al., 2005a).

Recently, TcpC, a Toll/interleukin-1 receptor (TIR) domain-containing protein of uropathogenic *E. coli* inhibiting Toll-like receptor (TIR) and MyD88-specific signaling, impairing the innate immune response was described (Cirl et al, 2008). The *tcpC* homologous sequences were found in about 40% of *E. coli* isolates from individuals with pyelonephritis, in 21% cystitis isolates, in 16% asymptomatic bacteriuria and in only 8% of commensal isolates therefore, TcpC is implicated in the severity of urinary tract infections (UTI) in humans (Cirl et al., 2008).

Among the 110 studied UPEC isolates (Table 1) 6 (5%) had the K1-capsule and 11 (10%) had the K5-capsule (Starčič Erjavec et al., 2007). The *traT* sequences were found in 63 (57%) (Rijavec et al., 2006) and the *tcpC* sequences were found in 23 (21%) (Starčič Erjavec et al., 2010) of studied UPEC isolates.

Analysis of the distribution of the studied immune system evading characteristics among the determined phylogenetic groups (Table 1) showed that, isolates with K1- and K5-capsules were the most prevalent in the B2 group, 4 (67%) and 8 (73%), respectively however, capsule possessing isolates also belonged to the A and B1 group, albeit at low prevalence. One (17%) K1-capsule coated strain was found in the A and one in the B1 group and 2 (18%) K5-capsule coated strains in the A group and one (9%) in the B1 group. The *traT* sequence was more evenly distributed among all four phylogenetic groups A, B1, B2 and D – the prevalence was 20 (32%), 4 (6%), 29 (46%) and 10 (16%), respectively. On the other hand, the *tcpC*-encoding strains were found only in the B2 group.

5. Antimicrobial susceptibility

An important task in clinical microbiology is the performance of antimicrobial susceptibility testing in order to detect possible drug resistance in common pathogens and to assure susceptibility to drugs of choice for particular infections (Jorgensen & Ferraro, 2009). Therefore, several studies on the subject of antimicrobial susceptibility and *E. coli* isolates from UTI have been performed (*e. g.* Karlowsky et al., 2003; Kahlmeter & Menday, 2003; Yilmaz et al., 2009).

In the year 2002, when the studied isolates were collected, treatment of UTI in outpatients in Slovenia was as follows: a course of antibiotics (therapy of choice - trimethoprim 160 mg or trimethoprim/sulfamethoxazole 160 mg/800 mg twice daily for 3 days) and advice to consume sufficient quantities of liquids (2–3 l per day) (Car et al., 2003).

The studied uropathogenic strains were screened for susceptibility to the following antibiotics: ampicillin, chloramphenicol, kanamycin, streptomycin, tetracycline, trimethoprim, trimethoprim-sulfamethoxazole, ciprofloxacin, norfloxacin, nalidixic acid, mezlocillin, amikacin, cefotaxime, cefotiame, cefoxitin, ceftazidime, and gentamicin. Susceptibilities to the tested antibiotics ranged from 109 (99%) susceptible to amikacin, cefotaxime, ceftazidime, to 47 (43%) susceptible to tetracycline. Antibiotics with the highest prevalence of susceptibility, apart from amikacin, cefotaxime, ceftazidime, were to cefotiame, cefoxitin, and gentamicin as 108 (98%), 103 (94%), and 101 (92%) of the studied strains, respectively, were susceptible. Antibiotics with the lowest prevalence of susceptibility, apart from tetracycline, were to chloramphenicol, ampicilin, mezlocillin and nalidixic acid, as 50 (45%), 57 (52%), 59 (54%) and 64 (58%), respectively, were susceptible (Rijavec et al., 2006).

Forty-six (42%) of the studied strains were resistant to more than three classes of the tested antimicrobial agents—beta lactams, quinolone/fluoroquinolone, trimethoprim/trimethoprim-sulfamethoxazole, tetracycline, chloramphenicol, aminoglycosides (streptomycin, kanamycin)—and were designated as multidrug resistant (MDR). Subsequently, the association between MDR and the phylogenetic group was examined. A statistically significant correlation between non-MDR and the B2 group was determined and a significant correlation between MDR and the D phylogenetic group was found. On the other hand, there were no statistically significant correlations between MDR or non-MDR strains and the A or B1 groups (Rijavec et al., 2006).

6. Mobile genetic elements

The loss and gain of mobile genetic elements has a pivotal role in shaping the genomes of pathogenic bacteria. Horizontal gene transfer is an important mechanism that rapidly disseminates new traits to recipient organisms. Acquiring these new traits is crucial in promoting the fitness and survival of a pathogen while it coevolves with its host (Croxen & Finlay, 2010).

Bacterial plasmids, self-replicating, extrachromosomal elements are key agents of change in microbial populations. They promote the dissemination of a variety of traits, including virulence, enhanced fitness, resistance to antimicrobial agents, and metabolism of rare substances (Johnson & Nolan, 2009). *E. coli* strains possess a variety of plasmid types, of different sizes, usually ranging in size from approximately 300 bp to 2400 kbp nevertheless, each plasmid must harbour a replication region (Kado, 1998). Plasmids are classified into incompatibility groups mostly on the basis of the replication region (Couturier et al., 1988).

Integrons are assembly platforms that incorporate exogenous open reading frames by site-specific recombination and convert them to functional genes by ensuring their correct expression. Integrons are composed of three key elements necessary for the capture of exogenous genes: a gene (*intI*) encoding an integrase belonging to the tyrosine-recombinase family; a primary recombination site (*attI*); and an outward-orientated promoter (Pc) that directs transcription of the captured genes. At present, five classes of mobile integrons are distinguished. These classes have been historically defined based on the sequence of the encoded integrases, which show 40–58% identity. All five classes are physically linked to mobile DNA elements, such as insertion sequences, transposons and conjugative plasmids, all of which can serve as vehicles for intraspecies and interspecies transmission of genetic material. Class 1 integrons are associated with functional and non-functional transposons derived from Tn*402* that can be embedded in larger transposons, such as Tn*21*. Class 2 integrons are exclusively associated with Tn*7* derivatives and class 3 integrons are thought to be located in a transposon inserted in a plasmid. The other two classes of mobile integrons, class 4 and class 5, have been associated only with *Vibrio* species; class 4 is a component of a subset of SXT elements found in *Vibrio cholerae*, and class 5 is located in a compound transposon carried on a plasmid in *Vibrio salmonicida* (Mazel, 2006).

The studied UTI strains were screened for replication regions of IncFI and IncFII plasmids. We found (Table 1) a high (62 strains, 56%) incidence of *rep* IncF sequences among the

examined UPEC strains. Particularly prevalent were RepFIB sequences that were detected in 57 (52%) of the strains while RepFIA and RepFIIA were found in 20 (18%) and 24 (22%) strains, respectively. *rep* sequences were found in all four phylogenetic groups. Of the 62 isolates harbouring at least one of the tested IncF replicons, 20 belonged to group A, 2 to B1, 27 to B2, and 13 to group D (Rijavec et al., 2006).
Since only class 1, 2 and 3 of integrons were shown to be associated with pathogenic *E. coli* in our study we focused only on these three classes. Analysis (Table 1) revealed that 29 (26%) of the strains harboured a class 1 integron, 1 strain (1%) contained a class 1 and a class 2 integron, and 4 strains (4%) a class 2 integron. Analysis of the distribution of integrons with regard to the phylogenetic group showed that integron sequences were found in all four groups. Of the 34 isolates harbouring integron sequences, 12 belonged to group A, 1 to B1, 12 to B2, and 9 to group D (Rijavec et al., 2006).

7. Colicins

Colicins are bacteriocins produced by *E. coli* strains. As other bacteriocins, colicins are extracellular bacterial toxic proteins that are active against the same, or closely related species as the producer cell (Daw & Falkiner, 1996). The mechanism of action of these compounds involves adsorption to specific receptors located on the external surface of sensitive bacteria followed by killing via one of three primary mechanisms: i) formation of channels in the cytoplasmic membrane, ii) degradation of cellular DNA or iii) inhibition of protein synthesis (Riley & Gordon, 1999). Because of their narrow range of activity, it has been proposed that the primary role of bacteriocins is to mediate intraspecific, or population level, interactions (Riley, 1998) however, bacteriocins have also been implicated in virulence determination, since many pathogenic strains harbour plasmid-encoded bacteriocins, for example the ColV plasmid of UPEC isolates (Johnson & Nolan, 2009). Typically, 25-50% of *E. coli* isolates are colicinogenic and usually, the percentages are higher among pathogenic than commensal strains (Riley & Gordon, 1996). Due to high levels of colicinogenity in natural *E. coli* populations, high levels of colicin resistance are known to occur (Feldgarden & Riley, 1998).

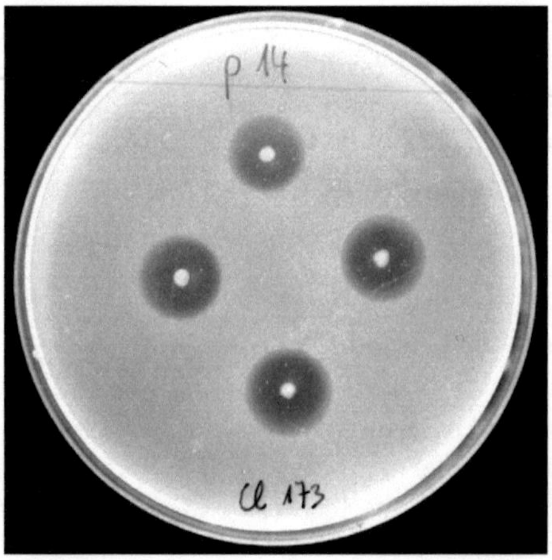

Fig. 2. A colicinogenic uropathogenic strain was stab inoculated on 4 points on an agar plate and overlaid with a sensitive *E. coli* strain.

Among the studied UPEC isolates 42 (38%) exhibited colicinogenic activity (Starčič Erjavec et al., 2006). Each of the 110 UPEC strains was resistant to at least 3 colicinogenic strains from Pugsley's collection of colicinogenic strains (Pugsley & Oudega, 1987), 23 UPEC strains (21%) were resistant to all 20 tested Pugsley's strains (our unpublished data). Colicinogenic strains were found in all four phylogenetic groups (Table 1) however, most colicinogenic strains, 20 (48%) belonged to the B2 group (our unpublished data).

8. Conclusion

Our investigation of UPEC isolates from Slovenia revealed a high prevalence of drug resistance and multidrug resistance. The virulence profile of the examined strains was comparable to that of strains from other geographic regions.

9. Acknowledgment

This work was supported by the by grant P1-0198 from the Slovenian Research Agency.

10. References

Alekshun, M. N. & Levy, S. B. (2007). Molecular mechanisms of antibacterial multidrug resistance. *Cell*, Vol.128, No.6, (March 2007), pp. 1037-1050, ISSN 0092-8674

Ananias, M. & Yano, T. (2008). Serogroups and virulence genotypes of *Escherichia coli* isolated from patients with sepsis. *Brazilian Journal of Medical and Biological Research*, Vol.41, No.10, (October 2008), pp. 877-883, ISSN 0100-879X

Bauer, R. J.; Zhang, L.; Foxman, B.; Siitonen, A.; Jantunen, M. E.; Saxen H. & Marrs, C. F. (2002). Molecular epidemiology of 3 putative virulence genes for *Escherichia coli* urinary tract infection – *usp*, *iha* and $iroN_{(E.\ coli)}$. *The Journal of Infectious Diseases*, Vol.185, No.10, (May 2002), pp. 1521-1524, ISSN 0022-1899

Binns, M. M.; Davies, D. L. & Hardy, K. G. (1979). Cloned fragments of the plasmid ColV,I-K94 specifying virulence and serum resistance. *Nature*, Vol.279, No.5716, (June 1979), pp. 778-781, ISSN 0028-0836

Boerlin, P. & Reid-Smith, R. J. (2008). Antimicrobial resistance: its emergence and transmision. *Animal Health Research Reviews*, Vol.9, No.2, (December 2008), pp. 115-126, ISSN 1466-2523

Bower, J. M.; Eto, D. S. & Mulvey, M. A. (2005). Covert operations of uropathogenic *Escherichia coli* within the urinary tract. *Traffic* Vol.6, No.1, (January 2005), pp. 18-31, ISSN 1398-9219

Braun, V. & Braun, M. (2002). Iron transport and signaling in *Escherichia coli*. *FEBS Letters*, Vol.529, No.1, (October 2002), pp. 78-85, ISSN 0014-5793

Car, J.; Švab, I.; Kersnik, J. & Vegnuti, M. (2003). Management of lower urinary tract infection in women by Slovene GPs. *Family Practice*, Vol.20, No.4, (August 2003), pp. 452-456, ISSN 0263-2136

Cirl, C.; Wieser, A.; Yadav, M.; Duerr, S.; Schubert, S.; Fischer, H.; Stappert, D.; Wantia, N.; Rodriguez, N.; Wagner, H.; Svanborg, C. & Miethke, T. (2008). Subversion of Toll-like receptor signaling by a unique family of bacterial Toll/interleukin-1 receptor domain–containing proteins. *Nature Medicine*, Vol.14, No.4, (April 2008), pp. 399–406, ISSN 1078-8956

Clermont, O.; Bonacorsi, S. & Bingen, E. (2000). Rapid and simple determination of the *Escherichia coli* phylogenetic group. *Applied and Environmental Microbiology*, Vol.66, No.10, (October 2010), pp. 4555-4558, ISSN 0099-2240

Croxen, M. A. & Finlay, B. B. (2010). Molecular mechanisms of *Escherichia coli* pathogenicity. *Nature Reviews Microbiology*, Vol.8, No.1, (January 2010), pp. 26-38, ISSN 1740-1526

Couturier, M.; Bex, F.; Bergquist, P. L. & Maas, W. K. (1988). Identification and classification of bacterial plasmids. *Microbiological Reviews*, Vol. 52, No.3, (September 1988), pp. 375-395, ISSN 0146-0749

Daw, M. A. & Falkiner, F. R. (1996). Bacteriocins: nature, function and structure. *Micron : The International Research and Review Journal for Microscopy*, Vol.27, No.6, (December 1996), pp. 467–479, ISSN 0968-4328

Dobrindt, U.; Chowdary, M. G.; Krumbholz, G. & Hacker, J. (2010). Genome dynamics and its impact on evolution of *Escherichia coli*. *Medical Microbiology and Immunology*, Vol.199, No.3, (August 2010), pp.145-154, ISSN 0300-8584

Escobar-Paramo, P.; Grenet, K.; Le Menac'h, A.; Rode, L.; Salgado, E.; Amorin, C.; Gouriou, S.; Picard, B.; Rahimy, M. C.; Andremont, A.; Denamur, E. & Ruimy, R. (2004). Large-scale population structure of human commensal *Escherichia coli* isolates. *Applied and Environmental Microbiology*, Vol.70, No.9, (September 2004), pp. 5698-700, ISSN 0099-2240

Feldgarden, M. & Riley, M. A. (1998). High levels of colicin resistance in *Escherichia coli*. *Evolution*, Vol.52, No.5, (October 1998), pp. 1270–1276, ISSN 0014-3820

Goller, C. C. & Seed, P. C. (2010). Revisiting the *Escherichia coli* polysaccharide capsule as a virulence factor during urinary tract infection: contribution to intracellular biofilm development. *Virulence*, Vol.1, No.4, (July-August 2010), pp. 337-337, ISSN 2150-5594

Grass, G. (2006). Iron transport in *Escherichia coli*: all has not been said and done. *Biometals : an International Journal on the Role of Metal Ions in Biology, Biochemistry, and Medicine*, Vol.19, No.2, (April 2006), pp. 159-172, ISSN 0966-0844

Henderson, I. R. & Nataro, J. P. (2001). Virulence functions of autotransporter proteins. *Infection and Immunity*, Vol.69, No.3, (March 2001), pp. 1231-1243, ISSN 0019-9567

Johnson, J. R. (1991). Virulence factors in *Escherichia coli* urinary tract infection. *Clinical Microbiology Reviews* Vol.4, No.1, (January 1991), pp. 80-128, ISSN 0893-8512

Johnson, J. R. & Stell, A. L. (2000). Extended virulence genotypes of *Escherichia coli* strains from patients with urosepsis in relation to phylogeny and host compromise. *The Journal of Infectious Diseases*, Vol.181, No.1, (January 2000), pp.261-272, ISSN 0022-1899

Johnson, J. R.; Kuskowski, M. A.; Gajewski, A.; Soto, S.; Horcajada, J. P.; Jimenez de Anta, M. T. & Vila, J. (2005a). Extended virulence genotypes and phylogenetic background of *Escherichia coli* isolates from patients with cystitis, pyelonephritis, or prostatitis. *The Journal of Infectious Diseases*, Vol.191, No.1, (January 2005), pp. 46-50, ISSN 0022-1899

Johnson, J. R.; Owens, K.; Gajewski, A. & Kuskowski, M. A. (2005). Bacterial characteristics in relation to clinical source of *Escherichia coli* isolates from women with acute cystitis or pyelonephritis and uninfected women. *Journal of Clinical Microbiology*, Vol.43, No.12, (December 2005), pp. 6064-72, ISSN 0095-1137

Johnson, T. J. & Nolan, L. K. (2009). Pathogenomics of the virulence plasmids of *Escherichia coli. Microbiology and Molecular Biology Reviews : MMBR,* Vol.73, No.4, (December 2009), pp. 750-774, ISSN 1092-2172

Jorgensen, J. H. & Ferraro, M. J. (2009). Antimicrobial susceptibility testing: a review of general principles and contemporary practices. *Clinical Infectious Diseases : an Official Publication of the Infectious Diseases Society of America,* Vol.49, No.11, (December 2009), pp. 1749-1755, ISSN 1058-4838

Kado, C. I. (1998). Origin and evolution of plasmids. *Antonie Van Leeuwenhoek,* Vol.73, No.1, (January 1998), pp. 117-126, ISSN 0003-6072

Kahlmeter, G. & Menday, P. (2003). Cross-resistance and associated resistance in 2478 *Escherichia coli* isolates from the Pan-European ECO.SENS Project surveying the antimicrobial susceptibility of pathogens from uncomplicated urinary tract infections. *The Journal of Antimicrobial Chemotherapy,* Vol.52, No.1, (July 2003), pp. 128-131, ISSN 0305-7453

Kaper, J. B.; Nataro, J. P. & Mobley, H. L. T. (2004). Pathogenic *Escherichia coli. Nature Reviews Microbiology,* Vol.2, No.2, (February, 2004), pp.123-140, ISSN 1740-1526

Karlowsky, J. A.; Thornsberry, C.; Jones, M. E. & Sahm, D. F. (2003). Susceptibility of antimicrobial-resistant urinary *Escherichia coli* isolates to fluoroquinolones and nitrofurantoin. *Clinical Infectious Diseases : an Official Publication of the Infectious Diseases Society of America,* Vol.36, No.2, (January 2003), pp. 183-187, ISSN 1058-4838

Kumarasamy, K. K.; Toleman, M. A.; Walsh, T. R.; Bagaria, J.; Butt, F.; Balakrishnan, R.; Chaudhary, U.; Doumith, M.; Giske, C. G.; Irfan, S.; Krishnan, P.; Kumar, A. V.; Maharjan, S.; Mushtaq, S.; Noorie, T.; Paterson, D. L.; Pearson, A.; Perry, C.; Pike, R.; Rao, B.; Ray, U.; Sarma, J. B.; Sharma, M.; Sheridan, E.; Thirunarayan, M. A.; Turton, J.; Upadhyay, S.; Warner, M.; Welfare, W.; Livermore, D. M.; & Woodford, N. (2010). Emergence of a new antibiotic resistance mechanism in India, Pakistan, and the UK: a molecular, biological, and epidemiological study. *The Lancet Infectious Diseases,* Vol.10, No. 9, (September 2010), pp. 597-602, ISSN 1473-3099

Kurazono, H.; Yamamoto, S.; Nakano, M.; Nair, G. B.; Terai, A.; Chaicumpa, W. & Hayashi, H. (2000). Characterization of a putative virulence island in the chromosome of uropathogenic *Escherichia coli* possessing a gene encoding a uropathogenic-specific protein. *Microbial Pathogenesis,* Vol.28, No.3, (March 2000), pp. 183-189, ISSN 0882-4010

Lindič, J. (2005). Pristop k bolniku z okužbo sečil.[Accession to a patient with urinary tract infection]. In: *Zbornik prispevkov /47. Tavčarjevi dnevi. [Proceedings / 47th Tavčar's days.,* Z Fras & P. Poredoš, (Eds.), pp. 137-148, University of Ljubljana, Medical Faculty, ISBN 961-6264-70-2, Ljubljana, Slovenia

Llobet, E.; Tomás, J. M. & Bengoechea, J. A. (2008). Capsule polysaccharide is a bacterial decoy for antimicrobial peptides. *Microbiology,* Vol.154, No.Pt 12, (December 2008), pp. 3877-3886, ISSN 1350-0872

Marrs, C. F.; Zhang, L. & Foxman, B. (2005). *Escherichia coli* mediated urinary tract infections: Are there distinct uropathogenic E. coli (UPEC) pathotypes? *FEMS Microbiology Letters,* Vol.252, No.2, (November 2005), pp. 183-190, ISSN 0378-1097

Martinez, J. J.; Mulvey, M. A.; Schilling, J. D.; Pinkner, J. S. & Hultgren, S. J. (2000). Type 1 pilus-mediated bacterial invasion of bladder epithelial cells. *The EMBO Journal,* Vol. 19, No.12, (June 2000), pp. 2803-2812, ISSN 0261-4189

Mazel, D. (2006). Integrons: agents of bacterial evolution. *Nature Reviews Microbiology*, Vol.4, No.8, (August 2006), pp. 608-620, ISSN 1740-1526

Moreno, E.; Prats, G.; Sabate, M.; Perez, T.; Johnson, J. R. & Andreu, A. (2006). Quinolone, fluroquinolone and trimethoprim/sulfamethoxazole resistance in relation to virulence determinants and phylogenetic background among uropahtogenic *Escherichia coli*. *The Journal of Antimicrobial Chemotherapy*, Vol.57, No.2, (February 2006), pp. 204-211, ISSN 0305-7453

Ochman, H.; Whittam, T. S.; Caugant, D. A. & Selander, R. K. (1983). Enzyme polymorphism and genetic population structure in *Escherichia coli* and *Shigella*. *Journal of General Microbiology*, Vol.129, No.9, (September 1983), pp. 2715–2726, ISSN 0022-1287

Oelschlaeger, T. A.; Dobrindt, U. & Hacker, J. (2002). Virulence factors of uropathogens. *Current Opinion in Urology*, Vol.12, No.1, (January 2002), pp. 33-38, ISSN 0963-0643

Orskov, F. & Orskov, I. (1992). *Escherichia coli* serotyping and disease in man and animals. *Canadian Journal of Microbiology*, Vol.38, No.7, (July 1992), pp. 699-704, ISSN 0008-4166

Otto, B. R.; van Dooren, S. J.; Dozois, C. M.; Luirink, J. & Oudega, B. (2002). *Escherichia coli* hemoglobin protease autotransporter contributes to synergistic abscess formation and heme-dependent growth of *Bacteroides fragilis*. *Infection and Immunity*, Vol.70, No.1 (January 2002), pp. 5-10, ISSN 0019-9567

Picard, B.; Garcia, J. S.; Gouriou, S.; Duriez, P.; Brahimi, N.; Bingen, E.; Elion, J. & Denamur, E. (1999). The link between phylogeny and virulence in *Escherichia coli* extraintestinal infection. *Infection and Immunity*, Vol.67, No.2, (February 1999), pp. 546-553, ISSN 0019-9567

Pugsley, A. P. & Oudega, B. (1987). Methods for studying colicins and their plasmids, In: *Plasmids, a practical approach*, K. G. Hardy (Ed.), 105-161. IRL Press Limited, ISBN 0-947946-81-0, Oxford, England

Rijavec, M.; Starčič Erjavec, M.; Ambrožič Avguštin, J.; Reissbrodt, R.; Fruth, A.; Križan-Hergouth, V. & Žgur-Bertok, D. (2006). High prevalence of multidrug resistance and random distribution of mobile genetic elements among uropathogenic *Escherichia coli* (UPEC) of the four major phylogenetic groups. *Current Microbiology*, Vol.53, No.2, (August 2006), pp. 158-162, ISSN 0343-8651

Rijavec, M.; Budič, M.; Mrak, P.; Müller-Premru, M.; Podlesek, Z. & Žgur-Bertok, D. (2007). Prevalence of ColE1-like plasmids and colicin K production among uropathogenic *Escherichia coli* strains and quantification of inhibitory activity of colicin K. *Applied and Environmental Microbiology*, Vol.73, No.3, (February 2007), pp. 1029-1032, ISSN 0099-2240

Riley, M. A. (1998). Molecular mechanisms of bacteriocin evolution. *Annual Review of Genetics*. Vol.32, pp. 255–278, ISSN 0066-4197

Riley, M. A. & Gordon, D. M. (1996). The ecology and evolution of bacteriocins. *Journal of Industrial Microbiology*, Vol.17, No.3-4, (September 1996), pp. 151–158, ISSN 0169-4146

Riley, M. A. & Gordon, D. M. (1999). The ecological role of bacteriocins in the bacterial competition. *Trends in Microbiology*, Vol.7, No.3, (March, 199), pp. 129–133, ISSN 0966-842X

Roberts, I. S. (1995). Bacterial polysaccharides in sickness and in health. The 1995 Fleming Lecture. *Microbiology,* Vol.141, No.Pt 9, (September 1995), pp. 2023-2031, ISSN 1350-0872

Roberts, I. S. (1996). The biochemistry and genetics of capsular polysaccharide production in bacteria. *Annual Review of Microbiology,* Vol.50, pp. 285–315, ISSN 0066-4227

Russo, T. A. & Johnson, J. R. (2000). Proposal for a new inclusive designation for extraintestinal pathogenic isolates of *Escherichia coli*: ExPEC. *The Journal of Infectious Diseases,* Vol.181, No.5, (May 2000), pp. 1753–1754, ISSN 0022-1899.

Russo, T. A. & Johnson, J. R. (2006). Extraintestinal isolates of *Escherichia coli*: identification and prospects for vaccine development. *Expert Review of Vaccines,* Vol.5, No.1, (Februar 2006), pp. 45-54, ISSN 1476-0584

Schaible, U. E. & Kaufmann, S. H. (2004). Iron and microbial infection. *Nature Reviews Microbiology,* Vol.2, No.12, (December 2004), pp. 946-953, ISSN 1740-1526

Schamberger, G. P.; Phillips, R. L.; Jacobs, J. L.; & Diez-Gonzalez, F. (2004). Reduction of *Escherichia coli* O157:H7 populations in cattle by addition of colicin E7-producing *E. coli* to feed. *Applied and Environmental Microbiology,* Vol.70, No.10, (October 2004), pp. 6053-6060, ISSN 0099-2240

Servin, A. L. (2005). Pathogenisis of Afa/Dr diffusely adhering *Escherichia coli. Clinical Microbiology Reviews,* Vol.18, No.2 (April 2005), pp. 264-292, ISSN 0893-8512

Stahl, C. H.; Callaway, T. R.; Lincoln, L. M.; Lonergan, S. M.; & Genovese, K. J. (2004). Inhibitory activities of colicins against *Escherichia coli* strains responsible for postweaning diarrhea and edema disease in swine. *Antimicrobial Agents and Chemotherapy,* Vol.48, No.8, (August 2004), pp. 3119-3121, ISSN 0066-4804

Starčič Erjavec, M.; Rijavec, M. & Žgur-Bertok, D. (2006). Colicins of the *Escherichia coli* uropathogenic strain collection. *Acta biologica slovenica,* Vol.49, No.2, pp. 13-21, ISSN 1408-3671

Starčič Erjavec, M.; Rijavec, M.; Križan-Hergouth, V.; Fruth, A. & Žgur-Bertok, D. (2007). Chloramphenicol- and tetracycline-resistant uropathogenic *Escherichia coli* (UPEC) exhibit reduced virulence potential. *International Journal of Antimicrobial Agents,* Vol.30, No.5, (November 2007), pp. 436-442, ISSN 0924-8579

Starčič Erjavec, M. & Žgur-Bertok, D. (2008). Prevalence, distribution and genetic association of adhesin gene sequences of *Escherichia coli* isolates from urinary tract infections in Slovenia. *Acta biologica slovenica,* Vol.51, No.1, pp. 21-31, ISSN 1408-3671

Starčič Erjavec, M.; Križan-Hergouth, V.; Gubina B. & Žgur-Bertok, D. (2008). Prevalence of toxin encoding genes in *Escherichia coli* isolates from urinary tract infections in Slovenia. *Zdravniški vestnik,* Vol.77,No.6/7, (June/July 2008), pp. 427-432. ISSN 1318-0347

Starčič Erjavec, M.; Arbiter, T. & Žgur-Bertok, D. (2009). Pathogenicity islands, plasmids and iron uptake systems in extraintestinal pathogenic *Escherichia coli* strains. *Acta biologica slovenica,* Vol.52, No.2, pp. 73-83, ISSN 1408-3671

Starčič Erjavec, M.; Jesenko, B.; Petkovšek, Ž. & Žgur-Bertok, D. (2010). Prevalence and associations of *tcpC,* a gene encoding a Toll/interleukin-1 receptor domain-containing protein, among *Escherichia coli* urinary tract infection, skin and soft tissue infection, and commensal isolates. *Journal of Clinical Microbiology,* Vol.48, No.3, (March 2010), pp. 966-968, ISSN 0095-1137

Thanassi, D. G.; Saulino, E. T. & Hultgren, S. J. (1998). The chaporene/usher pathway: a major terminal branch of the general secretory pathway. *Current Opinion in Microbiology* Vol.1, No.2, (April 1998), pp. 223-231, ISSN 1369-5274

Trautner, B. W.; Hull, R. A. & Darouiche, R. O. (2005). Colicins prevent colonization of urinary catheters. *The Journal of Antimicrobial Chemotherapy*, Vol.56, No.2, (August 2005), pp 413-415, ISSN 0305-7453

Whittam, T. S.; Ochman, H. & Selander, R. K. (1983). Multilocus genetic structure in natural populations of *Escherichia coli*. *Proceedings of the National Academy of Sciences of the United States of America*, Vol.80, No.6, (March 1983), pp. 1751–1755, ISSN 0027-8424

Xie, Y.; Kim, K. J. & Kim, K.S. (2004). Current concepts on *Escherichia coli* K1 translocation of the blood–brain barrier. *FEMS Immunology and Medical Microbiology*, Vol.42, No.3, (November, 2004), pp. 271-279, ISSN 0928-8244

Yilmaz, N.; Agus, N.; Yurtsever, S. G.; Pullukcu, H.; Gulay, Z.; Coskuner, A.; Kose, S.; Aydemir, S.; Gulenc, N. & Ozgenc, O. (2009). Prevalence and antimicrobial susceptibility of *Escherichia coli* in outpatient urinary isolates in Izmir, Turkey. *Medical Science Monitor : International Medical Journal of Experimental and Clinical Research*, Vol.15, No.11, (November 2009), pp. PI61-PI65, ISSN 1234-1010

Zhang, L. & Foxman, B. (2003). Molecular epidemiology of *Escherichia coli* mediated urinary tract infections. *Frontiers in Bioscience*, Vol.8, (January 2003), pp. e235-244, ISSN 1093-9946

4

Current Understanding of Streptococcal Urinary Tract Infection

Chee Keong Tan, Alison J Carey, Deepak Ipe and Glen C Ulett
Griffith University
Australia

1. Introduction

Group B streptococcus (GBS), also known as *Streptococcus agalactiae* is a Gram-positive, β-hemolytic, chain-forming bacterium and a commensal within the genital tract flora in approximately 25% of healthy adult women (Campbell et al., 2000). The organism is a leading cause of serious infection in newborns, pregnant women, and older persons with chronic medical illness (Baker et al., Edwards&Baker, 2005). In neonates GBS infection most commonly causes pneumonia, meningitis, and sepsis. In addition to maternal cervicovaginal colonization and neonatal infection that can result from vertical transmission of GBS from mothers to their infants, the bacterium can also cause urinary tract infection (UTI). The spectrum of GBS UTI includes asymptomatic bacteriuria (ABU), cystitis, pyelonephritis, urethritis, and urosepsis (Bronsema et al., 1993, Edwards&Baker, 2005, Farley et al., 1993, Lefevre et al., 1991, McKenna et al., 2003, Munoz et al., 1992, Ulett et al., 2009). GBS ABU is particularly common among pregnant women, although those most at risk for cystitis due to GBS appear to be elderly individuals (Edwards&Baker, 2005, Falagas et al., 2006, Muller et al., 2006). In addition to acute and asymptomatic UTI other invasive diseases caused by GBS infection include skin infections, bacteraemia, pneumonia, arthritis, and endocarditis (Liston et al., 1979, Patil&Martin, 2010, Tissi et al., 1997, Trivalle et al., 1998). Thus, GBS is considered unique in terms of its ability to cause a spectrum of diseases in newborns and adult humans and its ability to colonize the genital tract of healthy women in a commensal-type manner. In contrast to GBS disease conditions resulting from neonatal infection, the clinical and microbiological features of GBS UTI and asymptomatic genital tract colonization are not well characterized. Moreover, the risk factors for the various diseases caused by GBS including UTI and the pathogenesis of the different diseases caused as a result of GBS infection are not well defined.

Recent advances in the awareness, diagnosis and treatment of GBS infections, particularly in relation to vertical transmission and neonatal infection, have significantly reduced mortality in the newborn population. Establishment of preventative and treatment guidelines by the Centres for Disease Control (CDC) beginning in the 1990s has resulted in a reduction in mortality rates due to acute GBS infection in newborns from approximately 30-50% to 4–5% (Dermer et al., 2004). Guidelines for the prevention of GBS infections in newborns first published in 1992 and revised in 1997 include surveillance programs and administration of antibiotics during labour (intrapartum antibiotic chemoprophylaxis) (1992, 1997). Since the mid-1990s, most pregnant women in the United States have been screened for infection by

GBS and the success of intrapartum antibiotic chemoprophylaxis for the prevention of vertical transmission of GBS has been noted (Verani et al., 2010). However, preventive strategies to identify at-risk individuals are controversial and the rates of GBS-related stillbirths, prematurity, and late onset disease (LOD) have not decreased (Gibbs et al., 2004). The incidence of morbidities in newborn survivors of acute GBS infection ranges from 20–60% and includes neurological sequelae (Gibbs et al., 2004, Lukacs et al., 2004). The manner in which specific preventative strategies are implemented may also affect disease prevalence due to GBS in some areas (Krasnianin et al., 2009, Rausch et al., 2009). Thus, infections due to GBS and the ensuing diseases that result remain a significant cause of morbidity and mortality in newborns as well as healthy adults (Berner, 2004, van der Poll&Opal, 2008).

In addition to representing a major infection risk for neonates and pregnant women GBS is also a prominent pathogen of the elderly, immunocompromised, and individuals with diabetes and malignancies. These populations are particularly at risk for invasive GBS infection (Edwards&Baker, 2005, Farley, 2001). The manifestations of GBS infection in these populations are highly varied; however, some of the most common clinical presentations include skin and soft tissue infections, bacteraemia, pneumonia, arthritis, UTI, and endocarditis (Baker, 1997, Farley, 2001, Lee et al., 2007, Trivalle et al., 1998). The case fatality rate for GBS infection in elderly adults was estimated to be approximately 15% in the United States between 2001 and 2005 (Edwards&Baker, 2005, Farley, 2001). Importantly, there is no vaccine currently available to prevent GBS disease in neonates or adults despite a substantial research effort in identifying potential immunogens as vaccine candidates in immunization strategies (Doro et al., 2009).

The recent emergence of GBS strains that are resistant to multiple antibiotics represents a significant concern in the treatment of these infections in adults and children (Andrews et al., 2000, Bland et al., 2001, Dahesh et al., 2008, Heelan et al., 2004, Kimura et al., 2008, Nagano et al., 2008, Simoes et al., 2004). Penicillin-derived antibiotics remain the drugs of choice for treatment of GBS infections in infants and adults (Sendi et al., 2008, Verani&Schrag, 2010). These antibiotics inhibit cell wall synthesis during active growth of the bacteria. Vancomycin, cefezolin, clindamycin and telavancin are also used for the treatment of GBS infections. Trends of increasing antibiotic resistance (Edwards, 2006) may reflect clonal dissemination and horizontal transfer of resistance genes, which occurs among some GBS isolates (Puopolo et al., 2007). In addition, the identification of GBS strains resistant to penicillin, clindamycin and erythromycin represents a significant concern for the treatment of infections (Andrews et al., 2000, Bland et al., 2001, Dahesh et al., 2008, Heelan et al., 2004, Kimura et al., 2008, Nagano et al., 2008, Simoes et al., 2004). A large number of microbiological studies on GBS infection over the past two decades have underscored the importance of GBS as a major public health concern and a need for improvements in preventative and therapeutic strategies. An improved understanding of the mechanisms of GBS disease pathogenesis is vital for such strategies.

1.1 Host range and GBS serotypes

GBS was once seen only as a veterinary pathogen. The organism was originally isolated from cattle in the 1930s and prior to the 1980s was regarded as a prominent cause of bovine mastitis in dairy cows. Indeed, the species name, agalactiae, translates to "no milk" and reflects this history. Subsequently, epidemiology and prevalence studies indicated that GBS was associated with disease in neonates and the bacterium was increasingly recognized beginning in 1977 as a major cause of postpartum infection in human newborns (Ferrieri et al., 1977). GBS is now universally accepted as among the most common causes of neonatal sepsis and meningitis. Research in the mid-1980s demonstrated that GBS was carried in the genital tract and the gastrointestinal flora in up to 30% of healthy adult women, which reflected intermittent, transient, or persistent colonization (Boyer et al., 1983, Dillon et al., 1982). Over the last fifteen years studies have demonstrated that GBS is a significant cause of serious disease in non-pregnant adults including elderly people and immunocompromised individuals. Emerging trends in GBS disease incidence and prevalence strongly suggest that changes in the recognition and treatment of GBS infections are impacting the types of individuals affected by the bacterium and invasive disease in adults is now more common than in neonates (Baker, 2000. , Falagas et al., 2006, Muller et al., 2006).

There are ten different capsular serotypes of GBS, namely Ia, Ib, and II-IX. These are based on the structure of the surface polysaccharide capsule of the bacterium. Nontypeable GBS also exist and are associated with some infections in humans including UTI (Baker&Barrett, 1974, McKenna et al., 2003, Persson et al., 1985). Capsular serotyping of GBS can be performed by latex agglutination using commercial antisera (Slotved et al., 2003), which differentiates the major Lancefield groups (Facklam, 2002) based on serotype-specific antibody-based binding. Molecular serotyping (MS) methods have gained popularity and can provide additional insight into serotype traits that are not able to be derived from antisera-based approaches, possibly as a result of limited antigen expression in some strains (Ferrieri et al., 2004, Kong et al., 2002, Manning et al., 2008, Ramaswamy et al., 2006, Wen et al., 2006). MS identification of all ten serotypes is possible (MS Ia, Ib, and II-IX) with the use of a multiplex PCR and reverse line blot hybridization assay targeting a GBS species-specific gene (*cfb*) and serotype-specific sequences in various other capsular loci genes (Kong et al., 2005). Among the ten different types, the serotypes most frequently associated with serious disease are serotypes Ia, II, III, and V (Edwards&Baker, 2005). There is some evidence to suggest that switching can occur between capsular types in GBS (Martins et al., 2010).

1.2 GBS disease spectrum and Co-morbidities

GBS is a frequent cause of puerperal infections including pneumonia, sepsis, meningitis, amnionitis and endometritis. These infections are common in newborns, pregnant women, and adults with underlying medical conditions (Nizet et al., 2000, Pass et al., 1982). Diabetes mellitus and malignancy are among the most common underlying conditions associated with these GBS infections (Huang et al., 2006). Other co-morbidities that have been associated with GBS disease in adults include cardiovascular abnormalities, genitourinary disorders, neurologic deficits, cirrhosis, steroid use, AIDS, renal dysfunction, and peripheral vascular disease. Relapse of GBS disease in affected individuals is not uncommon, with approximately 5% of non-pregnant adults experiencing a second episode of GBS disease after resolution of the primary infection (Sendi et al., 2008). The pathogenic basis of this recurrence is unknown but it is nonetheless an important consideration clinically.

The nature of GBS as a frequent constituent of the resident vaginal bacterial microflora in healthy adult women means that the bacterium is regarded as a normal commensal under these circumstances. Colonized women often carry GBS for long periods of time and usually do not show clinical symptoms as a result of persistent genital tract infection. On the other hand, conditions during pregnancy may lead to increased GBS multiplication in the urogenital tract and GBS can grow to high numbers in human amniotic fluid. This may lead to serious consequences for both the colonized mother and the infant. Between 15%-45% of pregnant women harbour GBS in the gastrointestinal and or genitourinary tracts (Schuchat,

1998); neonates acquire the bacteria at birth from their asymptomatically colonized mothers in approximately 1% of all live births (Baker, 2000. , Nandyal, 2008, Schuchat, 1998). The neonatal lung can receive a substantial inoculum from infected amniotic fluid at birth (Nizet et al., 2000). In addition, GBS may be acquired by the growing fetus prior to birth *in utero*, which can trigger adverse pregnancy outcomes. Thus, GBS continues to be an important perinatal pathogen but causes a wide spectrum of diseases that is associated with various co-morbidities.

1.3 Detection and identification of GBS

The majority of GBS infections can be diagnosed through routine laboratory testing of clinical samples such as blood, cerebrospinal fluid, or aspirates from sites of local suppuration. In the majority of cases isolates are rapidly identified by typical colony morphology on agar medium such as tryptic soy agar-5% sheep blood, and are tested for catalase, which streptococci do not express. Isolates are grouped into the Lancefield B group (Facklam, 2002) using commercial typing antisera for latex agglutination assays. GBS antigens can occasionally be detected in blood, cerebrospinal fluid, and urine but are not routinely tested for in any diagnostic assays. A Gram stain of a clinical specimen can be useful in the detection of infection but is not specific and therefore not definitive for identification. Polymerase chain reaction and optical immunoassay may, on the other hand, provide rapid and specific results for the detection of GBS infection; however, optimization and validation of these assays to ensure sensitivity and specificity has limited their widespread application in the clinical laboratory (Daniels et al., 2009, Schwope et al., 2010).

1.4 GBS virulence factors and host cell responses

A number of GBS virulence factors that contribute to disease and infection in the host have been discovered. The role of these GBS virulence factors in UTI remains unexplored. A number of exotoxigenic virulence factors are produced by GBS, including hyaluronate lyase, Christine Atkins Munch Peterson (CAMP) factor, superoxide dismutase, proteases, nucleases, platelet-activating factor, collagenase/oligopeptidase, protein c, RIB, R protein, and C5a peptidase (Lindahl et al., 2005, Liu&Nizet, 2004, Nizet et al., 2000). The functions and structures of several of these virulence factors are reviewed elsewhere (Liu&Nizet, 2004). One of the major GBS virulence factor is the sialic acid-rich capsular polysaccharide, which has been extensively studied as a virulence factor for many years (Slotved et al., 2007). Capsular polysaccharide is anti-phagocytic and influences the pathogenicity of GBS by mediating evasion of phagocytes (Adderson et al., 2000). GBS lipotechoic acid (LTA) is another key virulence factor that contributes to successful infection in the host. GBS LTA is cytotoxic to human monocytes and induces inflammation including the production of pro-inflammatory cytokines such as TNF-α (Berner, 2002). Cytotoxicity including the ability to induce programmed cell death (PCD) in host cells may contribute to disease by promoting adhesion, invasion, and host immune-evasion (Nizet et al., 2000). β-hemolysin is produced in varying amounts by virtually all clinical isolates of GBS and has several known roles in virulence including cytotoxicity (Liu&Nizet, 2004, Nizet et al., 2000). β-hemolysin is expressed on the surface of GBS and is responsible for the characteristic β-hemolytic activity on blood agar (Nizet, 2002, Nizet et al., 2000). β-hemolysin has a role in early but not late PCD and its expression is abolished by glucose (Fettucciari et al., 2000, Ulett et al., 2003).

Several virulence factors of GBS including LTA, β-hemolysin, C5a peptidase and the R protein/antigen are involved in recognition by host cells and inducing or evading immune responses (Cheng et al., 2001, Fasola et al., 1996, Henneke et al., 2005, Liu et al., 2004). The proficiency of GBS recognition by macrophages is considered a crucial component of early immune responses against the bacteria (Chattopadhyay et al., 2011, Franke-Ullmann et al., 1996, Jonsson et al., 1985, Sherman et al., 1992, Sibille&Reynolds, 1990). However, GBS are able to persist inside macrophages for an extended period of time after nonopsonic phagocytosis and eventually trigger death of the host cell (Cornacchione et al., 1998, Fettucciari et al., 2000, Ulett et al., 2003, Valenti-Weigand et al., 1996). Intracellular persistence and manipulation of death pathways in macrophages may represent a virulence mechanism whereby GBS contributes to the characteristically poor inflammatory response in the neonatal lung. GBS-induced cell death is also a prominent feature of hepatocytes in a rabbit model of GBS sepsis (Ring et al., 2002) and in neurons of the dentate gyrus in GBS meningitis (Bogdan et al., 1997).

2. Bacterial UTI: general aspects

Ten to forty percent of adult women will contract at least one UTI in their lifetime, and approximately 3% will experience more than one infection per year (Andriole&Patterson, 1991, Patton et al., 1991, Foxman, 2002). UTI are the second most common infectious diseases in humans after respiratory tract infections, and contribute to approximately 60 million hospital visits per year. The costs to health care systems have been estimated at over $2 billion annually (Andriole&Patterson, 1991, Barnett&Stephens, 1997, Hooton&Stamm, 1997, Patton et al., 1991). Chronic UTI are difficult to prevent and treat, and infections are often recurrent. Over 80% of UTI are caused by uropathogenic *Escherichia coli* (UPEC) (Ronald, 2002). Approximately 2% of UTI are caused by GBS. Among an estimated 40% of all adult women who will experience a UTI episode in their lifetime almost 1% will suffer UTI caused by GBS (Foxman, 2002). The urinary tract is a distinct mucosal surface of the body and bacterial colonization of the uroepithelium is unique compared to other mucosal surfaces. Colonizing bacteria must overcome the normal flushing actions of urine flow and the physical barrier of the uroepithelial lining. This lining embodies a tightly interlaced latticework of proteins called uroplakins (Apodaca, 2004). These are closely associated with a collection of lipids, sphingolipids, and cholesterol referred to as lipid rafts that cumulatively constitute a surface that is highly impregnable to urine, solutes, and potential pathogens such as UPEC and GBS (Apodaca, 2004).

2.1 Prevalence of GBS in the urinary tract

The spectrum of UTI caused by GBS includes ABU, cystitis, pyenorephritis, urethritus, and urosepsis (Bronsema et al., 1993, Farley et al., 1993, Lefevre et al., 1991, McKenna et al., 2003, Munoz et al., 1992). In many cases, GBS colonization of the urinary tract in women probably occurs by an ascending route from the vagina, where GBS can persist asymptomatically. GBS is cultured from approximately 2% of all UTI cases (de Mouy et al., 2007, Munoz et al., 1992, Persson et al., 1988). In the most recent single-centre analysis of adult patients in the United States GBS was cultured from urine during routine assessment for UTI in 2% of patients; most of these represented ABU (Ulett et al., 2009). This is consistent with findings in other studies (Aungst et al., 2004, Le et al., 2004). However, several studies have reported high rates of GBS UTI in non-pregnant adults (Edwards&Baker, 2005, Falagas et al., 2006, Muller et al., 2006, Toumi et al., 2006). In one study, GBS was cultured from 39% of all cases of symptomatic UTI among nursing home residents >70 years of age (Trivalle et al., 1998).

Other studies have reported that GBS UTI may account for up to one-third of all invasive infections due to GBS in elderly adults (Falagas et al., 2006, Hernaiz et al., 2004, Lefebvre et al., 2007, Munoz et al., 1992) and up to 7% of late-onset disease in neonates (Yagupsky et al., 1991). Urinary tract abnormalities, chronic renal failure (Munoz et al., 1992), diabetes mellitus (Ronald, 2003), corticosteroid use (Falagas et al., 2006), and prior UTI (Ulett et al., 2009) are among risk factors for GBS UTI.

2.2 GBS ABU and UTI in pregnancy

While the overall prevalence of GBS UTI remains unclear, GBS bacteriuria during pregnancy occurs at rates of between 1 and 3.5% (Baker, 1997, McKenna et al., 2003, Whitney et al., 2004). Approximately 2-7% of pregnant women exhibit ABU caused by GBS and GBS ABU during pregnancy is considered a surrogate marker for heavy maternal genital tract colonization (Liston et al., 1979, McKenna et al., 2003, Moller et al., 1984, Persson et al., 1986a, Wood&Dillon, 1981) and is indicated for intrapartum antibiotic chemoprophylaxis (McKenna et al., 2003, Schrag et al., 2002). In addition, up to 7% of pregnancies may be complicated by GBS UTI, and GBS reportedly accounts for approximately 10% of all cases of pyelonephritis during pregnancy (Muller et al., 2006, Persson et al., 1986a, Persson et al., 1986b). GBS UTI may also contribute to chorioamnionitis (Anderson et al., 2007), premature onset of labour (Moller et al., 1984), and an increased risk of vertical transmission of GBS (Persson et al., 1985, Wood&Dillon, 1981). Stemming from this, maternal GBS ABU (including pure and predominant growth of GBS in the urine) has been associated with vertical transmission and an increased risk for early-onset disease (EOD) in newborn infants (Heath et al., 2009, Liston et al., 1979, Moller et al., 1984, Persson et al., 1986a, Persson et al., 1985, Wood&Dillon, 1981). One study found an elevated risk for EOD among infants born to women with low colony-count GBS ABU compared with mothers who did not have GBS ABU (Weng et al., 2010). However, studies have also demonstrated that some women with GBS ABU during the first trimester of pregnancy may not exhibit vaginal-rectal colonization at 35-37 weeks gestation (McKenna et al., 2003) or at the time of delivery (Edwards et al., 2002). Thus, while maternal ABU does not necessarily lead to vertical transmission, ABU at any point during pregnancy may be a risk factor for neonatal EOD and has therefore been an indication for intrapartum antibiotic chemoprophylaxis since 1996 (Schrag et al., 2002, Yancey et al., 1996). ABU may also be an indicator of potential preterm labour (Schrag et al., 2002, Yancey et al., 1996). The American College of Obstetricians and Gynecologists (ACOG) and CDC guidelines recommend the evaluation of pregnant women at 35-37 weeks gestation and antibiotic therapy for women with positive cultures for GBS ABU. The 1996 ACOG and CDC guidelines do not specify a colony-count threshold for defining GBS ABU. However, the 2002 and more recent guidelines recommend reporting of GBS at any concentration in urine (Lin&Fajardo, 2008). Finally, although pregnant women may receive antibiotics to treat GBS ABU this therapy may not eliminate GBS from the genitourinary tract, and recolonization after a course of antibiotics can occur (Baecher&Grobman, 2008, Gardner et al., 1979, Hall et al., 1976).

Most data on the risk for EOD among infants born to women with GBS ABU are derived from studies using thresholds $>10^5$ cfu/ml despite lower counts of 10^3 cfu/ml having been associated with acute GBS UTI (Persson et al., 1986b, Persson et al., 1985, Ulett et al., 2009, Wood&Dillon, 1981). Although low concentrations (10^3-10^4 cfu/ml) of GBS in urine can be associated with colonization (Centelles-Serrano et al., 2009) limited data support the risk for EOD among infants born to women with low colony-count GBS ABU (Persson et al., 1986a).

The recommendation to report any colony count of GBS in urine represents increased workload for clinical laboratories, which generally do not report bacterial growth in urine of other pathogens at concentrations $<10^4$ cfu/ml (McCarter et al., 2009) and rarely know whether urine samples are from pregnant women. In the context of universal late antenatal GBS screening, it is unclear how much EOD is prevented by screening for low colony-count GBS ABU and whether identification of low colony-count bacteriuria is cost-effective.

2.3 Diagnosis of GBS UTI

Diagnostic strategies for UTI vary substantially between clinicians (Hay&Fahey, 2002, Kaufmann&Modest, 2002, Libbus, 2002); however, patients with a combination of symptoms have a high probability of UTI (Bent et al., 2002, Nicolle, 2008). Pyuria concurrently with bacteriuria constitutes diagnostic criteria in some settings (Shaikh et al., 2007), although what constitutes clinically significant bacteriuria is not strictly defined; colony counts $>10^3$ cfu/ml of a uropathogen is however, now widely accepted diagnostic criteria for cystitis (Nicolle, 2008, Rubin et al., 1992). Clinically, UTI due to GBS may be indistinguishable from UTI caused by other uropathogens (Muller et al., 2006). A recent study of multiple uropathogens highlighted unique frequencies of host characteristics in UTI groups defined by the causal organism (Tabibian et al., 2008). This suggests that the clinical and microbiological features of UTI may differ depending on the infecting pathogen and the most ideal diagnostic approaches may depend on the causal organism. In one study the investigators regarded single-organism GBS bacteriuria and at least one UTI symptom as being a probable case of UTI and used urinary leukocyte esterase with pyuria as confirmatory for diagnosis (Ulett et al., 2009). Here, a provisional diagnosis was defined by the presence of single-organism GBS bacteriuria ($>10^4$ cfu/ml) with at least one symptom that included dysuria, increased urinary frequency and/or urgency, fever of >38°C, flank pain, and/or lumbar tenderness. In cases where urinalysis (UA) was performed, UTI was confirmed on the basis of positive urinary leukocyte esterase and significant pyuria ($\geq 10^7$ white blood cells/high-power field; non-spun). These are the generally accepted criteria for the diagnosis of UTI (Hay&Fahey, 2002, Kaufmann&Modest, 2002, Libbus, 2002) although inclusion of bacteriuria counts of $>10^3$ cfu/ml may provide additional clinical relevance. In this study group, patients were grouped into probable GBS UTI where UA was not performed and confirmed cases where (positive) UA data were available. Individuals defined as having GBS isolated from urine incidentally were selected on the basis of low-grade GBS bacteriuria ($<10^4$ cfu/ml) in the absence of symptoms. In this study, multiple patients were identified who had symptoms of UTI and positive UA findings but had GBS bacteriuria counts between 10^3-10^5 cfu/ml, which is consistent with reports that up to 30% of women with cystitis present with bacteriuria of $<10^5$ cfu/ml. Thus, the level of bacteriuria in GBS UTI may not correlate well with acute disease. The serotypes of GBS associated with UTI have not been well defined; however it appears that most serotypes can cause acute UTI. MS and antisera-based serotyping was used in one study to identify the serotypes associated with UTI (Ulett et al., 2009), and demonstrated a predominance of serotypes Ia, II, III, and V in patients with acute UTI. Other studies demonstrated that nontypeable GBS also cause acute UTI (McKenna et al., 2003, Persson et al., 1985).

2.4 How does GBS colonize the urogenital tract?

GBS infection often begins with binding to epithelial cells at mucosal surfaces, such as those lining the respiratory or urogenital tracts. GBS are able bind to human vaginal epithelial cells under low pH conditions, which are characteristic of vaginal mucosa. These interactions occur via low avidity interactions of cell-wall-associated LTA and via higher-affinity interactions mediated by hydrophobic GBS surface proteins (Tamura et al., 1994). Many of these host-cell interactions involve attachment of GBS to extracellular matrix molecules such as fibronectin, fibrinogen and laminin, which in turn bind host-cell-surface proteins such as integrins (Maisey et al., 2008). For example, ScpB, which is a GBS cell-surface protein previously characterised for its ability to cleave the complement-derived chemoattractant C5a (Beckmann et al., 2002), can bind fibronectin (Cheng et al., 2002). ScpB can bind to integrins, which may promote both binding to host cells and complement proteolysis (Brown et al., 2005). Naturally occurring ScpB variants with a deletion that destroys peptidase function retain the capacity to bind fibronectin (Cleary et al., 2004, Tamura et al., 2006). GBS attachment to fibrinogen is mediated by the surface-anchored protein FbsA (Schubert et al., 2004), and adherence to laminin involves the adhesin Lmb (Spellerberg et al., 1999). The serine-rich repeat domain protein Srr-1 binds human keratin 4 (Samen et al., 2007) and the GBS surface protein LrrG, containing the leucine-rich-repeat motif found in many invasins, binds to epithelial cells, suggesting that it serves as an adhesin during GBS infection (Seepersaud et al., 2005). In each of these examples, these binding interactions probably promote GBS adherence to epithelial cells.

GBS were also recently shown to express pili (Lauer et al., 2005), which typically facilitate Gram-negative bacterial attachment to host cells (Sauer et al., 2000). Among eight sequenced GBS genomes, two genetic loci encoding pili were identified, the second existing in one of two variants, although not all genomes contain both loci (Rosini et al., 2006). GBS pilus island 2′ includes the genes encoding PilB, an LP(x)TG-motif-containing protein that polymerises to form a pilus backbone, and accessory pilus proteins PilA and PilC (Dramsi et al., 2006, Maisey et al., 2007). Epithelial cell adherence is reduced in isogenic GBS mutants lacking PilA or PilC, but not those lacking PilB (Dramsi et al., 2006). The role of GBS pili in binding in the urogenital tract is unknown.

2.5 Modeling GBS UTI from clinical studies

Uropathogenic GBS (UPGBS) have been shown to bind to both murine and human bladder uroepithelium in in vivo (Figure 1) and in vitro (Figure 2) studies. These models were developed to study the pathogen-host interaction underlying GBS UTI. UPGBS bind more efficiently to bladder epithelial mucosa when compared with non-UPGBS (Ulett et al., 2010). Binding models of GBS UTI to study host cell interactions in vivo and in vitro have been derived from clinical studies conducted in the past five years. The largest of these clinical studies of GBS UTI to date was performed in the United States using a cohort of 387 patients with positive GBS cultures in urine. This study investigated the traits of UPGBS that cause acute UTI and ABU using detailed analysis of patients groups alongside serotyping comparisons, and risk factor analysis. The study also investigated the demographic data alongside standard diagnostic microbiological measures for the defined patient groups, which are summarized in Table 1. In this study, a total of 62 patients of the 387 patients with positive GBS urine culture had single-organism bacteriuria >10^4 cfu/ml concurrent with at least one UTI symptom and were defined as having probable GBS UTI. The most prevalent serotypes of GBS causing UTI in this study according to MS were serotypes V, Ia, and III, as shown in Table 2. Together, these serotypes accounted for 76% of GBS UTI cases. Serotype III GBS was the only serotype that was more frequently isolated from UTI case patients than from controls. Thus, in this study GBS UTI occurred mostly as uncomplicated cystitis in middle-aged women (>50 yrs) in the absence of chronic underlying disease but was associated with a prior history of UTI.

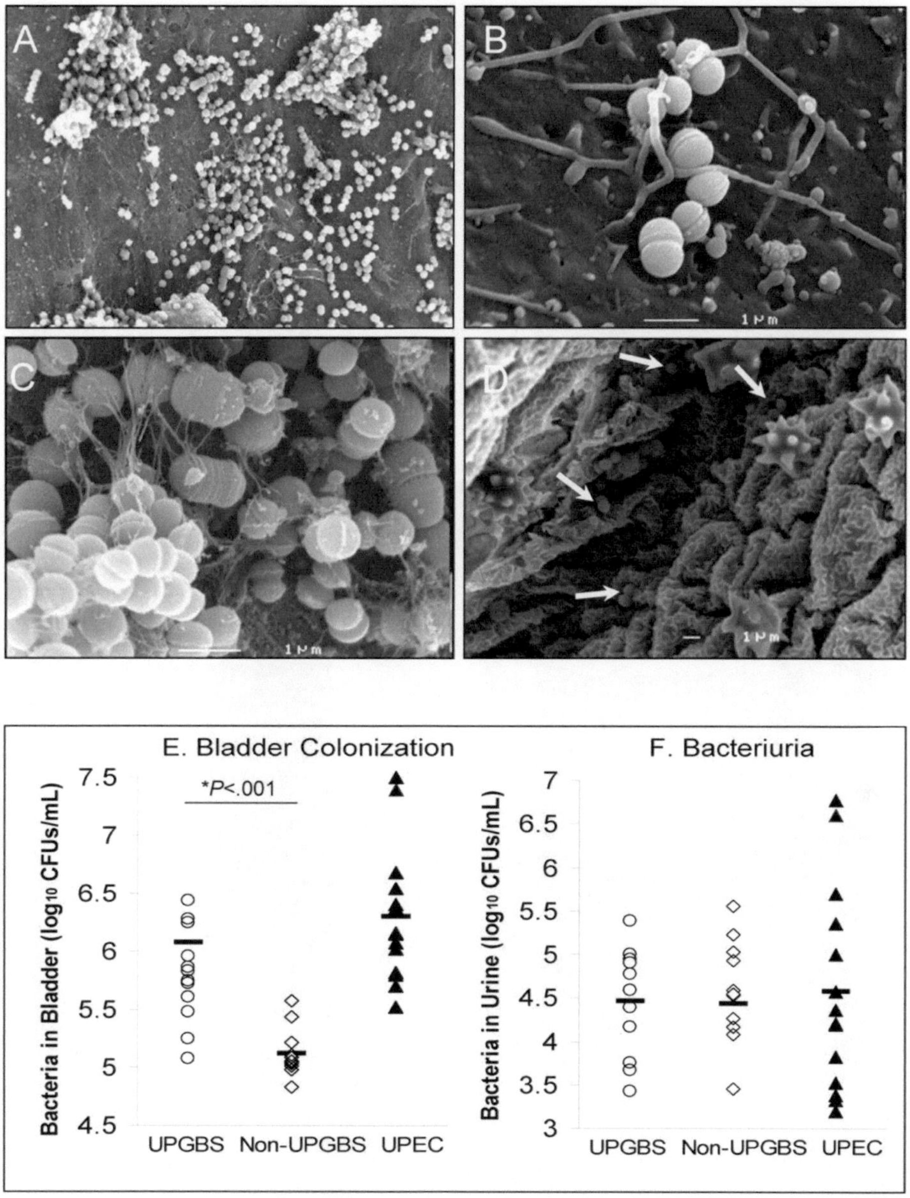

Fig. 1. UPGBS bound to bladder uroepithelium in a murine model of GBS cystitis (A–C, flattened bladder; D, native conformation). The arrows in panel *D* show bound UPGBS between folds of bladder uroepithelium. Panel E illustrates better bind of UPGBS to bladder mucosa compared with non-UPGBS although binding is not as efficient as uropathogenic *Escherichia coli* (UPEC) and levels of bacteriuria are simiular (F). Reproduced, along with Figure 2, with permission from (Ulett et al., 2010) courtesy of Oxford Journals.

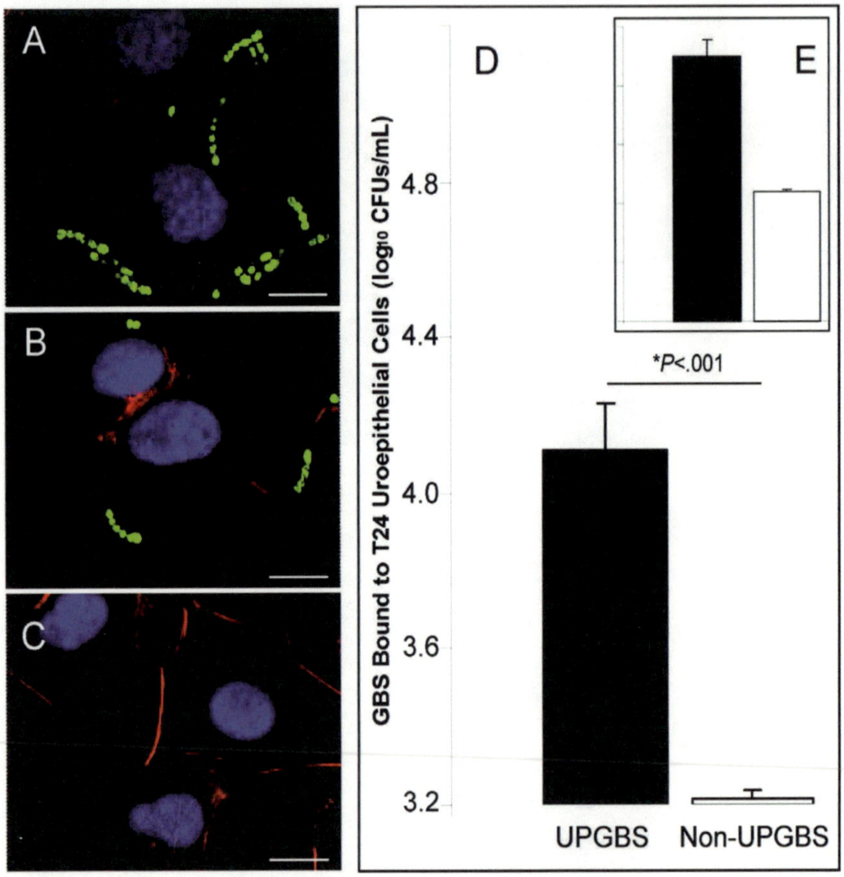

Fig. 2. UPGBS (green) bound to human bladder cells (blue, nuclei; red F-actin) at multiplicities of infection of 50 (A) and 5 (B). Uninfected cells in (C). Measures of binding of UPGBS and non-UPGBS to T24 (*D*) and 5637 (*E*) cells shows higher binding of UPGBS.

	Total Specimens (n=387)[a]	GBS UTI Cases[b]			Controls[d] (n=51)	P (All cases vs controls)
		UA +ve[c] (n=31)	UA ND[c] (n=31)	All (n=62)		
Age (mean years; range)	46; 18-95	54; 19-82	52; 19-93	53; 19-93	30; 18-64	< 0.001[g]
Female sex	322 (83)	25 (81)	27 (87)	52 (84)	46 (90)	0.002[h]
Symptoms						
- Dysuria	68 (17.6)	18 (58.1)	17 (54.8)	35 (56.5)	0 (0)	ND
- Frequency	57 (14.7)	11 (35.5)	12 (38.7)	23 (37.1)	0 (0)	ND
- Flank pain	35 (9.0)	7 (22.6)	7 (22.6)	14 (22.6)	0 (0)	ND
- Fever	15 (4.0)	4 (13.0)	2 (6.0)	6 (10.0)	0 (0)	ND
- C/W cystitis[e]	130 (33.6)	25 (80.6)	24 (77.4)	50 (81.0)	0 (0)	ND
- C/W pyleonphritis[f]	65 (16.8)	6 (19.4)	7 (22.6)	12 (19.0)	0 (0)	ND
Pregnant	99 (30.1)	1 (4)	5 (18.5)	6 (11.5)	35 (76)	
Possible Risk factors						
- Limited mobility	13 (3.4)	1 (3.2)	0 (0)	1 (1.6)	0 (0)	1.000
- Diabetes mellitus	91 (23.5)	5 (16.1)	4 (12.9)	9 (14.5)	9 (17.6)	0.651
- Chronic kidney disease	72 (18.6)	4 (12.9)	0 (0)	4 (6.5)	7 (13.7)	0.219
- Indwelling urinary catheter	4 (1.0)	0 (0)	0 (0)	0 (0)	0 (0)	ND
- Altered mental status	14 (3.6)	3 (9.7)	2 (6.5)	5 (8.1)	0 (0)	0.063[i]
- Prior History of UTI	76 (19.6)	9 (29.0)	9 (29.0)	18 (29.0)	6 (11.8)	0.032[j]
Pure GBS isolated	207 (53.5)	31 (100)	31 (100)	62 (100)	15 (29.4)	ND
GBS count >10^7 cfu/L	319 (82.4)	31 (100)	31 (100)	62 (100)	0 (0)	ND
Mean GBS count (x 10^7/L)	4.7 ± 3.6	7.4 ± 3.5	6.1 ± 3.1	6.7 ± 3.4	0.5 ± 0.3	ND
UA done	210 (54.3)	31 (100)	0 (0)	31 (50)	9 (17.3)	ND
- Pyuria	114 (54.3)	31 (100)	ND	31 (100)	0 (0)	ND
- Leukocyte esterase	122 (58.1)	31 (100)	ND	31 (100)	0 (0)	ND
- Hematuria	74 (35.2)	21 (67.7)	ND	21 (67.7)	2 (22)	ND
- +ve and C/W UTI[d-f]	91 (43.3)	31 (100)	ND	31 (100)	0 (0)	ND

Table 1. Patients who had GBS isolated from urine during routine assessement for UTI at University of Alabama Hospital between August 2007-2008. NOTE. Data are no. (%) of patients, unless otherwise indicated; [a.] Consecutive urine specimens sent for culture, from which GBS was isolated; [b.] Patients with ≥1 symptom(s) of UTI and pure growth of GBS >10^7 cfu/L; [c.] UA: +ve (consistent with UTI) positive leukocyte esterase and pyuria; ND not done; [d.] Subjects without symptoms from whose urine GBS was isolated in counts <10^7/L; [e.] Symptoms consistent with (C/W) cystitis: dysuria and/or frequency; [f.] Symptoms C/W pyelonephritis: dysuria and/or frequency plus flank pain and/or fever >38°C; [g.] By Mann-Whitney U test; [h.] By Pearson χ^2 analysis. Gender comparisons performed using population data (equal group sizes) from the US Census Bureau for Birmingham (male-female ratio 85.7); [i.] By Fisher's exact test; [j.] By forward stepwise logistic regression subsequent to Pearson χ^2 analysis; Reproduced, with Table 2, with permission from (Ulett et al., 2009) courtesy of The American Society for Microbiology.

GBS Serotype	All Specimens (n=387)[a]		GBS UTI Cases[b] *UA +ve*[c] (*n*=31)		*UA ND*[c] (*n*=31)		*All* (*n*=62)		Controls[d] (*n*=51)	
	n	(%)	*n*	(%)	*n*	(%)	*n*	(%)	*n*	(%)
Ia	81	(21)	6	(19)	8	(26)	14	(23)	8	(16)
Ib	31	(8)	2	(7)	3	(10)	5	(8)	5	(10)
II	69	(18)	5	(16)	3	(10)	7	(11)	12	(24)
III	48	(12)[e]	8	(26)	5	(16)	13	(21)[e]	5	(10)
IV	24	(6)	2	(7)	1	(3)	3	(5)	5	(10)
V	125	(32)	8	(26)	12	(37)	20	(32)	10	(20)
VI	0	(0)	0	(0)	0	(0)	0	(0)	0	(0)
VII	0	(0)	0	(0)	0	(0)	0	(0)	0	(0)
VIII	2	(1)	0	(0)	0	(0)	0	(0)	1	(2)
NT[f]	7	(2)	0	(0)	0	(0)	0	(0)	5	(10)
IX	0	(0)	0	(0)	0	(0)	0	(0)	0	(0)

Table 2. Molecular serotypes of GBS that cause UTI, from the largest study of 387 patients with positive urine cultures for GBS to date. NOTE. Data are no. (%) of GBS isolates, unless otherwise indicated; [a.] Consecutive urine specimens sent for culture, from which GBS was isolated; [b.] Patients with ≥1 symptom(s) of UTI and pure growth of GBS >10^7 cfu/L; [c.] UA: +ve (consistent with UTI) positive leukocyte esterase and pyuria; ND not done; [d.] Subjects without symptoms from whose urine GBS was isolated in counts <10^7/L; [e.] Difference between the prevalence of serotype III among all GBS UTI case patients and all other non-GBS UTI cases (*n*=325), significant by Pearson χ^2 analysis (P=0.026); [f.] Isolates were identified using antisera as: NT (3), II (2), IV (1) and V (1).

3. Conclusions

In summary, GBS is an important pathogen that causes serious infections in newborns, pregnant women, and elderly people with chronic illness. While early diagnosis and management of GBS among pregnant women can reduce the incidence of neonatal infection the prevalence of GBS disease in adult populations emphasizes the need for additional preventative and therapeutic measures. Moreover, the emergence of antibiotic-resistant strains of GBS imposes a significant threat to the successful treatment of these infections. This is particularly relevant to GBS UTI, which is associated with relatively high rates of treatment failure and poor clinical outcomes (Munoz et al., 1992). Screening pregnant mothers for GBS ABU appears to be important in relation to the vertical transmission of GBS to infants however more research is needed to clarify this aspect of GBS UTI. An overarching and intriguing theme with GBS infection in humans is that GBS can efficiently colonize the genital tract of healthy adult women long-term without triggering apparent disease but, on the other hand, can also cause acute disease in some individuals. How this occurs is unknown.

Research efforts to understand GBS pathogenesis should focus on the different strains of GBS that cause distinct clinical conditions of UTI such as ABU and cystitis in order to analyse the virulence traits that are associated with these infections. How these infections progress to disease in some individuals is completely unknown but acute inflammation in GBS UTI appears to differ mechanistically compared to that which occurs in other Gram-negative UTI. Further longer-term surveillance studies of GBS UTI and ABU will help to better define the clinical features and serotypes associated with these infections. The question of how GBS might adapt to the niche environment of the urinary tract is another intriguing and unanswered question. A better understanding of the molecular mechanisms used by GBS to colonise uroepithelium and persist in the bladder will be an important area for future investigation. Broader utilization of appropriate in vivo and in vitro models beyond those already characterized will help to answer these questions. One area for investigation, for example, would be to use human urine as a growth medium to study fitness traits of UPGBS as has been performed for other uropathogens to discover key elements of UTI disease pathogenesis and how some successful uropathogens persist within the urinary tract in the absence of direct binding to cellular targets. Such studies will pave the way to develop new preventive and perhaps therapeutic strategies for GBS UTI. While many of the current strategies have focused on the development of vaccines for prevention of GBS disease (Maione et al., 2005) their potential for reducing GBS disease burden due to UTI is unknown. Identification of alternate drug targets would also be a goal of future research. Elucidation of the mechanisms that underlie GBS disease pathogenesis is pivotal for the identification of such alternate drug targets and also in the development of novel vaccines. A better understanding of how GBS regulates expression of its virulence survival factors is imperative. Finally, the underlying phenotypic basis for UPGBS could be gained by comparing GBS isolated from asymptomatic infection to cystitis strains by comparative genome sequencing approaches. Discoveries from such research may challenge the existing paradigms and reveal surprising insights into the versatile nature of this important human pathogen.

4. Acknowledgment

This work was supported with grants from the Australian National Health and Medical Research Council (grant 569674) and a Griffith Health Institute Grant.

5. References

AAPC 1992. American Academy of Pediatrics Committee on Infectious Diseases and Committee on Fetus and Newborn: Guidelines for prevention of group B streptococcal (GBS) infection by chemoprophylaxis. *Pediatrics,* 90, 775-778.

AAPC 1997. Revised guidelines for prevention of early-onset group B streptococcal (GBS) infection. American Academy of Pediatrics Committee on Infectious Diseases and Committee on Fetus and Newborn. *Pediatrics,* 99, 489-496.

Adderson, E. E., et al. 2000. Bacterial genetics and human immunity to group B streptococci. *Mol Genet Metab,* 71, 451-454.

Anderson, B. L., et al. 2007. Untreated asymptomatic group B streptococcal bacteriuria early in pregnancy and chorioamnionitis at delivery. *Am J Obstet Gynecol,* 196, 524 e521-525.

Andrews, J. I., et al. 2000. Group B streptococci causing neonatal bloodstream infection: antimicrobial susceptibility and serotyping results from SENTRY centers in the Western Hemisphere. *Am J Obstet Gynecol,* 183, 859-862.

Andriole, V. T. & Patterson, T. F. 1991. Epidemiology, natural history, and management of urinary tract infections in pregnancy. *Med Clin North Am,* 75, 359-373.

Apodaca, G. 2004. The uroepithelium: not just a passive barrier. *Traffic,* 5, 117-128.

Aungst, M., et al. 2004. Low colony counts of asymptomatic group B streptococcus bacteriuria: a survey of practice patterns. *Am J Perinatol,* 21, 403-407.

Baecher, L. & Grobman, W. 2008. Prenatal antibiotic treatment does not decrease group B streptococcus colonization at delivery. *Int J Gynaecol Obstet,* 101, 125-128.

Baker, C. 2000. . Group B Streptococcal infections. . *Streptococcal Infections. Clinical aspects, microbiology, and molecular pathogenesis.* . New York:: Oxford University Press; .

Baker, C. J. 1997. Group B streptococcal infections. *Clin Perinatol,* 24, 59-70.

Baker, C. J. & Barrett, F. F. 1974. Group B streptococcal infections in infants. The importance of the various serotypes. *JAMA,* 230, 1158-1160.

Baker, C. J., et al. 1973. Suppurative meningitis due to streptococci of Lancefield group B: a study of 33 infants. *J Pediatr,* 82, 724-729.

Barnett, B. J. & Stephens, D. S. 1997. Urinary tract infection: an overview. *Am J Med Sci,* 314, 245-249.

Beckmann, C., et al. 2002. Identification of novel adhesins from Group B streptococci by use of phage display reveals that C5a peptidase mediates fibronectin binding. *Infect Immun,* 70, 2869-2876.

Bent, S., et al. 2002. Does this woman have an acute uncomplicated urinary tract infection? *JAMA,* 287, 2701-2710.

Berner, R. 2002. Group B streptococci during pregnancy and infancy. *Curr Opin Infect Dis,* 15, 307-313.

Berner, R. 2004. Significance, management and prevention of Streptococcus agalactiae infection during the perinatal period. *Expert Rev Anti Infect Ther,* 2, 427-437.

Bland, M. L., et al. 2001. Antibiotic resistance patterns of group B streptococci in late third-trimester rectovaginal cultures. *Am J Obstet Gynecol,* 184, 1125-1126.

Bogdan, I., et al. 1997. Tumor necrosis factor-alpha contributes to apoptosis in hippocampal neurons during experimental group B streptococcal meningitis. *J Infect Dis,* 176, 693-697.

Boyer, K. M., et al. 1983. Selective intrapartum chemoprophylaxis of neonatal group B streptococcal early-onset disease. II. Predictive value of prenatal cultures. *Journal of Infectious Diseases,* 148, 802-809.

Bronsema, D. A., et al. 1993. Secular trends in rates and etiology of nosocomial urinary tract infections at a university hospital. *J Urol,* 150, 414-416.

Brown, C. K., et al. 2005. Structure of the streptococcal cell wall C5a peptidase. *Proc Natl Acad Sci U S A,* 102, 18391-18396.

Campbell, J. R., et al. 2000. Group B streptococcal colonization and serotype-specific immunity in pregnant women at delivery. *Obstet Gynecol,* 96, 498-503.

Centelles-Serrano, M. J., et al. 2009. [Effectiveness of systematic investigation for Group B Streptococcus in urine samples to identify colonized pregnant women]. *Enferm Infecc Microbiol Clin,* 27, 394-398.

Chattopadhyay, D., et al. 2011. Phylogenetic lineage and pilus protein Spb1/SAN1518 affect opsonin-independent phagocytosis and intracellular survival of Group B Streptococcus. *Microbes and infection / Institut Pasteur,* 13, 369-382.

Cheng, Q., et al. 2001. Antibody against surface-bound C5a peptidase is opsonic and initiates macrophage killing of group B streptococci. *Infection and immunity,* 69, 2302-2308.

Cheng, Q., et al. 2002. The group B streptococcal C5a peptidase is both a specific protease and an invasin. *Infect Immun,* 70, 2408-2413.

Cleary, P. P., et al. 2004. Immunization with C5a peptidase from either group A or B streptococci enhances clearance of group A streptococci from intranasally infected mice. *Vaccine,* 22, 4332-4341.

Cornacchione, P., et al. 1998. Group B streptococci persist inside macrophages. *Immunology,* 93, 86-95.

Dahesh, S., et al. 2008. Point mutation in the group B streptococcal pbp2x gene conferring decreased susceptibility to beta-lactam antibiotics. *Antimicrob Agents Chemother,* 52, 2915-2918.

Daniels, J., et al. 2009. Rapid testing for group B streptococcus during labour: a test accuracy study with evaluation of acceptability and cost-effectiveness. *Health Technol Assess,* 13, 1-154, iii-iv.

De Mouy, D., et al. 2007. [Community-acquired urinary tract infections in 15 to 65 years old female patients in France. Susceptibility of E. coli according to history: AFORCOPI-BIO network 2003]. *Med Mal Infect,* 37, 594-598.

Dermer, P., et al. 2004. A history of neonatal group B streptococcus with its related morbidity and mortality rates in the United States. *J Pediatr Nurs,* 19, 357-363.

Dillon, H. C., JR., et al. 1982. Anorectal and vaginal carriage of group B streptococci during pregnancy. *J Infect Dis,* 145, 794-799.

Doro, F., et al. 2009. Surfome analysis as a fast track to vaccine discovery: identification of a novel protective antigen for Group B Streptococcus hypervirulent strain COH1. *Mol Cell Proteomics,* 8, 1728-1737.

Dramsi, S., et al. 2006. Assembly and role of pili in group B streptococci. *Mol Microbiol,* 60, 1401-1413.

Edwards, M. S. 2006. Issues of antimicrobial resistance in group B streptococcus in the era of intrapartum antibiotic prophylaxis. *Semin Pediatr Infect Dis,* 17, 149-152.

Edwards, M. S. & Baker, C. J. 2005. Group B streptococcal infections in elderly adults. *Clin Infect Dis,* 41, 839-847.

Edwards, R. K., et al. 2002. Intrapartum antibiotic prophylaxis 2: positive predictive value of antenatal group B streptococci cultures and antibiotic susceptibility of clinical isolates. *Obstet Gynecol,* 100, 540-544.

Facklam, R. 2002. What happened to the streptococci: overview of taxonomic and nomenclature changes. *Clinical microbiology reviews,* 15, 613-630.

Falagas, M. E., et al. 2006. Streptococcus agalactiae infections in non-pregnant adults: single center experience of a growing clinical problem. *Medical Science Monitor,* 12, CR447-451.

Farley, M. M. 2001. Group B streptococcal disease in nonpregnant adults. *Clin Infect Dis,* 33, 556-561.

Farley, M. M., et al. 1993. A population-based assessment of invasive disease due to group B Streptococcus in nonpregnant adults. *N Engl J Med,* 328, 1807-1811.

Fasola, E. L., et al. 1996. Immune responses to the R4 protein antigen of group B streptococci and its relationship to other streptococcal R4 proteins. *Clinical and diagnostic laboratory immunology,* 3, 321-325.

Ferrieri, P., et al. 1977. Epidemiology of group-B streptococcal carriage in pregnant women and newborn infants. *Journal of Medical Microbiology,* 10, 103-114.

Ferrieri, P., et al. 2004. Characterization of vaginal & rectal colonization with multiple serotypes of group B streptococci using multiple colony picks. *Indian Journal of Medical Research,* 119 Suppl, 208-212.

Fettucciari, K., et al. 2000. Group B Streptococcus induces apoptosis in macrophages. *J Immunol,* 165, 3923-3933.

Foxman, B. 2002. Epidemiology of urinary tract infections: incidence, morbidity, and economic costs. *Am J Med,* 113 Suppl 1A, 5S-13S.

Franke-Ullmann, G., et al. 1996. Characterization of murine lung interstitial macrophages in comparison with alveolar macrophages in vitro. *J Immunol,* 157, 3097-3104.

Gardner, S. E., et al. 1979. Failure of penicillin to eradicate group B streptococcal colonization in the pregnant woman. A couple study. *Am J Obstet Gynecol,* 135, 1062-1065.

Gibbs, R. S., et al. 2004. Perinatal infections due to group B streptococci. *Obstet Gynecol,* 104, 1062-1076.

Hall, R. T., et al. 1976. Antibiotic treatment of parturient women colonized with group B streptococci. *Am J Obstet Gynecol,* 124, 630-634.

Hay, A. D. & Fahey, T. 2002. Clinical diagnosis of urinary tract infection. *JAMA,* 288, 1229; author reply 1230-1221.

Heath, P. T., et al. 2009. Group B streptococcal disease in infants: a case control study. *Arch Dis Child,* 94, 674-680.

Heelan, J. S., et al. 2004. Resistance of group B streptococcus to selected antibiotics, including erythromycin and clindamycin. *J Clin Microbiol,* 42, 1263-1264.

Henneke, P., et al. 2005. Role of lipoteichoic acid in the phagocyte response to group B streptococcus. *Journal of immunology,* 174, 6449-6455.

Hernaiz, C., et al. 2004. [Clinical significance of Streptococcus agalactiae isolation from urine samples of outpatients from health care centers]. *Enferm Infecc Microbiol Clin,* 22, 89-91.

Hooton, T. M. & Stamm, W. E. 1997. Diagnosis and treatment of uncomplicated urinary tract infection. *Infect Dis Clin North Am,* 11, 551-581.

Huang, P. Y., et al. 2006. Group B streptococcal bacteremia in non-pregnant adults. *J Microbiol Immunol Infect,* 39, 237-241.

Jonsson, S., et al. 1985. Phagocytosis and killing of common bacterial pathogens of the lung by human alveolar macrophages. *J Infect Dis,* 152, 4-13.

Kaufmann, J. & Modest, G. A. 2002. Clinical diagnosis of urinary tract infection. *JAMA,* 288, 1229-1230; author reply 1230-1221.

Kimura, K., et al. 2008. First molecular characterization of group B streptococci with reduced penicillin susceptibility. *Antimicrob Agents Chemother,* 52, 2890-2897.

Kong, F., et al. 2002. Serotype identification of group B streptococci by PCR and sequencing. *J Clin Microbiol,* 40, 216-226.

Kong, F., et al. 2005. Simultaneous detection and serotype identification of Streptococcus agalactiae using multiplex PCR and reverse line blot hybridization. *J Med Microbiol,* 54, 1133-1138.

Krasnianin, E., et al. 2009. The incidence of Streptococcus Group B in 100 parturient women and the transmission of pathogens to the newborn. *Ginekol Pol,* 80, 285-289.

Lauer, P., et al. 2005. Genome analysis reveals pili in Group B Streptococcus. *Science,* 309, 105.

Le, J., et al. 2004. Urinary tract infections during pregnancy. *Ann Pharmacother,* 38, 1692-1701.

Lee, H. C., et al. 2007. Invasive Streptococcus agalactiae septic arthritis as an initial presentation of tonsillar carcinoma. *Singapore Med J,* 48, 678-681.

Lefebvre, N., et al. 2007. Invasive Streptococcus agalactiae infections in non-pregnant adults. *Med Mal Infect,* 37, 796-801.

Lefevre, J. C., et al. 1991. Clinical and microbiologic features of urethritis in men in Toulouse, France. *Sex Transm Dis,* 18, 76-79.

Libbus, M. K. 2002. Review: specific combinations of symptoms effectively rule in the diagnosis of urinary tract infection based on history alone. *Evid Based Nurs,* 5, 119.

Lin, K. & Fajardo, K. 2008. Screening for asymptomatic bacteriuria in adults: evidence for the U.S. Preventive Services Task Force reaffirmation recommendation statement. *Ann Intern Med,* 149, W20-24.

Lindahl, G., et al. 2005. Surface proteins of Streptococcus agalactiae and related proteins in other bacterial pathogens. *Clin Microbiol Rev,* 18, 102-127.

Liston, T. E., et al. 1979. Relationship of neonatal pneumonia to maternal urinary and neonatal isolates of group B streptococci. *Southern Medical Journal,* 72, 1410-1412.

Liu, G. Y., et al. 2004. Sword and shield: linked group B streptococcal beta-hemolysin/cytolysin and carotenoid pigment function to subvert host phagocyte defense. *Proc Natl Acad Sci U S A,* 101, 14491-14496.

Liu, G. Y. & NIZET, V. 2004. Extracellular virulence factors of group B Streptococci. *Front Biosci,* 9, 1794-1802.

Lukacs, S. L., et al. 2004. Trends in sepsis-related neonatal mortality in the United States, 1985-1998. *Pediatr Infect Dis J,* 23, 599-603.

Maione, D., et al. 2005. Identification of a universal Group B streptococcus vaccine by multiple genome screen. *Science,* 309, 148-150.

Maisey, H. C., et al. 2008. Recent advances in understanding the molecular basis of group B Streptococcus virulence. *Expert Rev Mol Med,* 10, e27.

Maisey, H. C., et al. 2007. Group B streptococcal pilus proteins contribute to adherence to and invasion of brain microvascular endothelial cells. *J Bacteriol,* 189, 1464-1467.

Manning, S. D., et al. 2008. Genotypic diversity and serotype distribution of group B streptococcus isolated from women before and after delivery. *Clinical Infectious Diseases,* 46, 1829-1837.

Martins, E. R., et al. 2010. Evidence for rare capsular switching in Streptococcus agalactiae. *J Bacteriol,* 192, 1361-1369.

Mccarter, Y., et al. 2009. *Cumitech 2C: laboratory diagnosis of urinary tract infections.,* Washington, DC, ASM Press.

Mckenna, D. S., et al. 2003. Maternal group B streptococcal (GBS) genital tract colonization at term in women who have asymptomatic GBS bacteriuria. *Infectious Diseases in Obstetrics & Gynecology,* 11, 203-207.

Moller, M., et al. 1984. Rupture of fetal membranes and premature delivery associated with group B streptococci in urine of pregnant women. *Lancet,* 2, 69-70.

Muller, A. E., et al. 2006. Morbidity related to maternal group B streptococcal infections. *Acta Obstet Gynecol Scand,* 85, 1027-1037.

Munoz, P., et al. 1992. Group B Streptococcus: a cause of urinary tract infection in nonpregnant adults. *Clin Infect Dis,* 14, 492-496.

Nagano, N., et al. 2008. Genetic heterogeneity in pbp genes among clinically isolated group B Streptococci with reduced penicillin susceptibility. *Antimicrob Agents Chemother,* 52, 4258-4267.

Nandyal, R. R. 2008. Update on group B streptococcal infections: perinatal and neonatal periods. *J Perinat Neonatal Nurs,* 22, 230-237.

Nicolle, L. E. 2008. Uncomplicated urinary tract infection in adults including uncomplicated pyelonephritis. *Urol Clin North Am,* 35, 1-12, v.

Nizet, V. 2002. Streptococcal beta-hemolysins: genetics and role in disease pathogenesis. *Trends Microbiol,* 10, 575-580.

Nizet, V., et al. 2000. Molecular pathogenesis of Group B Streptococcal disease in newborns. *Streptococcal Infections. Clinical aspects, microbiology, and molecular pathogenesis.* New York: Oxford University Press.

Pass, M. A., et al. 1982. Puerperal and perinatal infections with group B streptococci. *Am J Obstet Gynecol,* 143, 147-152.

Patil, N. & Martin, R. E. 2010. Native aortic valve infective endocarditis caused by Streptococcus agalactiae in a renal transplant recipient. *Am J Med Sci,* 340, 518-520.

Patton, J. P., et al. 1991. Urinary tract infection: economic considerations. *Med Clin North Am,* 75, 495-513.

Persson, K., et al. 1986a. Group B streptococci at delivery: high count in urine increases risk for neonatal colonization. *Scandinavian Journal of Infectious Diseases,* 18, 525-531.

Persson, K., et al. 1986b. Group B streptococci at delivery: high count in urine increases risk for neonatal colonization. *Scand J Infect Dis,* 18, 525-531.

Persson, K., et al. 1985. Asymptomatic bacteriuria during pregnancy with special reference to group B streptococci. *Scand J Infect Dis,* 17, 195-199.

Persson, K. M., et al. 1988. Significance of group B streptococci in urine cultures from males and non-pregnant females. *Scand J Infect Dis,* 20, 47-53.

Puopolo, K. M., et al. 2007. A composite transposon associated with erythromycin and clindamycin resistance in group B Streptococcus. *J Med Microbiol,* 56, 947-955.

Ramaswamy, S. V., et al. 2006. Molecular characterization of nontypeable group B streptococcus. *Journal of Clinical Microbiology,* 44, 2398-2403.

Rausch, A. V., et al. 2009. Group B Streptococcus colonization in pregnancy: prevalence and prevention strategies of neonatal sepsis. *J Perinat Med,* 37, 124-129.

Ring, A., et al. 2002. Group B streptococcal beta-hemolysin induces mortality and liver injury in experimental sepsis. *J Infect Dis,* 185, 1745-1753.

Ronald, A. 2002. The etiology of urinary tract infection: traditional and emerging pathogens. *Am J Med,* 113 Suppl 1A, 14S-19S.

Ronald, A. 2003. The etiology of urinary tract infection: traditional and emerging pathogens. *Dis Mon,* 49, 71-82.

Rosini, R., et al. 2006. Identification of novel genomic islands coding for antigenic pilus-like structures in Streptococcus agalactiae. *Mol Microbiol,* 61, 126-141.

Rubin, R. H., et al. 1992. Evaluation of new anti-infective drugs for the treatment of urinary tract infection. Infectious Diseases Society of America and the Food and Drug Administration. *Clin Infect Dis,* 15 Suppl 1, S216-227.

Samen, U., et al. 2007. The surface protein Srr-1 of Streptococcus agalactiae binds human keratin 4 and promotes adherence to epithelial HEp-2 cells. *Infect Immun,* 75, 5405-5414.

Sauer, F. G., et al. 2000. Bacterial pili: molecular mechanisms of pathogenesis. *Curr Opin Microbiol,* 3, 65-72.

Schrag, S., et al. 2002. Prevention of perinatal group B streptococcal disease. Revised guidelines from CDC. *MMWR Recomm Rep,* 51, 1-22.

Schubert, A., et al. 2004. The fibrinogen receptor FbsA promotes adherence of Streptococcus agalactiae to human epithelial cells. *Infect Immun,* 72, 6197-6205.

Schuchat, A. 1998. Epidemiology of group B streptococcal disease in the United States: shifting paradigms. *Clin Microbiol Rev,* 11, 497-513.

Schwope, O. I., et al. 2010. The effect of a chlorhexidine-based surgical lubricant during pelvic examination on the detection of group B Streptococcus. *American Journal of Obstetrics & Gynecology,* 202, 276.e271-273.

Seepersaud, R., et al. 2005. Characterization of a novel leucine-rich repeat protein antigen from group B streptococci that elicits protective immunity. *Infect Immun,* 73, 1671-1683.

Sendi, P., et al. 2008. Invasive group B Streptococcal disease in non-pregnant adults : a review with emphasis on skin and soft-tissue infections. *Infection,* 36, 100-111.

Shaikh, N., et al. 2007. Does this child have a urinary tract infection? *JAMA,* 298, 2895-2904.

Sherman, M. P., et al. 1992. Role of pulmonary phagocytes in host defense against group B streptococci in preterm versus term rabbit lung. *J Infect Dis,* 166, 818-826.

Sibille, Y. & Reynolds, H. Y. 1990. Macrophages and polymorphonuclear neutrophils in lung defense and injury. *Am Rev Respir Dis,* 141, 471-501.

Simoes, J. A., et al. 2004. Antibiotic resistance patterns of group B streptococcal clinical isolates. *Infect Dis Obstet Gynecol,* 12, 1-8.

Slotved, H. C., et al. 2003. Latex assay for serotyping of group B Streptococcus isolates. *J Clin Microbiol,* 41, 4445-4447.

Slotved, H. C., et al. 2007. Serotype IX, a Proposed New Streptococcus agalactiae Serotype. *J Clin Microbiol,* 45, 2929-2936.

Spellerberg, B., et al. 1999. Lmb, a protein with similarities to the LraI adhesin family, mediates attachment of Streptococcus agalactiae to human laminin. *Infect Immun,* 67, 871-878.

Tabibian, J. H., et al. 2008. Uropathogens and host characteristics. *J Clin Microbiol,* 46, 3980-3986.

Tamura, G. S., et al. 2006. High-affinity interaction between fibronectin and the group B streptococcal C5a peptidase is unaffected by a naturally occurring four-amino-acid deletion that eliminates peptidase activity. *Infect Immun,* 74, 5739-5746.

Tamura, G. S., et al. 1994. Adherence of group B streptococci to cultured epithelial cells: roles of environmental factors and bacterial surface components. *Infect Immun,* 62, 2450-2458.

Tissi, L., et al. 1997. Group B streptococci. Role of capsular polysaccharide on virulence and induction of septic arthritis. *Adv Exp Med Biol,* 418, 817-818.

Toumi, A., et al. 2006. [Streptococcus agalactiae in nonpregnant adults]. *Tunis Med,* 84, 161-164.

Trivalle, C., et al. 1998. Group B streptococcal bacteraemia in the elderly. *J Med Microbiol,* 47, 649-652.

Ulett, G. C., et al. 2003. Beta-hemolysin-independent induction of apoptosis of macrophages infected with serotype III group B streptococcus. *J Infect Dis,* 188, 1049-1053.

Ulett, G. C., et al. 2010. Group B Streptococcus (GBS) urinary tract infection involves binding of GBS to bladder uroepithelium and potent but GBS-specific induction of interleukin 1alpha. *Journal of Infectious Diseases,* 201, 866-870.

Ulett, K. B., et al. 2009. Diversity of group B streptococcus serotypes causing urinary tract infection in adults. *Journal of Clinical Microbiology,* 47, 2055-2060.

Valenti-Weigand, P., et al. 1996. Entry and intracellular survival of group B streptococci in J774 macrophages. *Infect Immun,* 64, 2467-2473.

Van Der Poll, T. & Opal, S. M. 2008. Host-pathogen interactions in sepsis. *Lancet Infect Dis,* 8, 32-43.

Verani, J. R., et al. 2010. Prevention of perinatal group B streptococcal disease--revised guidelines from CDC, 2010. *MMWR Recomm Rep,* 59, 1-36.

Verani, J. R. & SCHRAG, S. J. 2010. Group B streptococcal disease in infants: progress in prevention and continued challenges. *Clin Perinatol,* 37, 375-392.

Wen, L., et al. 2006. Use of a serotype-specific DNA microarray for identification of group B Streptococcus (Streptococcus agalactiae). *Journal of Clinical Microbiology,* 44, 1447-1452.

Weng, C., et al. 2010. Pregnancy outcomes in women with group B streptococcal bacteriuria. *Annual Meeting of the Pediatric Academic Societies.* Vancouver, Canada.

Whitney, C. G., et al. 2004. The international infections in pregnancy study: group B streptococcal colonization in pregnant women. *J Matern Fetal Neonatal Med,* 15, 267-274.

Wood, E. G. & Dillon, H. C., JR. 1981. A prospective study of group B streptococcal bacteriuria in pregnancy. *American Journal of Obstetrics & Gynecology,* 140, 515-520.

Yagupsky, P., et al. 1991. The changing spectrum of group B streptococcal disease in infants: an eleven-year experience in a tertiary care hospital. *Pediatr Infect Dis J,* 10, 801-808.

Yancey, M. K., et al. 1996. The accuracy of late antenatal screening cultures in predicting genital group B streptococcal colonization at delivery. *Obstetrics & Gynecology,* 88, 811-815.

5

Chlamydia Trachomatis in Non-Specific Urethritis

Okoror Lawrence
Department of Microbiology, Joseph Ayo Babalola University,
Ikeji-Arakeji, Ilesha, Osun State
Nigeria

1. Introduction

The Chlamydiae belongs to the order Chlamydiales with one family Chlamydiaceae one genus *Chlamydia* and three species that infect man *Chlamydia trachomatis, Chlamydia psittacci* and *Chlamydia pneumoniae* (Thylefers et al. 1987; Zhang and Stephens, 1992; Peeling et al. 1998). Chlamydiae were first cultured in the 1950s. The wide spread importance and frequencies of genital tract *Chlamydia* infections were first appreciated in the 1960s. *Chlamydia* were first thought to be viruses and were referred to as large viruses (Peeling et al. 1998). They look like bacteria by having cell wall which lack muramunic acid and are like viruses by being filterable (Koh et al. 2002).

Chlamydia includes organisms previously called the psittacisis- lymphogranuloma venereum-trachoma group (PLT organisms) or the trachoma-inclusion conjunctivitis (TRIC organisms). *Chlamydia* are non-motile, coccoid looking like gram-negative bacteria ranging in size from 0.2 to 1.5μ. For years *Chlamydia* were considered to be viruses but they are now considered to be a special kind of Gram negative bacteria. They also differ from viruses by containing both DNA and RNA (Strickland, 1994). They can only reproduce in the cytoplasmic vesicle of the host cell by a unique developmental life cycle involving the formation of elementary and reticulate bodies (Miyuashita et al. 1993).

Chlamydia are rapidly inactivated by heat. They lose their infectivity completely after 10 minutes at 60°C and partly after 3 to 12 hours at 37°C. They can maintain infectivity for years at 5°C and 7°C. During the process of freeze-drying, much of the infectivity is lost, but successfully lyophylised preparations are stable for a long period. Chlamydiae are rapidly inactivated in the presence of phenols (Koh et al. 2002).

Chlamydia psittaci is a diverse species that has poorly been characterized. Strains that infect psittacine birds seem to differ from those that infect poultry. Several mammals and marsupials have species-specific strains (Prescott et al. 1999). Generally humans are not susceptible to infection with most mammalian strains of *Chlamydia psittaci.* A major problem with *Chlamydia psittaci* is that it is zoonotic in nature. In birds *Chlamydia psittaci* may present as an upper respiratory infection with nasal and ocular discharge, diarrhea or a combination of both. In some cases birds may be infected with no sign. These cases are of importance because birds are carriers and shed the organism. Psittacosis in humans can result in mild and severe disease. In several cases, humans that are infected often have severe fever with night sweats leading to pneumonia. It is very important that pet birds owners and handlers of poultry become aware of this disease in order to prevent outbreak (McPhee and Harrignton, 1987).

The first *Chlamydia pneumoniae* case which was formally called Taiwanese acute respiratory (TWAR) agent strain was first cultured in 1960s in chick embryo sac but was thought to be a member of the species *Chlamydia psittaci. Chlamydia pneumoniae* as an important respiratory pathogen has led to the reappraisal of our concept chlamydia respiratory infections (Grayston et al. 1990 and Grayston, 1992). *Chlamydia pneumoniae* is mainly unique to man and in man infection may vary from mild to severe cases. Result of surveys indicated that sub clinical chlamydial infections occur, which often remains undiagnosed because of their similarity to other respiratory infections. The onset of pneumonia may be sudden with chills, fever, anorexia, sore throat, severe headache and photophobia or the disease may develop gradually. In severe cases, nausea, vomiting and diarrhea or constipation may be observed. The fever remains high in severe cases while it may fall to normal within a week in milder cases. Cyanoids and low blood pressure may be observed. Generally, *Chlamydia pneumoniae* causes pneumonia, bronchitis and pharyngitis in school children (Karvonem et al. 1992). Some physicians have reported *Chlamydia pneumoniae* infection in patients with asthma.

A mention of *Chlamydia* is often referred to a disease caused by *Chlamydia trachomatis. Chlamydia trachomatis* infections are mainly spread through sexual contact and most times neonatal. This includes from penis to vagina, penis to rectum and also from mother to child during birth (Lin et al. 1992) the sexually transmitted disease usually comes with no clear-cut symptoms. *Chlamydia trachomatis* threatens to cause reproductive damage and infertility in as many as 3 to 5 million people in America alone each year (Lin et al. 1992). This makes *Chlamydia trachomatis* the most prevalent sexually transmitted diseases worldwide (Macaulay et al. 1990; Azenabor and Eghafona, 1997; Azenabor et al. 2007). Due to its latent infection *Chlamydia trachomatis* is rarely diagnosed especially in developing countries, which is why this study sought to establish the prevalence of *Chlamydia trachomatis* in non-specific urethritis. *Chlamydia trachomatis* still remains ahead of gonorrhea and syphilis in the list of most commonly transmitted sexual disease. *Chlamydia trachomatis* may result in urethritis, epididymitis, cervicitis, pelvic inflammatory disease (PID) and other conditions. Men and women infected with *Chlamydia* may have discharge from the penis or vagina and may notice burning urination. Infections in the rectum may cause problems or pains. In many instances, both men and women will not notice any symptoms (50% of women and 25% of men). If symptoms do occur, they usually show up within 1 to 2 weeks after been exposed. A person can be infected at any age, the age group been mostly affected being 15-19 years of age but Okoror et al. (2008) reported age group 30-36 being mostly exposed but this they attributed to the fact that they sampled only women of child bearing age and their spouses. Okoror et al. (2007) also reported that *Chlamydia trachomatis* infect all age groups. The discrepancies in their reports would have been because of difference in the populations sampled. Johnson et al. (Johnson et al. 1994) reported that the adolescents are at high risk. In a study by Agbonlahor et al. (2009) in North West zone of Nigeria, 75% of the total samples cultured were positive to *Chlamydia trachomatis* although the diseases were not stratified. They also reported that most of the subjects whose samples were positive had difficulty urinating and that most of the positive women had symptoms looking like that of PID as confirmed by a clinician. They also confirmed the endemicity of *Chlamydia trachomatis* in the population studied. However, there could be prevalence of *Chlamydia trachomatis* in asymptomatic individuals. Baud et al. (2008) reported low prevalence of *Chlamydia trachomatis* in asymptomatic Swiss males. They also reported that the prevalence of *Chlamydia trachomatis* is low compared to other countries.

Urinary tract infections (UTI) could be defined as the persistent presence within the urinary tract of actively multiplying microorganisms. UTI implies both microbial colonization of the urine and invasion of the lower or upper urinary tract by microorganisms (Reld and Spied, 1987). It is an infection with more than 100,000 organisms per millilitres in the mid-stream samples of urine (Macleod *et al.*, 1984).

Urinary tract infection is the most common disease of the urinary tract and it is a major cause of morbidity in both the hospital and the community (Hannan *et al.*, 1993). The most common cause of UTI are bacteria, and less often viruses, yeasts or other intracellular microorganisms (Cattell, 1985). According to Bohnson (1986), bacteriuria may be completely asymptomatic or remain localised in the bladder without the development of renal infection. Urine secreted by normal kidney is sterile and remain so while it travels to the bladder, however, normal urine is known to have a microbial flora and any voided urine in normal persons may therefore contain thousands of bacteria per millilitre derived from this normal flora. In other to differentiate this smaller number of microorganisms from the larger number of microorganisms commonly found in infections of the urinary tract, it is essential to count the number of bacteria present in fresh properly collected specimens by appropriate methods (Schroeder, *et al.*, 1990).

In Nigeria, UTI is prevalent among men and women, but more common among women, especially during pregnancy (Eke *et al.*, 1987). Unrecognised UTI in infancy and childhood may have serious long-term effects and chronic pyelonephritis may occur in adults. However, the infection occurs in all persons regardless of sex or age with particular impact on the young and the very elderly (Rubin *et. al.*, 1986). Sexually active females are also predisposed to UTI than their male counterparts (Wiswell and Smith, 1985; Johnson *et al.*, 1995). In later life, UTI is more among men until the age of prostatic hypertrophy (above 40 years of age) (Schroeder *et al.*, 1990).

For many years, pathogens associated with uncomplicated UTI have remained constant, with *E. coli* identified as the etiological agent in about 75-90% of infections (Hooton and Stamm, 1997). Five to ten percent of uncomplicated cases are caused by *S. saprophyticus* (Gupta *et al.*, 1999) with *Klebsiella, Proteus, Enterococcus* and *Pseudomonas* species seen in much smaller percentages. (Kahlmeter, 2001; Gupta., 2001; Wright *et. al.*, 2000).

In women, signs can include unusual vaginal discharge or bleeding, burning during urination or lower abdominal pain. Men like women, may in addition to pain during urination develop swellings in the testicles. Without treatment 40% of infected women develop pelvic inflammatory disease (PID) which affects the fallopian tubes and causes damage to the ovaries (Delpiano et al. 1994). *Chlamydia trachomatis* have human as their only natural host primates may be susceptible to experimental infection (Orienston, 1998) . *Chlamydia trachomatis* causes about 40% non-gonococcal urethritis in men and occur concurrently with *Niesseria gonorrheae* in as many as 50% of the later in women. *Chlamydia trachomatis* causes muco-purulent cervicitis, urethritis, endometritis, salpingitis, perihepatitis and later post partum endometritis (Okoror, 2010). At least a third of infected females have no symptom (Orienston, 1998). Young children are particularly vulnerable to the infection. Transmission is usually by contact with formitis where it causes pharyngitis in children. Approximately 75% of neonates born by vaginal infected mothers become infected. The infection may remain latent for several months after birth (Schachter and Dawson, 1978). Less commonly infants born with caesarian sections may also be infected. The anatomic sites most commonly infected in infants are the conjunctiva which often manifest as purulent conjunctivitis and nasopharynx. Serious manifestation of post-natal chlamydial infection is pneumonia, which may range in severity. Reports have it that the male urethral and the female cervix serves as a reservoir for *Chlamydia trachomatis* (Chernesky et al. 1994) and that if symptoms are present in the lower urinogenital genital tract they are expressed as cervicitis or urethritis. A major involvement of *Chlamydia trachomatis* in urethritis was studied by Chernesky et al. (1994b) when they tested first void urine in both males and females in Canada using the Ligase Chain reaction of which 6% females and 18.4% males were positive to *Chlamydia trachomatis.*

Age groups	Total Tested		Number Positive (%)		Total Positive
	Male	Female	Male	Female	
10-15	10	15	2 (8)	6 (24)	8 (32)
16-21	72	108	49 (27.2)	69 (38.3)	118 (65.6)
22-27	56	99	52 (35.5)	54 (34.8)	106 (68.4)
28-33	49	71	33 (27.5)	40 (33.3)	73 (60.8)
34-39	40	71	23 (20.7)	40 (36)	63 (56.8)
40-45	42	66	25 (23.1)	37 (34.3)	62 (57.4)
46-51	32	59	20 (22)	26 (28.6)	46 (50.5)
52-57	29	42	19 (26.8)	24 (33.8)	43 (60.6)
58-63	36	38	22 (29.7)	23 (31.1)	45 (60.8)
64-69	29	40	18 (26.1)	19 (27.5)	37 (53.6)
Total	**395 (39.3)**	**609 (60.7)**	**263 (43.8)**	**338 (56.2)**	**601 (59)**

Table 1. Distribution of subjects tested for multiple infection (non-specific urethritis) with bacteria associated with UTI.

This study sought to establish the involvement of *Chlamydia trachomatis* in non-specific urethritis so as to make treatment of the disease easier and quicker by knowing the likely organisms that are involved in urethritis especially when multiple organisms are involved which might make treatment and management of disease more complex.

2. Materials and methods

2.1 Sample collection

Mid urine samples (1004) were collected from both male (467) and females (537) as well as urethral swabs were from males and endocervical and high vaginal swabs from females visiting various clinics for cases of urethritis. Blood samples were also collected from all the patients. The blood samples were aseptically collected into sterile vacutaniers, centrifuged at 3000 rpm (hetituch), sera separated, collected into sterile vials and stored at -20°C until used. The endocervical swab and the urethral swabs were collected into modified Ringer's solution as transport medium. Ringer's solution has been modified by the addition of calf serum and addition of vancomycin, streptomycin and nystatin. The samples were then transported to the laboratory. Clinical information of the patients sampled were collected which included pain during urination, penal and vaginal discharge, urethral and vaginal itching, foul vaginal smell and urethral irritation. Only those samples that gave a growth of more than one bacteria were further screened for *Chlamydia trachomatis.* Sample size was calculated using the online sample size calculator from sample survey network using the 2005 National Census figure available in the Nigerian Population Commission.

2.2 Procedure

The urine samples were immediately cultured onto, Nutrient agar, McConkey agar, Blood agar, Chocolate agar, Mannitol salt agar, Thayer Martins media and CLED agar plates (Oxoid). All the samples were cultured in duplicates and incubated both aerobically an anaerobically at 37°C (Gallenkamp, UK) for 24 hours. Bacterial count and identification were done according to the standard methods of *Bergey's manual* (1997), Harrigan and McCane (1976) and Cowan and Steel (1993). Endocervical swabs and urethral swabs were cultured into the yolk sac of chicken's embryonated eggs (Krivoshein 1998). The blood samples were analysed using the complement fixation test (Okoror, 2010) using the positive culture material from embryonated eggs as antigen. The antigen was then titetrated to the required concentration. The sheep red blood cells used was obtained by bleeding the jugular vein of a sheep and then washed in Alseveir's solution. The sheep red blood cells were stored at 4°C until used. Guinea pig serum was obtained by cardiac puncture of guinea pigs to obtain blood and the blood centrifuged to obtain the serum which was later mixed with required concentration of streptomycin and stored at 4°C until used as complements. Sheep red blood cells was used to vaccinate rabbit for at least two weeks, the blood of the rabbit was obtained by jugular vein, centrifuged and titerated to the required concentration and used as heamolytic serum. The swabs were emulsified in sterile phosphate buffered saline before inoculating into yolk sac of 7 days old chicken's embryonated eggs as described by Krivoshein (1998). The eggs were harvested after 10 days of incubation. The eggs were candled before and after incubation prior to harvesting. Upon harvesting a portion of the harvest materials were fixed with pure ethanol on a clean grease free slide, Romanoesky-Giemsa staining technique carried out and observed for species-specific inclusion bodies under the oil immersion objectives. Statistical analysis was done using the SPSS version 17 by carrying out the regression analysis using the total positive result as the dependent variable and other individual results (CCFA, Culture into chicken's embryonated eggs and monoclonal antibody tests) as the explanatory variable.

3. Results

Of the 1004 mid stream urine samples collected from patients with symptoms of urethritis in Nigeria and tested for bacteria involved in urethritis, only 601 were positive for multiple infections with UTI organisms. This included 56 samples positive for *Pseudomonas aeruginosa* and *Staphyloccocus aureus,* 129 positive for *Proteus mirabilis, Pseudomonas aeruginosa, Staph aureus* and *E. coli.* 97 were positive for *Klebsellia* sp and *Pseudomonas* sp, 21 for *Enteroccocus* sp and *Staph aureus,* 102 for *E. coli* and *Staph aureus* while 196 were positive for *E. coli, Staph aureus, Streptoccocus* sp and *Proteus* sp. From the 601 positive for different UTI organisms, 263 (43.8%) were males while 338 (56.2%) were females. Age group distribution shows that age group 16-21 had the highest number of individuals visiting hospitals for UTI cases which was followed by 22-27 with the highest number of individuals positive to non-specific urethritis (Table 1). A total of 395 (39.3%) males and 609 (60.7%) females visitied the hospitals for UTI. The 601 positive samples for non-specific urethritis were screened for *Chlamydia* complement fixing antibody (CCFA) with 205 (34.1%) positive for males and 278 (46.3%) positive for females. Distribution of CCFA according to age group (table 2) shows that age group 22-27 had the highest positive case which was closely followed by 16-21. More females had the CCFA (272) as compared to males (227). Females also had the highest positive individuals across the age groups with the exception of 22-27 age groups where more males had the CCFA.

Age groups	Number positive (%) Males	Females	Total
10-15	2	5	7
16-21	33	56	89
22-27	50	47	97
28-33	31	46	77
34-39	30	45	75
40-45	17	30	47
46-51	16	26	38
52-57	17	24	41
58-63	17	25	42
64-69	14	14	28
Total	**227**	**272**	**541**

Table 2. Distribution of samples positive to CCFA across the age groups.

Antibody titeration shows that 66% of the subjects positive to CCFA had antibody titre higher than 1:16. Age group 16-21 had the highest number of subjects with anti body titre higher than 1:16 Culture of samples into chicken's embryonated eggs shows that 499 of the total samples positive to CCFA were positive to *Chlamydia trachomatis* specific inclusion bodies with age groups 16-21 and 22-27 having the highest positive results. Also the result from the embryonated eggs culture was 31 less than those CCFA with antibody titre of 1:16 and above. Regression analysis showed that there was no significant (t=0.111, p=0.915, -18.797-20.587; CI=99%) difference between the result obtained by culture into chicken's embryonated eggs and CCFA as well as test using the monoclonal antibodies kits (CCFA t=1.176, p=0.284, -2.756-7.854; Culture t=2.410, p=0.053, -0.122-16.282; Monoclonal antibody t=-1.921, p=0.103, -21.415-2.576; CI=99%) however, the monoclonal antibody kits varied differently while culture into chicken's embryonated eggs and CCFA varied in the same direction (table 5). ANOVA reveal a significant difference within groups of all the positive results by comparing the sum of squares (F=35.17).

Age Groups	Antibody titre 1:8	1:16	1:32	1:64	1:128	1:256	1:512	1:1024	Total
10-15	-	2	2	2	1	-	-	-	7
16-21	20	20	13	11	9	10	6	-	69
22-27	31	19	42	-	-	-	5	-	66
28-33	11	29	17	5	5	5	-	5	66
34-39	21	18	13	3	10	5	5	-	54
40-45	5	5	10	11	13	1	-	2	42
46-51	3	8	8	5	5	4	4	1	35
52-57	21	9	10	10	-	-	-	-	30
58-63	5	32	3	-	1	1	-	-	37
64-69	3	3	3	1	6	6	6	-	25
Total	**120**	**145**	**121**	**48**	**50**	**32**	**26**	**9**	**431**

Table 3. Antibody titeration of sera positive to CCFA.

Age Groups		Test Performed	
	CFT	Culture	Monoclonal
10-15	7	6	7
16-21	89	80	82
22-27	97	89	91
28-33	77	66	69
34-39	75	67	71
40-45	47	47	47
46-51	38	38	38
52-57	41	38	39
58-63	42	40	40
64-69	28	28	28
Total		**499**	**501**

Table 4. Distribution of *Chlamydia* in different test performed (CFT, Culture and Monoclonal antibodies).

4. Discussion

Infection of the genital with *Chlamydia trachomatis* cannot be overemphasized. Reports have it that the organism has been involved in both female and male urinogenital infection with the females worse hit in both mild and chronic infections [Okoror et al 2008). *Chlamydia trachomatis* have also been reported to cause about 40% non-gonoccocal urethritis and occur concurrently with about 25% cases with *Niesseria gonorrheae* with sparse report of *Chlamydia trachomatis* in non-specific urethritis especially in developing countries where *Chlamydia trachomatis* is not currently been screened for in the day to day clinical diagnosis (Okoror, 2010). Reports also has it that relative frequency of *Chlamydia trachomatis* infections in developing countries is sparse and that infections could be higher than have been reported which is largely due to lack of diagnosis for *Chlamydia trachomatis* in developing countries which justifies this study. The lack of information on relative frequencies of *Chlamydia trachomatis* infection have let to lack of diagnosis in routine clinical diagnosis and therefore difficulty in treatment of *Chlamydia trachomatis* diseases like urethritis. This study is particularly concerned with the involvement of *Chlamydia trachomatis* in non-specific urethritis.

The lack of treatment of *Chlamydia trachomatis* infections may be the reason why there was a high positive result for *Chlamydia trachomatis* in this study (59.9%) which is similar to earlier reports but the percentage positivity was far higher than an earlier report by Chernesky et al. (1994) This could be because Chernesky et al. (1994) carried out their study in Canada a developed country with routine clinical diagnosis for *Chlamydia* as opposed to this study in Nigeria where there is no routine clinical diagnosis for *Chlamydia* and hence no opportunity for treatment of the infection except the infection has come up with serious sequelae. Other bacteria involved in UTI were identified in order to establish the fact that infection were actually caused by multiple organism. De Jongh et al. (2009) screened 253 males with urethritis using PCR for *Chlamydia trachomatis, Neisseria gonorrheae* and *Trichomonas vaginalis* where they reported 15% positive samples for *Chlamydia trachomatis* and 7.5% co-infection with *Neisseria gonorrheae* in South African males a result similar with the one observed in this study though with a higher positive result which is also a reflection of lack of screening for *Chlamydia trachomatis* and most probably because they screened only males. Complement fixation test though cumbersome and not very specific for *Chlamydia trachomatis* because of the group reactive antigen of *Chlamydia* spp still remains one of the most reliable serological tests (Okoror, 2010). However, the use of culture into embryonated eggs for examination of species-specific *Chlamydia* inclusion bodies helped to distinguish *Chlamydia trachomatis* form other *Chlamydia* spp that may have a cross-reaction with *Chlamydia trachomatis*. To further act as quality control, *Chlamydia trachomatis* monoclonal antibody spot test immunochromatographic kits were used to further enhance or validated the results confirmed with the culture into chicken's embryonated eggs especially to take care of human error while observing for *Chlamydia trachomatis* inclusion bodies. Reports also have it that a titre of ≤1:16 are diagnostic. Though convalescence sera might affect the result of CFT which is why a combination of other tests was involved in this study with the CFT being the primary test. The difference in the results from culture in chicken's embryonated eggs and that of complement fixation test as well as the spot test kit may be as a result of the fact that since CFT measures antibodies, infected individuals are detected even while still convalescing. Since both CFT and the spot test kit measure antibodies, there could be possibilities of an individual shedding the organism at convalescent stage without having the disease. The fact that CFT captures antibodies in convalescent stage of infection may be the reason while the culture result is lower than that of the CCFA, although the difference is insignificant (t=0.111, p=0.915, -18.797-20.587; CI=99%) (Table 6) statistically. The result from the monoclonal antibody test kit varies in the opposite direction as compared with that of the culture and CCFA is suggestive of the more sensitivity of the monoclonal antibody test kit and then justifies its use as confirmatory test. The significant difference within the age groups shows that though *Chlamydia trachomatis* UTI is more in the sexual active age of the adolescents and though the older ages may have the infection significantly, may have contacted the infection in their adolescent age since the organism is found of latent infection. Adults involved in indiscriminate sexual activities may also have contacted UTI which involved *Chlamydia trachomatis* which also accounts to why a high percentage of adults were positive to *Chlamydia trachomatis* UTI and also other organisms involved in non-specific urethritis.

Model			Mono	CFT	Culture
1	Correlations	Mono	1.000	-.823	-.907
		CFT	-.823	1.000	.508
		Culture	-.907	.508	1.000
	Covariances	Mono	24.033	-8.743	-14.912
		CFT	-8.743	4.700	3.695
		Culture	-14.912	3.695	11.235

[a]Dependent Variable: Total positive
Key: Mono=Monoclonal antibody test

Table 5. Coefficient correlations[a].

Age is a factor to UTI especially as it involves the early age groups with lesser number as well as lower percentage of individuals with UTI and also non-specific urethritis involving *Chlamydia trachomatis* as most individuals in this age group are not yet sexually active. The high percentage of females which is significantly different from those of their male counterparts both in the UTI generally, as well as multiple infection with *Chlamydia trachomatis* is not unconnected with the short urethral of the female genital organ which makes them more prone to UTI both in unhygienic environment as well as sexually as earlier reported. This study, however establish the fact that *Chlamydia trachomatis* is highly involved in UTI at the same time with other organisms. This makes treatment of UTI difficult especially in developing countries where *Chlamydia trachomatis* is not screened for in cases of UTI and hence the infection remains to lead to more serious sequelae.

	Unstandardized Coefficients		Standardized Coefficients	t	Sig.	95.0% Confidence Interval for B	
	B	Std. Error	P			Lower Bound	Upper Bound
(Constant)	.895	8.048		.111	.915	-18.797	20.587
CFT	2.549	2.168	2.245	1.176	.284	-2.756	7.854
Culture	8.080	3.352	6.228	2.410	.053	-.122	16.282
Mono	-9.420	4.902	-7.518	-1.921	.103	-21.415	2.576

Key: Mono=Monoclonal antibody test

Table 6. Statistical coefficients.

5. References

Agbonlahor DE, Okoror LE and Esumeh FI (2009) Seroepidemiological survey of *Chlamydia* in North West zone of Nigeria. *Asian-Pacific Journal of Tropical Medicine* 2(4) 58-63

Azenabor A.A., and Eghafona N.O (1997). Association of *Chlamydia trachomatis* antibodies with genital contact disease in women in Benin City, Nigeria. Tropical Medicine and International Health. ;2: 389-392.

Azenabor A, Kennedy P and Balistreri S (2007) *Chlamydia trachomatis* infection of human trophoblast alters estrogen and progesterome biosynthesis: an insight into the role of infection in pregnancy sequelae. *Int. J. Med. Sci.* 4 (4): 223-231

Baud D, Jaton K, Bertelli C, Kullin J and Greub G (2008) Low prevalence of *Chlamydia trachomatis* infection is asymptomatic young Swiss men. *BMC Infec Dis.* 8-45.

Bohnson, R.R. (1986). Urosepsis. *Urol. Clin. North Am.* 13: 627.

Cattell, W.R. (1985). Urinary tract infections in adults. *Postgrad. Med. J.* 61: 907 – 913.

Chernesky, MA, H Lee, J Schachter, JD. Burczak, WE. Stamm, WM McCormack, and TC Quinn. (1994). Diagnosis of *Chlamydia trachomatis* urethral infection in symptomatic and asymptomatic men by testing firstvoid urine in a ligase chain reaction assay. *J. Infect. Dis.* 170:1308–1311.

Chernesky, MA, D Jang, H Lee, J D Burczak, H Hu, J Sellors, SJ Tomazic-Allen, and JB Mahony, (1994). Diagnosis of *Chlamydia trachomatis* infections in men and women by testing first-void urine by ligase chain reaction. *J. Clin. Microbiol.* 32:2682–2685.

Cheesbrough, M. (2000). Biochemical tests to identify bacteria. In: *District Laboratory Practice in Tropical Countries*, Part 2. Cambridge University Press, Cambridge, UK; Pp 63 – 70.

Cowan, S.T. (1993). *Cowan and Steel's Manual for the Identification of Medical Bacteria*. Burrow, G.I. and Feltham, R.K.A. (eds.), 3rd edition. Cambridge University Press, Cambridge, UK; 331pp.

De Jongh M, M Le Roux, A. Adam, A.M. Caliendo and A.A. Hoosen (2009) Co-Infection with *Neisseria gonorrhoeae, Chlamydia trachomatis* and*Trichomonas vaginalis* in Symptomatic South African Men with Urethritis: Implications for Syndromic Management. *The Open Tropical Medicine Journal* 2, 13-16.

Del piano M, Magliano EM, Latino MA, Nicosia R, Pustorine R, Sanitino I, Gordini C, Clerici P, Colombo R and Sessa R. (1994) Epidemiology of urinogenital infection caused by *Chlamydia trachomatis* and outline characteristic features of the patients at risk. *J. of Med. Microbiol.* 41: 168-172.

Eke, P.I and Rotimi, V.O (1987). Resistance of Pathogenic Bacteria to antibiotics, *Afr. J. Med. Sci*. 16: 1 - 8.

Grayston JT, Campbell LA and Kuo CC. (1990) A new respiratory tract pathogen: *Chlamydia pneumoniae* strain TWAR K. *Infect. Dis.* 161: 618-625.

Grayston JT. (1992) Infections caused by *Chlamydia pneumoniae* strain TWAR. *Clin. Infect. Dis.* 15: 757-763.

Gupta K, Scholes D, Stamm W.E (1999). Increasing prevalence of antimicrobial resistance among uropathogens causing acute uncomplicated cystitis in women. *JAMA* 281: 736 - 738.

Gupta K, (2001). Antimicrobial resistance among uropathogens that cause community-acquired urinary tract infection in women: a nationwide analysis *Clin. Infect. Dis.* 33: 89 - 94.

Harrigan, W.F. and McCane, M.E. (1976). *Laboratory Methods in Microbiology*. Academic Press, New York; 553pp.

Hannan, M.M. Cormican and Flynn, J. (1993). A comparison of antimicrobial sensitivities of urinary pathogens for the years 1980 and 1990. *Ir. J. Med. Sci*, 162: 499 - 501.

Hooton, T.M. and Stamm W.E. (1997). Diagnosis and treatment of uncomplicated urinary tract infections. *Infect. Dis. Clin. North. Am.* 11: 551 - 581.

Johnson J, B Neas, DE Parker, JD Forteberry and LD Cowan. (1994) Screening for urethral infection in adolescent and young adult males. .*J. Adolesc. Health* 1994. 14: 233-237.

Johnson, J.R., Tiu, F.S. and Stamm, W.E. (1995). Direct antimicrobial susceptibility testing for acute urinary tract infections in women *J. Clin. Microbiol.* 33: 2316 - 2323.

Kahlmeter G. (2001). The ECO* SENS project: A prospective, multinational, multicentre epidemiology survey of the prevalence and antimicrobial susceptibility of urinary tract pathogens - interim report. *J. Antimicrob. Chemother.* 46 (suppl. A): 15 - 22.

Karvonen M, Tuonilento J, Naukkarinem A, Saikku P (1992). The regional distribution of antibodies against *Chlamydia pneumoniae* (strain TWAR) in Finland in 1958. *Intern. J. of epidemiol.* 21: 391-397.

Koh, W.P., Taylor, M.B., Hughes, K., Chew, S.K., Fong, C.W., Phoon, M.C., Kang, K.I. and Chow, V.T. (2002): Seroprevalence of *Chlamydia pneumoniae* in Chinese Malays, and Asian Indians in Singapore. *Int. J. Epidemiology. 31*(95): 1001-1007.

Krivoshein YS (1989). *Handbook on Microbiology Laboratory Diagnosis of Infectious Diseases.* 319pp. Mir publishers Moscow.

Lin JS, WE Jones, L Yan, KA Wirthwein, EE Flaherty, RM Haivanis and PA Rice (1992). Under diagnosis of *Chlamydia trachomatis* infection. Diagnostic limitations in patients with low level infection. *Sex. Transm. Dis.* 259-265.

Macleod J., Edward, C. and Bouchier, I., (1984). *Principles and Practice of Medicine.* 15th edition. English Language Book Society/Churchill Livingstone, London. Pp 382 - 395.

Macauley M.E., Riordan T., James J.M., Laventhall P.A., Morris E.M., Neal B.R, et al. (1990) A prospective study of genital infections in a family planning clinic. *Epidemiol. Infect.* 104: 55-61.

McPhee S.J. and Harrington W (1987) Psittacosis. *West Afri J Med;* 196: 285-309.

Miyuashita, N., Y. Kanamoto and A. Matsumoto (1993). The morphology of Chlamydia Pseumoniae *J.Med. Microbiol* 38:418 – 425.

Okoror LE, SA Omilabu, PO Orhue and G Ajayi. (2008)Seroepidemiological survey of *Chlamydia trachomatis* in patients attending pre and post natal clinics in Lagos Nigeria. *The open trop. Med. J.* 1: 83-86.

Okoror LE, Agbonlahor DE, Esumeh FI and Umolu PI. (2007)Prevalence of *Chlamydia* in patients attending gynaecological clinics in south eastern Nigeria. *Afri. Health sci.* 7 (1):18-24.

Okoror LE (2010) Geograpical/Season distribution and characterization of *Chlamydia* in Nigeria. . VDM publishers Germany. ISBN 978-3-639-24237-9, 198pp

Orienston E (1998) Chlamydiae. In: Medical Microbiology 21st ed USA: Appleton and Lange Publishers. 310-318

Peeling, R.W., Bailey, R.L., Conway, D.J., Holland, A.E.C., Ousman J., Hilton, C.W. and David, C.W.M.

(1998):Antibody resistance to the 60KDA Chlamydia heat shocked protein is as associated with scaring trachoma.

Journal of infectious diseases 177:256-9.

Prescott, L.M., Harley, J.P. and Aklein, D.(1999): Human diseases caused by other bacteria (Chlamydia, Mycoplasma, Rickettsia), Dental and nosocomial infections. In: *Microbiology.* 4th edn. WBC/Mc-graw hill companies USA.8002.

Reld, G. and Spied, J.D. (1987). "Bacterial adherences in pathogenesis of urinary tract infection" *Rev. Infect Dis.* 9: 490.

Rubin, R.H., Tolkoff, R.N.E. and Contran, R.S. (1986). Urinary tract infections: pyelonephritis and reflux nephropathy. *Pediatrics;* 83: 1085 - 1141.

Schroeder, S.A., Krupp, J.A., Tierney, L.M. and Mephee, S.J. (1990). *Current Medical Diagnosis and Treatment.* Appleton and Lange, New York, Pp 622 - 628.

Strickland, T.G. (1994) Trachoma. In: *Hunters tropical Medicine.* 7th Ed. 1001 1003.

Thylefers, B., Dawson, C.R. and Jones B.R.(1987): A simple system for the assessment of trachoma and its complications. *Bull WHO* 65, 485.

Wiswell, T.E. and Smith, F.R. (1985). Decreased incidence of urinary tract infections *Paediatrics* 75: 901 - 903.

Zhang, J.P. and Stephens, R.S. (1992): Mechanism of *Chlamydia trachomatis* attachment to host cell. *Cell 69*: 861.

6

Catheters and Infections

S. Siracusano, S. Ciciliato, G. Ollandini and F. Visalli
Department of Urology – Trieste University
Italy

1. Introduction

Catheters are used for effective drainage of the bladder, either temporally or permanently, in the presence of physiological and anatomical defects or obstruction of the lower urinary tract. Catheters are used for a variety of reasons, as follows, to maintain bladder drainage during and following surgery or epidurals anesthesia for minimizing and prevention of the risk of distension injuries; investigations, for accurate urine output measurement, and measurement of post-micturition residuals; treatments, to relieve urinary retention or for chemotherapy instillation; intractable incontinence, as the final option for containment.

2. Urethral catheterization

Urethral catheterization is a routine medical procedure that allows direct drainage of the urinary bladder into an attached bag or container. It consists in the insertion of a catheter into a patient's bladder.

Urinary catheterization is employed in hospital and nursing home settings to maintain urine output in patients who are undergoing surgery, or who are confined to the bed and physically unable to use a bedpan. Critically ill patients who require strict monitoring of the urinary output are also frequently catheterized. Urethral catheterization may be performed as either a therapeutic or a diagnostic procedure. Therapeutically, catheters may be placed to decompress the bladder in patients with acute or chronic urinary retention. In addition, catheters may be placed to facilitate bladder irrigation in patients with gross hematuria. Diagnostically, urinary catheters may be placed to obtain an uncontaminated urine sample for microbiologic testing, to measure urinary output in critically ill patients or during surgical procedures, or to measure post-void residuals. The only absolute contraindication to urethral catheterization is known or suspected urethral injury, usually in the setting of a pelvic fracture.

Surely these interventions were performed already long time before recorded history. Although in the most ancient medical writings, such the code of Hammurabi -1700 B.C.- (1), there is no clear mention of catheterism, the condition of urinary retention is well described in an ancient Chinese medical text, the Huang Ti Nei Chingh Su Wen (mentioned in the Annals of the Former Han Dinasty- 206 B.C. to 25 A.C., but referred to a much earlier origin). It is a sort of dialogue where the emperor (Huang Ti) poses questions to a minister, whose answers convey a clear sense of organ-based pathology: "(…) When the bladder does not function efficiently, it causes retention of urine; when it functions without restraint, it causes copious urination" (2). If urinary retention was so specifically identified and described, it is likely that it was treated with catheterization: the technology was available. For instance, hollow leaves of Allium Fistolosum, an onion plant, coated with laquer, were used as catheters in China around 100 B.C (3). The Sushruta Samhita, an early Indian surgical text dated approximately around 1000 B.C: describes tubes of gold, silver, iron and wood smeared with ghee (liquid butter) for evacuation of urine, management of strictures, instillation of medication and for assistance in lithotomy. Sushruta suggest also that "wine should be used before operation to produce insensibility to pain" (4).

Urethral catheterization is then always well described among the medical writings of the first millennium and the Renaissance, even if it was not even mentioned by one of the most famous scientists ever, Leonardo da Vinci. During this period the main factor driving the need for diagnostic and therapeutic catheterization was the bladder stone. Even Benjamin Franklin, in a letter written on December 8th, 1752, described a flexible silver catheter he designed for his older brother John, who suffered from bladder stone. This device was made from a flat silver wire, wound spirally and then covered with waxed threadbound parchment (5). In 1756 Heuermann provided a good description of catheter therapy for benign prostatic hypertrophy, and during the next 150 years, according to Laurisden, this method was "absolutely Paramount" (6).

Industrialization brought about the manufacturing ability to make better surgical instruments as well as the scientific means to fit the tool to the task: the configuration of the catheter was investigated by anatomical studies, and the designs of past millennia were for the most part found appropriate. The Goodyear patent for moldable hard rubber in 1851 permitted faster and cheaper production of catheters: Auguste Nelaton, physician to Napoleon III, introduced a flexible rubber catheter in 1860 (7). Mercier the coudé catheter in 1836 and the bicoudé in approximately 1841, with one or two bends near the tip respectively. By the late 19th century a wide armamentarium of catheters was available to the practitioner. George Tiemann's catalogue of surgical instruments listed nearly 80 different types of catheters. Special types were used for various purposes in cases of urethral strictures, stones or foreign bodies, and for evacuation of urinary retention, irrigating and distending the bladder (8). The development of the balloon catheter has been documented by Zorgniotti, who traced it back to Reybard's device in 1853. Foley (1891 to 1966), an ingenious American urologist, devised a balloon catheter for haemostatis in prostatic surgery (9). He demonstrated the first production model at the annual meeting of the AUA in 1935. Although a different company (the Davol Rubber Company) retained the rights to the balloon catheter after applying a key patent five months later, the "Foley" name has become universally synonymous of self-retaining balloon catheter.

By these times, lacking the scientific justification of the germ theory, medical practitioners, except for a few ones, had little interest in cleanliness around wounds. Joseph Lister experimented with urine putrefaction, and found out that was normally sterile and had an uncanny sense of host resistance (10). After his studies and the similar ones performed by Roberts, clean techniques and antiseptic principles became standard practice, and urethral catheterization thereby achieved another degree of safety (11).

3. Diagnostic uses

Bladder catheterization facilitates obtaining a specimen for urinalysis or culture (e.g. in children), measuring post-void residual volume, and undertaking more extensive urodynamic studies to diagnose causes of urinary incontinence. Radiographic contrast may be instilled through a catheter to visualize bladder or urethral pathology, and document vesicoureteric reflux. The bladder may be distended with a saline solution to form a sonoluscent structure, prior to a pelvic ultrasound.

4. Short-term (0-2 weeks) or intermediate term (2-6 weeks) therapeutic uses

Indwelling catheters are used during labor following epidural anesthesia, and in the fluid management and tocolysis of patients with pre-eclampsia and eclampsia. An empty bladder facilitates pelvic dissection in patients undergoing hip and abdominopelvic surgical procedures. Moreover urethral catheterization enables measurement of intra- and post-operative urine output and eases post-procedure patient care. Intermittent or short-term catheterization may be helpful in treating bladder neoplasms (Cytotoxic drugs and BCG may be administered intravesically), and mycotic infections (Amphotericin in fungal cystitis).

Surely the primary care of any patient with acute urinary retention (that may arise from a variety of causes) is urethral catheterization: temporary decompression of the bladder through an indwelling catheter may be necessary until resolution of the primary cause of the retention.

Short term or intermittent catheterization may be required following urethropexy or a sling procedure for bladder neck obstruction, when swelling and pain may cause retention. Other organic causes of obstructed voiding in women (neoplastic, inflammatory) may also be managed with clean intermittent or indwelling catheter drainage until the underlying condition is treated. Incomplete pelvic floor relaxation with resulting dysfunctional voiding may also be treated with catheterization.

Gluteal, sacral or trochanteric skin trauma or decubitus ulcers contaminated by urine in an incontinent patient will respond to temporary urinary diversion through catheterization to maintain a moist and infection-free environment.11

5. Long-term therapeutic uses (> 6 weeks)

In selected cases of urinary incontinence not responding to conservative treatments Clean Intermittent Catheterization (CIC) may be carried out. This will maintain mobility and renal function, and minimize residual urine, infectious complications and calculus disease. In this setting another application of CIC is represented by the presence of a poorly contractile bladder that is usually unresponsive to behavioral or pharmacologic therapy. Surgery is generally not indicated for men with this condition, and in most cases, patients are required to perform CIC.

During the last ten years CIC has become the standard care in patients with spinal cord injuries. Continuous or intermittent catheterization should be established immediately in a hypotonic bladder to prevent over-distention, infection and detrusor muscle damage. Spastic bladder following spinal injury may require condom catheter or long-term suprapubic drainage. In these cases CIC or continuous bladder drainage may also be helpful for incontinent patients, immobile subjects due to aging or finally in cases of terminal illness. However, continuous drainage should be used rarely, and only as a last resort.

6. Catheter characteristics

Urethral catheterization is the most frequent retrograde manipulation performed on the urinary tract. Catheters are placed to drain the bladder during and after surgical procedures, to assess urinary output in critically ill patients, to collect reliable urine specimen and to assess post voiding residual urine. Such catheters can be left indwelling with a self-retaining balloon or used for clean intermittent catheterization procedure.

The choice of a specific type of catheter depends upon the reasoning of catheterization. Large-caliber catheters are used to evacuate potential blood clots or to assess urinary output. Other catheter variables include balloon size and construction materials. In this way large balloons can be inflated to help hemostasis after transurethral resection of the prostate or in case of open prostatectomy. Sometimes the standard latex catheter can result in severe reactions in patients with latex allergies and silicone varieties are good alternatives in such situations. In particular the silicone catheters are usually manufactured with several grooves placed on the surface of catheter itself to allow an interface between the catheters and the urethra and thus avoiding the possibility of infection in the short term (1). Therefore the catheters can be distinguished by the shape of the tip, the characteristics, the diameter, the number of ways and the materials.

Straight rubber or latex catheters often referred to as Robinson catheters, are straight catheters used for short-term catheterization, as in measurement of residual urine and instillation of medication chemotherapeutic agents or in case of radiological evaluation of the bladder. The tip of the Robinson catheter is rounded, with one or two drainage ports along the side. Self-retaining catheters like the Pezzer and Malecot catheters, are shaped in such a way that after placement at open surgery the catheter configuration maintains the catheter within a hollow viscus (Fig.1a). The advantage of these catheters include the excellent urinary drainage and the tip design, which make them ideal for use as cystostomy or nefrostomy tubes. Foley-types catheters are most often used for long-term urethral catheterization.

The catheters are often named according to the characteristics of the proximal tip as follows:

1. The Nelaton catheter is the standard catheter and has a rounded and straight proximal end. It has two lateral eyes for drainage (Fig.1b).
2. The Mercier catheter has a rounded and angular (30-45°) tip. The angle helps the introduction of the catheter in the membranous or prostatic urethra (Fig.1c).
3. The Tiemann catheter can have a cone shaped tip, which can be straight (olive-tip catheter) or angular (Fig.1d).
4. Couvelaire catheter is used in case of bladder hemorrhage or after a urologic surgical intervention because it guarantees an efficient drainage. The structure can be rigid or semi-rigid and it has one drainage eye at the end and two lateral eyes (Fig.1e).
5. Dufour catheter (semi-rigid, self-retaining) has three ways. The tip has a 30° curve, is open and with two staggered drainage eyes. It is used in case of gross haematuria (Fig.1f).

External diameter is sized by Charrièr (1CH=1/3mm). The size of the catheter is selected according to specific clinical use. The length of catheter is usually 420mm for male, 260mm for female and a shorter for pediatric patients. In clinical use the size of the catheter should guarantee a safe urine drainage without damaging the urethral mucosa and avoiding infections, stricture or scarring causing stenosis. The use of smaller than 14Ch is recommended in contrast with large catheter that increases the risk of blockage of paraurethral glands causing urethritis or other ascending infection. Silicon or silicon-coated catheters produce less tissue reaction and less encrustation than rubber catheters(2). They also have a larger lumen diameter than catheters made of rubber and thus are preferred by some for long-term indwelling catheterization.

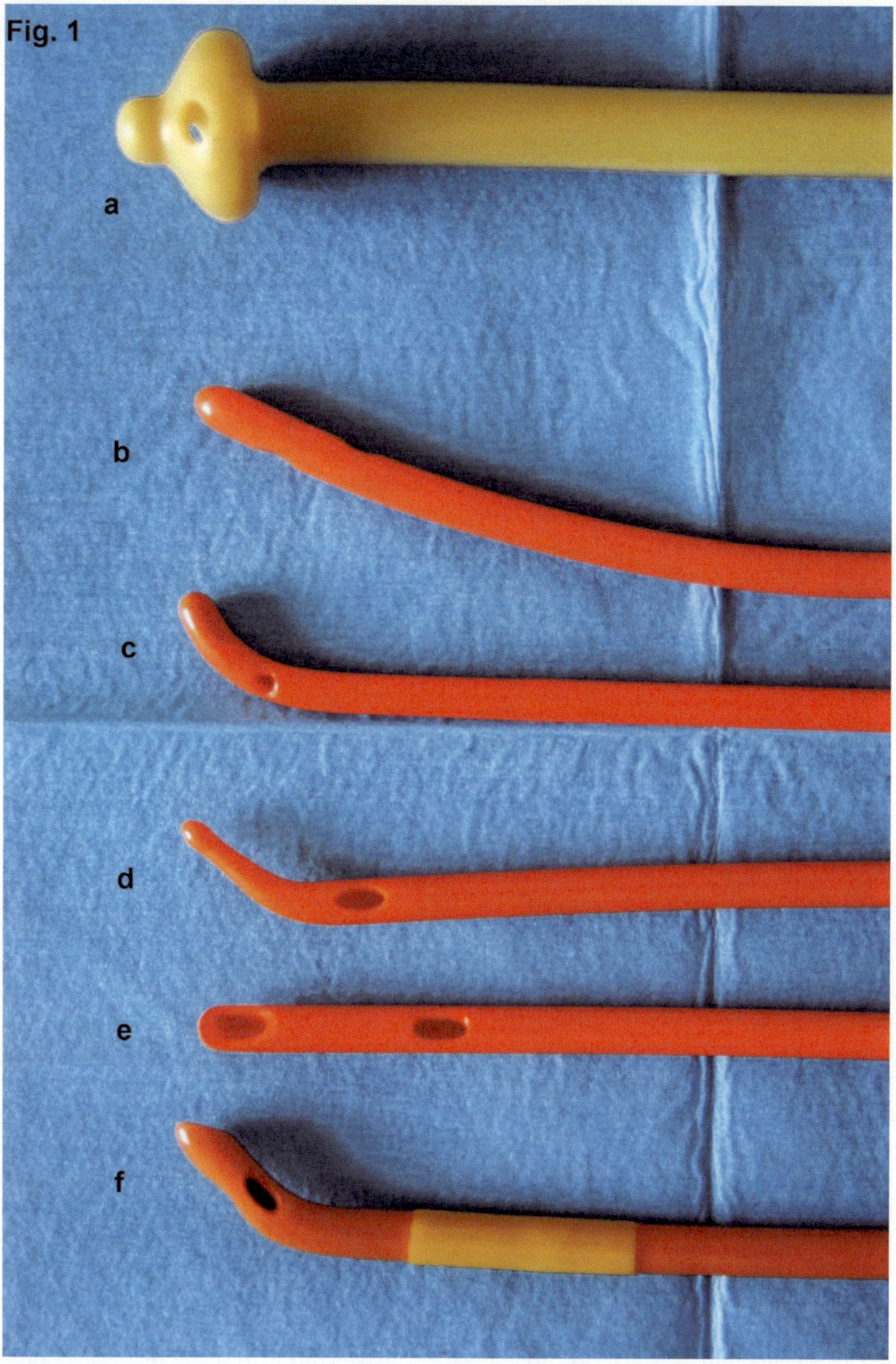

Fig. 1. Types of urinary catheters : a) Pezzer self-retaining catheter; b) Nelaton catheter; c) Mercier catheter; d) Tiemann catheter; e) Couvelaire catheter; f) Dufour catheter.

Catheters can have one, two or three ways. In two ways catheters, one way provides urine drainage, the other way which is provided with a valve allows the inflation of a balloon that is inserted in the bladder to keep the catheter securely in place. Three-way catheters have a small lumen inflating the balloon mechanism, a lumen for instilling irrigant and a larger lumen for bladder drainage. Silicone, PVC and latex are the most used materials to produce catheters. Latex and PVC are mostly used for short-term catheters or in intermittent catheterization. Silicone is more used for long-term catheters because it is considered to be biocompatible and it is recommended for patients who are allergic to latex. Different catheter surfaces, such as latex, silicone, or Teflon, have not been shown to alter the frequency of urinary infection. Silicone catheters may be less likely to become blocked by encrustations due to prolonged use (3,4). In this way it seems to be evident that the use of silicone catheters are less prone to infections. Thus, silicone catheters, which tend to be more expensive, should be reserved for residents shown to have a consistent problem with repeated catheter obstruction. In this context P aeruginosa had a higher rate of adherence to Teflon or silicon catheters than other gram-negative species. (5) Conflicting results describing the effectiveness of antimicrobial-coated catheters, including silver-coated catheters, in preventing infection for short-term catheters have been reported. These materials are likely to be less effective for long-term catheters, because duration of catheter use is such an overwhelming determinant for infection. Catheters available today have a roughly engineered surface that is extremely vulnerable to blockage by crystalline biofilms and therefore we hope that in the future new biomaterials, which limit biofilm formation, will be developed.

7. Urethral catheter and related infections

7.1 Epidemiology

The catheterization is widely used to relieve anatomic or physiologic obstructions, to provide a dry environment for comatose or incontinent patients, and to permit the accurate measurement of urine output in severely ill patients. Unfortunately, when catheters are used inappropriately or when left in place too long they increase the risk of asymptomatic bacteriuria and urinary tract infection (UTI). The catheter-associated urinary infections (CAUTIs) have been reported to increase mortality and have a considerable economic impact. For these reasons catheter should be removed as soon as possible in order to prevent the risk of infection. Urinary tract infections account for 20 to 40% of hospital-associated infections, and an estimated 80% are associated with urinary catheter. The majority of studies say that 10 to 30% of people who are catheterized for a short period develop bacteriuria (often asymptomatic) and that after 30 days of catheterization bacteria can be found in the urine of all patients. The infections provoked by the use of a short-term catheter may prolong hospitalization by 2.4 to 4.5 days, and are likely to be associated to an increase in nosocomial mortality. Asymptomatic bacteriuria converts to symptomatic in approximately 24% of patients(7). Long-term urinary catheters are a leading cause of morbidity in acute care settings, accounting for up to 40% of hospital-associated infections (8,9). Within the hospital environment, the intensive care unit has the highest prevalence of nosocomial infections with estimated rates of 8–21% for nosocomial UTI of which 95% are catheter-associated(10). The daily incidence of bacteriuria in catheterized patients is approximately 3–10%. Among patients with bacteriuria, up to 25% will develop symptoms of local UTI, and about 3% will develop bacteremia (11). Catheter-associated UTI is the second most common cause of nosocomial bloodstream infection. Patients who develop nosocomial UTI have their hospital stay extended by approximately 3 days and are nearly three times more likely to die during hospitalization than patients without such an infection. The case-fatality rate from UTI-associated bacteremia is approximately 13% within severely ill patients at highest risk (12,13).

It Deserves a mention the CIC has emerged as the most practical to ménage urinary emptying dysfunction and reduces significant lower urinary tract infection. CIC has been effective in managing patients with spinal cord injury, diabetes, multiple sclerosis, outlet obstruction and continent urinary diversion. This management technique is not without complications, including urethral trauma, increased urinary infection, stone disease and even progression of the upper urinary tract deterioration that the management technique is attempting to prevent. A controversy has surrounded the concept of CIC vs. sterile technique from the beginning of its use. Regarding bacteriology and urinary tract infections and even for CIC most authors conclude that in the still existing light of many controversies in bacteriology and management of infections, CIC is an acceptable way of voiding a neuropathic bladder, enabling a voluntarily induced balanced micturition within a shorter period of bladder training, having less aggressive urinary tract infections by reducing the residual urine volume and last but not least assisting continence and avoiding unaesthetic leg-bags, aggressive indwelling catheters or irritating external urine collecting devices such as diapers. In his publication Kuhn observe that after CIC, in 13 out of 46 patients (28%) the type of bacteria in the urine did not change from that of the first bacteriological control. Antibiotic prophylaxis is probably ineffective in preventing symptomatic urinary tract infections. Recent Cochrane library reviews conclude that the current strength of evidence is weak and well-designed studies are strongly recommended. Based on the current evidence, it is not possible to state that any catheter type, technique or strategy of self-catheterization is better than another in prevention of infections. The sterile versus clean technique question is of relatively low importance because in community settings (where most IC takes place) a sterile technique is not practical. In hospital settings rising concerns about infection control indicate that a sterile technique would be needed for safety (14,15) In any case intermittent catheterization is a commonly recommended procedure for people with incomplete bladder emptying not satisfactorily managed by other methods.

7.2 Pathogenesis

Indwelling urinary catheters are used for short-term (<14 days mainly in hospitals) and long-term (>30 days mainly in nursing homes and home care) urinary drainage (16). Short-term catheterization usually results in bacteriuria that rapidly clears after removal of the catheter, especially with antibiotic therapy. Symptomatic urinary infection or febrile episodes are more commonly associated with long-term catheterization. An indwelling catheter impairs normal host defenses both by promoting increased access of microorganisms to the bladder and by compromising complete voiding. Generally, infection is introduced via two routes after catheterization: the intraluminal route via the inside lumen of the catheter, or the trans-urethral route between the catheter and the urethra. The infections that arise with catheterization are caused by bacteria from patient's body or colonic flora and by bacteria found in the hospital setting. Bacteria can invade the lower urinary tract along the surface of the catheter or by its lumen. Bacteriuria that occurs during short-term catheterization is usually caused by a single organism. The most commonly isolated pathogen its *Escherichia-coli* and *enterococci, pseudomonas, enterobacter, staphylococcus aureus* or *epidermidis, klebsiella* and *serratia.* In the long-term catheterization common urophatogens include *Escherichia-coli, Pseudomonas aeruginosa* and *proteus mirabilis(17,18).* Many of these pathogens develop a multiple antibiotic resistance and they could adhere to the catheter surface, in these case the catheter becomes a reservoir for the pathogens. The reason why bacteria migrate through the catheter into the bladder without being expelled by the urine is still not clear. Urine has a cleaning action that protects the bladder from backwards invasion of skin pathogens, which is why healthy subjects do not get an infection if bacteria is injected in the bladder. Most probably the reason why bacteria are not expelled in UTIs associated with catheterization is the adhesion of bacteria to the bladder urothelium. Epithelial cells in the bladder usually are coated with Lactobacillus that are not invasive nor virulent but can prevent virulent organisms from sticking to the bladder wall (19). When the coat of the cells is missing, colonization of bacteria and infections of the lower urinary tract begin. The mechanism is therefore strictly related to the adhesion of bacteria to the bladder during catheterization. Analysis with electron microscope of the surface of catheters show that indwelling catheters are rapidly colonized by a thick layer of microorganisms included in a protein matrix of the host, and by polysaccharides produced by bacteria that form a biofilm (20).

The risk of urinary tract infection is related to the length of time that the catheter is in place. Most patients catheterized for a week or less should escape infection, but for the elderly and disabled patients who are catheterized for several months or years, bacteriuria is inevitable (21). Risk factors other than the duration of catheterization include contamination of the drainage-bag, diabetes mellitus, female patient, antibiotic usage and a compromised status of renal function. The risk of CAUTIs is increased in patients who are in urinary retention, in patients catheterized peripartum, in debilitated patients (22). In this case organisms that colonize the periurethral skin can migrate into the bladder through the mucoid film that forms between the epithelial surface of the urethra and the catheter. In addition, contamination of the urine in the drainage bag can allow organisms to access the bladder through the drainage tube and the catheter lumen (23). The initial bacteria that cause the urinary tract infections are usually *Staphylococcus epidermidis, Escherichia coli* or *Enterococcus faecalis.* As time goes by, other species appear in the residual bladder urine, including *Pseudomonas aeruginosa, Proteus mirabilis, Providencia stuartii, Morganella morganii* and *Klebsiella pneumoniae.*(8,23). Biofilms containing 5 × 109 viable cells per centimeter can be found on long-term indwelling catheters removed from patients.(20) The biofilm populations, therefore are often outnumber than those in the urine. The most common species present in the mixed-population biofilms are *E. faecalis, P. aeruginosa, E. coli, and P. mirabilis.* The biofilms formed are generally sparse, and because the catheter is removed within a few days, they cause few problems. By contrast, long-term catheters become colonized by extensive biofilms, which can have profound effects on the health of the patient. By far the most troublesome biofilms are those that become crystalline in nature (24,25). These biofilms may be present on the outer surface of the catheter around the balloon and catheter tip, and can cause trauma to the bladder and urethral epithelia. The crystalline deposits on catheters have a similar composition to infection-induced kidney and bladder stones. Struvite (magnesium ammonium phosphate) and a poorly crystalline form of apatite (a hydroxylated calcium phosphate, in which a variable proportion of the phosphate groups are replaced by carbonate) are the principle crystalline components (23,26). Urease is the driving force of crystallization: it hydrolyzes urea, leading to the formation of ammonium and carbonate ions and an increase in urinary pH. As the urine becomes alkaline, magnesium and calcium phosphate crystals are precipitated. Aggregates of this crystalline material accumulate in the urine and in the biofilm that develops on the catheter surfaces. The continued accumulation of crystalline bacterial biofilm blocks the flow of urine through the catheter (2) causing bladder over-distension and damaging the urothelium aiding the attachment of bacteria to epithelial surface. *P. mirabilis* is not usually a pioneer colonizer of the catheterized urinary tract, and is not commonly found in patients undergoing short-term catheterization(26). *P. mirabilis* is considered to be an ingenious organism capable of initiating crystalline biofilms. Microorganisms that grow in biofilm are less likely to respond to antibiotic treatments. The majority of catheters removed within the seventh day of catheterization are already colonized by a bacterial biofilm. The presence of a urinary catheter impairs the normal protective mechanisms of the bladder. The duration of catheterization is the important factor of bacteriuria (27) but important risk factors are also the microbial colonization of the periurethral area and perineum providing a route for bacterial entry along both the internal and the external surfaces. In addition, urine often pools in the bladder or in the catheter itself and urinary stasis encourages bacterial multiplication.

8. Fungal urinary tract infections

Fungal urinary tract infections (funguria) are rare in community medicine, but common in hospitals where 10 to 30% of urine cultures isolate Candida species Funguria, or candiduria, may develop as early as the first 2 weeks of hospitalization. An indwelling urinary catheter is a known risk factor for funguria. Candida albicans is the most commonly isolated fungal species (40–65%) from the urine, but other species such as Candida glabrata and Candida tropicalis, also may occur. Candida as well as staphylococci can reach the hub site via the hands of health personal (26) . Non-pharmacologic measures, such as removing unnecessary antibiotics, and removing the urinary catheter, are typically beneficial but generally inadequate without additional pharmacologic therapy. The most serious complication of untreated asymptomatic funguria is candidemia, which occurs in less than 10% of cases. (28).

8.1 Diagnosis

Patients with CAUTIs are usually asymptomatic. The presence of bacteria in the urine does trigger an inflammatory response in terms of pyuria and urinary interleukins. The most common presentation of symptomatic infection is fever often associated with haematuria. Symptomatic bacteriuria is characterized by the presence of dysuria, urgency, frequency and hematuria (28). Symptomatic UTI occurs when bacteriuria leads to either local symptoms of infection, or systemic symptoms. Urinary catheter-related bacteremia is diagnosed when the same organism is isolated from both the urine and the blood cultures in the absence of other likely sources of infection. The risk of asymptomatic bacteriuria to bacteremia conversion is approximately 3–4%, and the estimated attributable mortality of urinary tract-related bacteremia is approximately 13%. Catheter associated UTI is diagnosed at a lower level of bacteriuria (>102 or >103 CFU/ml) for asymptomatic infections, plus associated symptoms for the symptomatic infections (29,30). The wide spectrum of potential infecting organism and increased likelihood of resistance means microbiological confirmation of the infecting organism and susceptibility testing are essential for determining optimal therapy. A positive urine culture supports a diagnosis of UTI but it is not sufficient to distinguish symptomatic from asymptomatic infection. Thus, urine culture result must always be interpreted in the clinical context. In patients with short term indwelling catheter the specimen should be obtained by sampling through the catheter port. In patients with chronic indwelling catheter the preferred specimen is obtained from a new catheter placed immediately prior to initiating antimicrobial therapy (26). The urine specimen obtained through the new placed catheter reflects the bacteriology of the urine, rather than the biofilm.

9. Prevention and treatment of catheter-associated urinary infections

Prevention of UTI is therefore one of the most important tools in the treatment of catheterized subjects. The procedure of catheterization has to be done in order to avoid contamination of the intra or extra lumen drainage system. In accordance with the 2009 guidelines of the English Department of Health to prevent urinary tract infections in catheterized subjects, it is well know that closed drainage is infection free for the first 15 days and that after this period bacteria begin to spread in the bladder. In this context it seems that there are no differences in the infection rate between short-term sterile and short-term clean catheterization techniques based on recent literature reviews(31,32). The first review compared sterile catheterization with clean catheterization. No difference was shown between the two groups of patients, even if the sample was too limited to show any possible differences. The second review based on 436 women in labor compared genital cleaning before catheterization using chlorhexidine with the one using tap water alone showing also in this case no significant differences. The conclusion was that antiseptics do not reduce the bacteriuria rate. On the contrary open catheter drainage systems lead to bacteriuria in virtually all patients in few days, and this system is not recommended. (Grade of recommendation: A)(33).

Since as biofilm is the central factor in the pathogenesis of CAUTI, strategies designed to prevent biofilm formation with novel catheter material or coating are currently being investigated as shown in randomized trials reporting antimicrobial-impregnated catheters containing either nitrofurazone (34) or the combination of the broad-spectrum antibiotics minocycline and rifampin (35). This report demonstrated significant reductions in bacterial CAUTIs even if these results need further confirmations. In this way the advantage from the use of coated urinary catheters is not clear. In fact clinical trials have shown conflicting results as to the efficacy of silver oxide-coated catheters compared with uncoated catheters. In a prospective clinical trial involving hospitalized patients, silver oxide-coated catheters reduced the incidence of UTI only among women without antimicrobial agents administration compared with a control silicone catheter (36). A randomized study of 1,309 patients catheterized longer than 24h failed to demonstrate the effectiveness of a silicone catheter coated externally with silver oxide compared to a standard silicone coated latex catheter. However, these silver oxide catheters showed a significantly increased incidence of bacteriuria (37). With regard to this, literature on silver alloy latex catheters has failed to resolve the controversy over their efficacy and at present there is insufficient evidence to recommend the use of silver alloy catheters (Grade of recommendation: B)(33). Therefore it is evident that the use of indwelling urinary catheters, due to their complications, should be strictly related to specific and inalienable clinical conditions. Current data do not support the treatment of asymptomatic bacteriuria, either during short-term catheterization or during long-term catheterization, because it will promote the emergence of resistant strains (33). In short-term catheterization, antibiotics may delay the onset of bacteriuria, but do not reduce complications (33). A symptomatic complicated UTI associated with an indwelling catheter is treated with an agent with as narrow a spectrum as possible, based on culture and sensitivity results. The optimal duration is not well established. Treatment durations that are both too short as well as too long may cause the emergence of resistant strains. A 7-day course may be a reasonable compromise (33).

Finally in case of treatment of fungal urinary tract infection we know that it is recommended only when funguria is symptomatic or in cases of fungal colonization when host factors increase the risk of fungemia. The antifungal agents used for funguria are mainly fluconazole and amphotericin B deoxycholate, because other drugs have extremely low concentrations in urine. Intravesical amphotericin B and oral fluconazole therapy are each effective in treatment of funguria (28).

10. Antibiotic prophylaxis and invasive urodynamics in female

Invasive urodynamics involving catheterization of the lower urinary tract is an essential part in the evaluation of detrusor filling and voiding phase in patients needing assessment of bladder function(1).

Urinary tract infections (UTI) are a recognized complication of urodynamic study. The natural history of bacteriuria after urodynamics is not completely known. The overall incidence of bacteriuria after urodynamic studies is not yet clear. In fact bacteriuria occurs in 1-5% of hospitalized patients after single short-term catheterization and in ambulatory ones lower than 1%. After cystometry, the reported incidence of bacteriuria varies from 1.5% to 30%, showing that the incidence of UTI in patients who underwent invasive urodynamics is present in most cases (2,3). In this context, the opinions on the safety of urodynamic studies differ among the authors. At present, published data on prophylaxis in urodynamics have showed contradictory results with a limited predictive value. Some investigators concluded that antibiotic prophylaxis seems to reduce the incidence of urinary tract infections and to protect patients from the risk of bacterial contamination from urethral catheterization, especially for those with high risk of infection(4). In this setting it was reported an overall infection rate of 15%, so concluding that antibiotic prophylaxis should be considered(5). Subsequently other authors reported that after invasive urodynamics the patients had UTI in 4% of cases, recommending the use of antibiotic before the procedure(4). In this way others reported an incidence of significant bacteriuria in less than of 1% of patients with antibiotic prophylaxis, so this approach is considered useful (6,). Similarly it was described that invasive urodynamics in postmenopausal female subjects are safe procedures without the necessity to perform it(1).

Antimicrobial prophylaxis entails treatment with an antimicrobial agent before and for a limited time after a procedure to prevent local or systemic postprocedural infections. For most procedures, prophylaxis should be initiated between 30 minutes and 120 minutes before the procedure. Efficacious levels should be maintained for the duration of the procedure and, in special circumstances, a limited time (24 hours, at most) after the procedure(7).

In this scenario several conditions are associated with a major risk of UTI with particular regard to women. In this setting many studies have revealed that for women presenting urogynecologic units to undergo an invasive urodynamic examination, there is a relatevely low incidence of bacteriuria (8%) after few days(8,9). Other series of a comparable number of women have shown incidences ranging from 1.6% to 17%(3). These discrepancies may be due to variability in age of patients, kwowing well that advancing age is associated with a higher rate of UTI, or with different catheterization techniques (the trauma caused by catheterization itself may leave the lower urinary tract more susceptible to a later infection)(10). Recently it showed that the low vascularization of soft tissues in bladder and urethra in postmenopausal female is associated with a higher risk of UTI perhaps because this condition could delay or prevent the effect of an antibiotic prophylactic drug, which probably cannot reach these tissues in an adequate manner and concentration(11).

Recently some authors revealed that in postmenopausal women there is a slightly higher incidence rate of UTI after invasive urodynamics compared to the studies previously published in literature and this trend is not affected by the administration of an antibiotic prophylaxis. Urodynamic testing however remains a safe investigative procedure with low morbidity and infection rate in postmenopausal women when performed by sterile catheterization, even without any antibiotic prophylaxis(5).

In conclusion, we could stop administering antibiotic prophylaxis to postmenopausal patients undergoing invasive urodynamics

11. Conclusions

Urinary tract infections represent the second most often observed infectious diseases in community, following the respiratory tract infections. In nosocomial setting, UTIs represent the most frequent diseases, whose incidence equates 40% of nosocomial infections overall considered; about 80% of UTIs is related to urinary catheterization. Therefore it is strongly suggested the opportunity to increase any prevention strategy able to reduce the incidence of infections related to urinary catheterization and its consequences, as a more rational length and modality of catheterization, in addition to the use of innovative catheters: recently the use of newborn materials, such as antibiotic-impregnated catheters or silver-coated ones has started. By now, though, there was not enough evidence to suggest whether or not any standard catheter was better than another in terms of reducing the risk of urinary tract infection in hospitalised adults catheterised short-term. Siliconised catheters may be less likely to cause urethral side effects however, these results should be interpreted with some caution as the trials were small and the outcomes are still under investigation.

12. Appendix: standard catheterization procedure

1. Gather equipment.
2. Explain procedure to the patient.
3. Assist patient into supine position with legs spread and feet together.
4. Open catheterization kit and catheter.
5. Prepare sterile field, apply sterile gloves.
6. Check balloon for patency.
7. Generously coat the distal portion (2-5 cm) of the catheter with lubricant.
8. Apply sterile drape.
9. If female, separate labia using non-dominant hand. If male, hold the penis with the non-dominant hand. Maintain hand position until preparing to inflate balloon.
10. Using dominant hand to handle forceps, cleanse peri-urethral mucosa with cleansing solution. Cleanse anterior to posterior, inner to outer, one swipe per swab, discard swab away from sterile field.

11. Pick up catheter with gloved (and still sterile) dominant hand. Hold end of catheter loosely coiled in palm of dominant hand.
12. In the male, lift the penis to a position perpendicular to patient's body and apply light upward traction (with non-dominant hand).
13. Identify the urinary meatus and gently insert until 1 to 2 inches beyond where urine is noted.
14. Inflate balloon, using correct amount of sterile liquid (usually 10 cc but check actual balloon size).
15. Gently pull catheter until inflation balloon is snug against bladder neck.
16. Connect catheter to drainage system.
17. Secure catheter to abdomen or thigh, without tension on tubing.
18. Place drainage bag below level of bladder.
19. Evaluate catheter function and amount, color, odor, and quality of urine.
20. Remove gloves, dispose of equipment appropriately, wash hands.
21. Document size of catheter inserted, amount of water in balloon, patient's response to procedure, and assessment of urine

13. References

Urethral catheterization

[1] Lyons, A.A. and Petrucelli, R.J., II: Medicine: An illustrated History. New York: Harry S. Abrams, Inc., pp. 65-67, 1978.

[2] Veith, I: Huang Ti Nei Ching Su Wen: The Yellow Emperor's Classic of Internal Medicine. Berkeley: University of California Press, pp. 206-207, 1970.

[3] Tucker, R. A.: History of sizing of genitourinary instruments. Urology, 20: 346, 1982. Das, S.: Shusruta of India, the pioneer in the treatment of urethral stricture. Surg. Gynec. & Obst., 157:581, 1983

[4] Corner, G. W. and Goodwin, W. E.: Benjamin Franklin's bladder stone. J. Hist. Med. Allied Sci., (: 359, 1953.

[5] Laurisden, L.: From the history of prostatic hypertrophy. A medico-historical investigation of its pathology and palliative surgical treatment up to the beginning of the 20th century. Danish Med. Bull., 16: 77, 1969.

[6] Castiglioni, A.: A history of Medicine. New York: Knopf, pp. 202 and 715, 1947. Hambrecht, F.T. and Endmonson, J.M.: American Armamentarium Chirurgicum: George Tiemann & Co. San Francisco: Norman Publishing and The Printer's Devil, pp. 57, 390 and 781-782, 1989.

[7] Ellis, H.: Therapeutic milestones. The Foley catheter. Brit. J. clin. Pract., 42: 248, 1988.

[8] Roberts, W.: On the occurrence of micro-organisms in fresh urine. Brit. Med. J., 1: 623, 1881.

[9] Bloom, D.A., McGuire, E.J. and Lapides, J.: A Brief history of urethral catheterization. J. Urol., 151:317-325, 1994.

Catheter characheteristics/Urethral catheter and related infections/Fungal urinary tract infections/Prevention and treatment of catheter-associated urinary infections

[1] Schumm K, Lam TB. Types of urethral catheters for management of short-term voiding problems in hospitalised adults. Cochrane Database Syst Rev. 2008 Apr 16;(2):CD004013.

[2] Toughhill E. "Indwelling urinary catheters: Common mechanical and pathogenic problems," AJN,2005; 105 (5): 35–37.Toughhill E. "Indwelling urinary catheters: Common mechanical and pathogenic problems," AJN,2005; 105 (5): 35–37.

[3] Trautner BW, Darouiche RO. "Role of biofilm in catheter-associated urinary tract infection," Am J Infect Control, 2004; 32:177–183.

[4] Brosnahan CM, Chin QF, Tracy C. Type of urethral catheter for management of short term voiding problems in hospitalized patients. Cochrane Database Sys Rev 2004;(1): CD004013.

[5] Kunin CM, Chin QF, Chambers ST. Formation of encrustations on indwelling urinary catheters in the elderly: comparison of different types of catheter materials in "blockers" and "nonblockers." J Urol 1987;138:899-902.

[6] Stickler DJ, Clayton CL, Harber MJ, Chawla JC. Pseudomonas aeruginosa and long-term indwelling bladder catheters. Arch Phys Med Rehab 1988;69:25-28.

[7] Breitenbucher RB. Bacterial changes in the urine samples of patients with long-term indwelling catheters. Arch Intern Med 1984;144:1585-1588.

[8] Warren JW, Tenney JH, Hoopes JM, Muncie HL, Anthony WC. A prospective microbiologic study of bacteriuria in patients with chronic indwelling urethral catheters. J Infect Dis 1982;146:719-723.

[9] Smith PW, Seip CW, Schaefer SC, Bell-Dixon C. Microbiologic survey of long term care facilities. Am J Infect Control 2000;28:8-13

[10] Wilde MH. "Urinary tract infection in people with long-term urinary catheters," J WOCN, 2003;30:314–323.

[11] Saint S, Kaufman SR, Thompson M, Rogers MA, Chenowith CE. "A reminder reduces urinary catheterization in hospitalized patients," Joint Commision Journal on Quality and Patient Safety, 2005; 31 (8):455–462.

[12] Richards M, Edwards J, Culver D, Gaynes R. Nosocomial infections in medical intensive care units in the United States. National Nosocomial Infections Surveillance System. Crit Care Med 1999;27:887–892.

[13] Trautner BW, Hull RA, Darouiche RO: Prevention of catheter-associated urinary tract infection, Curr Opin Infect Dis 2005;18(1):37-41

[14] Kuhn W, Rist M, Zaech GA. Intermittent urethral self-catheterisation: long term results (bacteriological evolution, continence, acceptance, complications). Paraplegia. 1991 May;29(4):222-32..

15] Moore KN, Fader M, Getliffe K. Long-term bladder management by intermittent catheterisation in adults and children. Cochrane Database Syst Rev. 2007 Oct 17;(4):CD006008

[16] Tambyah PA, Halvorson KT, Maki DG.. A prospective study of pathogenesis of catheter-associated urinary tract infections. Mayo Clin Proc 1999; 74: 131–136

[17] Matsukawa M, Kunishima Y, Takahashi S, Takeyama K, Tsukamoto T.. Bacterial colonization on intraluminal surface of urethral catheter. Urology 2005;65: 440–444

[18] Howard RJ Host defense against infection. Curr Probl Surg 1980;27:267-316

[19] Ganderton L, Chawla J, Winters C, Wimpenny J, Stickler D.. Scanning electron microscopy of bacterial biofilms on indwelling bladder catheters. Eur J Clin Microbiol Infect Dis 1992; 11: 789–796

[20] Liedl B) Catheter-associated urinary tract infections. Curr Opin Urol 2001;11: 75–79

[21] Stickler DJ Bacterial biofilms in patients with indwelling urinary catheters Nature Clin Pract Urology; 2008; 5(11):598-608
[22] Kunin CM, MkCormar RC: Prevention of catheter-induced urinary tract infections by sterile by sterile closed drainage. N Engl J Med 274:1115,1966
[23] Morris NS et al. The development of bacterial biofilms on indwelling urethral catheters. World J Urol 1999; 17: 345–350
[24] Macleod SM and Stickler DJ Species interactions in mixed-community crystalline biofilms on urinary catheters. J Med Microbiol 2007; 56: 1549–1557
[25] Cox AJ and Hukins DW Morphology of mineral deposits on encrusted urinary catheters investigated by scanning electron microscopy. J Urol 1989;142:1347–1350
[26] Lindsay EN, Catheter-related urinary tract infection Drugs Aging 2005:22(8); 627-639
[27] Chenoweth CE, Saint S. Urinary tract unfection. Infect Dis Clin North Am 2011;25(1):103-15
[28] Etienne M, Caron F Management of fungal urinary tract infections Presse Med. 2007;36:1899-906
[28] Schumm K, Lam TLB. Types of Urethral Catheters for Management of Short-Term Voiding Problems in Hospitalized Adults: A Short Version Cochrane Review Neurourology and Urodynamics 2008; 27:738–746
[29] Horan TC, Andrus M, Dudeck MA. CDC/NHSN surveillance definition of health care-associated infection and criteria for specific types of infections in the acute care setting. Am J Infect Control 2008 Jun;36(5):309–32
[30] Trautner BW Management of catheter-associated urinary tract infection (CAUTI). Curr Opin Infect Dis 2010; 23(1):76-82
[31] Joanna Briggs Institute. Management of short term indwelling urethral catheters to prevent urinarytract infections. Best Practice 2000;4:1-6.
[32] Webster G, Hood RH, Burridge CA et al. Water or antiseptic for periurethral cleaning before urinarycatheterisation: a randomized controlled trial. American Journal Infection Control 2001; 29:389-94.
[33] M. Grabe , M.C. Bishop, T.E. Bjerklund-Johansen, H. Botto, M. Çek, B. Lobel, K.G. Naber, J. Palou, P. Tenke, F. Wagenlehner Guidelines on Urological Infections. EAU guidelines 2009
[34] Maki, D. G., V. Knasinski, K. T. Halvorson, P. A. Tambyah, and R. G. Holcomb. 1997. A prospective, randomized, investigator-blinded trial of a novel nitrofurazone-impregnated urinary catheter. infect. Control Hosp. Epidemiol. 18:50
[35] Darouiche, R. O., J. A. Smith, Jr., H. Hanna, C. B. Dhabuwala, M. S. Steiner, R. J. Babaian, T. B. Boone, P. T. Scardino, J. I. Thornby, and I. I. Raad. 1999. Efficacy of antimicrobial-impregnated bladder catheters in reducing catheter-associated bacteriuria: a prospective, randomized, multicenter clinical trial. Urology 54:976–981.
[36] Johnson, J. R., P. L. Roberts, R. J. Olsen, K. A. Moyer, and W. E. Stamm. 1990. Prevention of catheter-associated urinary tract infection with a silver oxide-coated urinary catheter: clinical and microbiologic correlates. J. Infect. Dis. 162:1145–1150.
[37] Riley, D. K., D. C. Classen, L. E. Stevens, and J. P. Burke. 1995. A large randomized clinical trial of a silver-impregnated urinary catheter: lack of efficacy and staphylococcal superinfection. Am. J. Med. 98:349–356.

Antibiotic prophylaxis and invasive urodynamics

[1] Siracusano S, Knez R, Tiberio A, Alfano V, Giannantoni A, Pappagallo G (2008) The usefulness of antibiotic prophylaxis in invasive urodynamics in postmenopausal female subjects. Int Urogynecol J 19:939-94

[2] Cutinha PE, Potts LK, Fleet C, Rosario D, Chapple CR (1996) Morbidity following pressure flow studies-are prophylactic antibiotics necessary? Neurourol Urodyn 15:304-305

[3] Kingler HC, Madersbacher S, Djavan B, Schatzl G, Marberger M, Schidbauer CP (1998) Morbidity of the evaluation of the lower urinary tract with transurethral multichannel pressure-flow studies. J Urol 159:191-194

[4] Porru D, Madeddu G, Campus G, Montisci I, Scarpa RM, Usai E (1999) Evaluation of morbidity of multichannel pressure-flow studies. Neurourol Urodyn 18:647-652

[5] Payne SR, Timoney AG, McKenning ST, den Hollander D, Pead LJ, Maskell RM (1988) Microbiological look at urodynamic studies. Lancet 2:1123-1126

[6] Kartal ED, Yenilmez A, Kiremitci A, Meric H, Kale M, Usluer G (2006) Effectiveness of ciprofloxacin prophylaxis in preventing bacteriuria caused by urodynamic study: a blind, randomized study of 192 patients. Urology

[7] Campbell-Walsh (2007) Urology. Saunders IX Edizione Volume I

[8] Raz R (2001) Postmenopausal women with recurrent UTI. Int J Antimicrob Agents 17:269-271

[9] Stamm W, Raz R (1999) Factors contributing to susceptibility of postmenopausal women to recurrent urinary tract infections. Clin Infect Dis 28:723-725

[10] Bombieri L, Dance DAB, Rienhart GW, Waterfield A, Freeman RM (1999) Urinary tract infection after urodynamic studies in women: incidence and natural history. BJU Int 83:392-39

[11] Siracusano S, Bertolotto M, Cucchi A, Lampropoulou N, Tiberio A, Gasparini C (2006) Application of ultrasound contrast agents for characterization of female urethra vascularization in healthy pre- and postmenopausal volunteers: preliminary report. Int Urogynecol J 19:939-942

[12] Jarmy-DiBella ZI, Girao MG, Sartori MF, DiBella Junior V, Ledermann HM, Barcat EC et al (2000) Power Doppler of the urethra in continent or incontinent, pre- and postmenopausal women. Int Urogynecol J 11(3):148-154

Part 3

Immunology

7

The Pathogenesis of Urinary Tract Infections

Niall F. Davis and Hugh D. Flood
Department of Urology, Mid-Western Regional Hospital,
Dooradoyle, Co. Limerick,
Ireland

1. Introduction

Urinary tract infections (UTIs) are among the most common conditions requiring medical treatment with 6-10% of all young females demonstrating bacteriuria (Raz 2001). The incidence of UTIs increases with age and 25-50% of females aged 80 or more have bacteriuria (Abrutyn et al. 1988). UTIs occur as a result of interactions between the uropathogen and host and their pathogenesis involves several processes. Initially the uropathogen attaches to the epithelial surface; it subsequently colonises and disseminates throughout the mucosa causing tissue damage. After the initial colonisation period, pathogens can ascend into the urinary bladder resulting in symptomatic or asymptomatic bacteriuria. Further progression may lead to pyelonephritis and renal impairment. Specific virulence factors residing on the uropathogen's membrane are responsible for bacterial resistance to the normally effective defence mechanisms of the host. Recently, bacterial adhesins and their associated epithelial binding sites have been identified and natural anti-adherence mechanisms are currently under investigation.

An understanding of pathogenic and anti-adherence mechanisms may allow physicians to develop appropriate strategies for UTI prevention and adequate management protocols. In the present chapter we discuss current concepts on the pathogenesis of UTIs with particular emphasis on pathogenic bacteria, virulence factors, predisposing factors, natural defences within genitourinary tract and consequences when these defence mechanisms are altered.

2. Routes of infection

In healthy patients most uropathogens originate from rectal flora and enter the urinary tract via the urethra into the bladder (Handley et al. 2002). This is known as the ascending route and uropathogens initially adhere to and colonise urothelium of the distal urethra (Fig.1). Enhancement of this route is exacerbated in patients with soiling around the perineum, in patients with urinary catheters and in females that use spermicidal agents (Foxman 2002). In patients with established cystitis up to 50% of infections may ascend into the upper urinary tracts and most episodes of pyelonephritis are caused by ascension of bacteria from the bladder through the ureter and into the renal pelvis (Busch and Huland 1984). Bacterial ascent is aided by conditions such as pregnancy and ureteral obstruction as these conditions inhibit ureteral peristalsis. Bacteria that reach the renal pelvis can penetrate the renal parenchyma through the collecting ducts and disrupt the renal tubules.

In healthy individuals infection of the kidney through the haematogenous route is uncommon. Occasionally, the renal parenchyma may be breeched in patients with Staphylococcus aureus bacteraemia or Candida fungaemia that originate from oral sources in immunosuppressed patients (Smellie et al. 1975). On rare occasions bacteria from adjacent organs may penetrate the urinary tract via the lymphatics. Conditions associated with the lymphatic route are retroperitoneal abscesses and severe bowel infections.

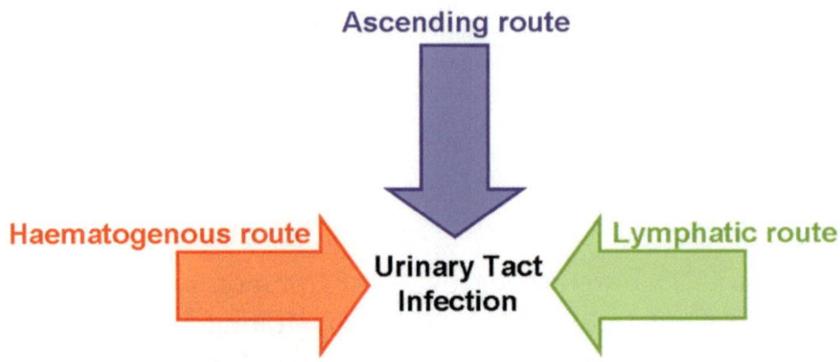

Fig. 1. Urinary tract infections may arise from ascending, haematogenous or lymphatic routes. Ascending routes of infection are most common among patients with an established UTI.

3. Urinary pathogens

3.1 Pathogenic bacteria

E. coli accounts for 85% of community acquired and 50% of hospital acquired urinary tract infections. Within the E.coli species a number of subgroups (O1, O2, O4, O6, O7, O8, O18, O25, O68 and O75) are frequently isolated from patients with UTI (Brooks et al. 1981, Gruneberg 1969, Roberts and Phillips 1979, Vosti et al. 1964). Gram negative bacteria such as Klebsiella and Proteus; and Gram positive Enterococcus faecalis and Staphylococcus saprophiticus are causative agents for the remainder of community acquired infections (Kennedy et al. 1965). The remainder of hospital acquired infections usually occur after colonisation with Klebsiella, Enterobacter, Citrobacter, Serratia, Pseudomonas aeruginosa, Providencia, E. faecalis, or S. epidermidis (Kennedy et al. 1965). Notably, the patient's age may influence they type of infective organism present with Staphylococcus saprophiticus now accounting for 10% of UTIs in young females compared to less than 1% in elderly female patients.

3.2 Uncomplicated UTIs

UTIs can be classified as either complicated or uncomplicated depending on underlying host factors and on underlying uropathogens as illustrated in table 1. The aetiology of uncomplicated UTIs has remained constant over the last 2 to 3 decades with E. coli accounting for the vast majority of cases. Previously, female patients with uncomplicated UTIs generally remained sensitive to a trimethoprim-sulfamethoxazole combination and the traditional approach to therapy had been an empirical short-course treatment with this antibiotic regimen (Hooton and Stamm 1997, Stamm and Hooton 1993). Unfortunately, a number of more recent studies have demonstrated increasing antimicrobial resistance among uropathogens causing uncomplicated cystitis and traditional antibiotic regimens have been questioned (Gupta et al. 1999). One study investigated antimicrobial resistance among 4000 female petients with UTI isolates over a 5 year experimental time period. Results from this study demonstrated an increase in antimicrobial (E. coli) resistance from 9% to 18% in patients treated with trimethoprim-sulfamethoxazole (Gupta et al. 1999). In addition, resistance to cephalothin (a first generation cephalosporin) increased from 20% to 28% and resistance to ampicillin increased from 26% to 34%. Notably, resistance to nitrofrantoin and ciprofloxacin remained <1% after the 5 year period. This increase in bacterial resistance has been attributed to recent administration of trimethoprim-sulfamethoxazole, diabetes mellitus, recent hospitalisation and recent administration of any other antibiotic (Wright et al. 1999).

Clinical implications for increasing resistance trends include a potential alteration to antibiotic regimens commonly administered for treating uncomplicated UTIs. One study demonstrated a greater cure rate after a 7-day course of ciprofloxacin compared to a 14-day course of trimethprim-sulfamethoxazole in premenopausal females with uncomplicated pyelonephritis (Talan et al. 2000). In this study it is also notable that E. coli resistance to trimethoprim-sulfamethoxazole was significantly greater (18%) compared to ciprofloxacin (0%). Lower cure rates for uncomplicated UTIs in females treated with trimethoprim-sulfamethoxazole have also been demonstrated in another study where failure rates increased from 3% to 13% in sensitive E.coli strains and from 27% to 40% in resistant strains (McCarty et al. 1999). Based on these studies antimicrobial treatment with either a fluoroquinolone, nitrofurantoin or fosfomycin are currently recommended for uncomplicated UTIs. Importantly, clincians should also be aware of the antimicrobial spectrum for these agents prior to administration as nitrofurantoin is not effective for treating uncomplicated pyelonephritis but highly effective for treating acute cystitis. Recurrent uncomplicated UTIs occur after 3 to 6 months in 25% to 35% of patients after their initial UTI. The second strain is caused by an identical strain to the first UTI in up to 60% of patients with recurrent UTI (Ronald 2003).

3.3 Complicated UTIs

Underlying host factors such as age, catheterisation, diabetes mellitus and spinal cord injury predispose to complicated UTIs (Fig. 2). In complicated UTIs less virulent uropathogens (that rarely cause disease in a normal urinary tract) can cause significant damage to an abnormal urinary tract. Studies have demonstrated associations between Group B streptococcal bacteraemia, Candida and Enterococci with complicated UTIs in the elderly population (Khan and Ahmed 2001, Munoz et al. 1997).

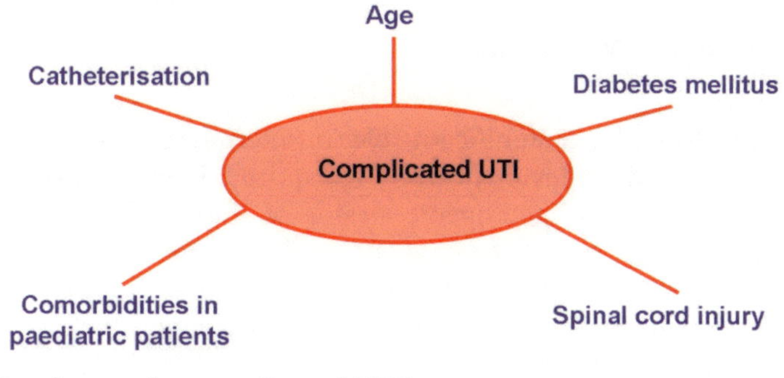

Fig. 2. Predisposing factors for complicated UTIs.

Children with comorbidities are more likely to develop complicated UTIs and Staphylococcus aureus is the most frequently isolated micro-organism in paediatric patients with indwelling catheters (Schlager 2001). Candida and coagulase-negative staphylococci are associated with complicated UTIs after instrumentation of the paediatric urinary tract. Of note, enterobacteriaceae are the most frequently isolated uropathogen in children with uncomplicated UTIs (Schlager 2001).

UTIs are among the top 10 complicating illnesses in patients with diabetes mellitus with E. coli, Klebsiella, Group B Streptococci and Enterococcus among the common uropathogens (Ronald and Ludwig 2001). In fact, Group B Streptococcus and Klebsiella are 2-3 times more common in patients with diabetes mellitus than in patients without the condition (Ronald and Ludwig 2001). However, E. coli remains the most causative uropathogen for UTIs in patients with diabetes as demonstrated in one prospective study where E. coli was isolated in 56.1% of diabetic patients with a UTI (Bonadio et al. 1999). There is a higher rate of bladder catheterisation in patients with diabetes and this factor may partially account for the higher incidence in this patient cohort (Ronald 2003).

Common uropathogens causing complicated UTIs among patients with spinal cord injuries and indwelling catheters include E. coli, Pseudomonas and Proteus mirabilis (Mobley et al. 1994). The latter is particularly associated with complicated UTIs as it possesses unique virulence factors that enhance its invasive potential (Coker et al. 2000). One study demonstrated a significant increase in nosocomial UTIs from 2.63 of 1000 patient days to 4.35 of 1000 patient days over a 9 year period ($p<0.003$). Notably, 88% of nosocomial UTIs in this study were catheter related (Bronsema et al. 1993).

Pathogens in uncomplicated UTIs	Pathogens in complicated UTIs
Escherichia coli Staphylococcus saprophyticus Kelbsiella Enterococcus faecalis	Escherichia coli Kelbsiella Enetrobacter cloacae Serratia marcescens Proteus mirabilis Pseudomonas aeruginosa Enterococcus faecalis Group B streptococci

Table 1. Underlying uropathogens commonly isoloated in complicated and uncomplicated urinary tract infection (UTI) (Ronald 2003).

4. Bacterial adherence mechanisms

4.1 Virulence factors

Bacterial virulence factors play a significant role in determining whether an organism will invade the urinary tract and the level of infection acquired. Uropathogenic E. coli (UPEC) is present within bowel flora and pathogenic strains of this microorganism can infect the urinary tract by expressing specific virulence factors that permit adherence and colonisation of the lower urinary tract (Schlager et al. 2002, Yamamoto et al. 1997). Adherence of the micro-organism is dependent on 3 important environmental characteristics; firstly the bacteria's own adhesive characteristics, secondly the receptive features of the urothelium and finally the fluid that is present between both surfaces (Schaeffer et al. 1981). Bacteria will migrate proximally and precipitate a host derived inflammatory response after adhering to the mucosal surface.

Adhesins found on the surface of the bacterial membrane are responsible for initial attachment onto urinary tract tissues (Mulvey 2002) (Fig. 3).

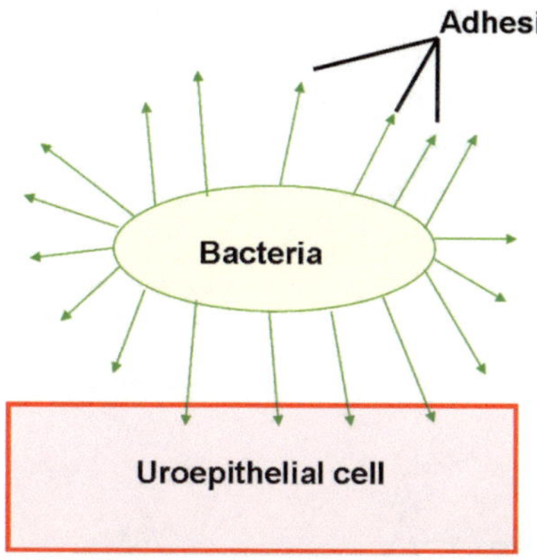

Fig. 3. Adhesins on the uropathogen are responsible for attachment of the bacteria to the uroepithelial cell membrane of the host.

Adhesins are classified as fimbrial or afimbrial, depending on whether the adhesin is displayed as part of a rigid fimbria or pilus. Fimbriae and pili are surface glycoproteins that function as ligands for glycolipid and glycoprotein receptors on uroepithelial cells. Bacteria may produce 100-400 pili on the same cell and other cells can produce the same pilus type. Each pilus is 5-10 μm in diameter and up to 2 μm in length (Klemm 1985). A pilus is composed of subunits referred to as pilin and they are classified as either mannose sensitive or mannose resistant, based on their ability to mediate haemagglutination of erythrocytes. The most common types of pili are types 1, P and S. Assemblance of pili within the urinary tract is mediated by the 'chaperone/ usher pathway' where periplasmic chaperones such as P pilus chaperone 'PapD' and type 1 pilus chaperone 'FimC' possess two immunoglobulin (Ig)-like domains that are oriented to form a boomerang like shape (Kau et al. 2005, Kuehn et al. 1993, Lau et al. 2005). These chaperones are important for binding with pilus subunits to form stable complexes. The FimC chaperone accelerates the folding of type 1 pilus subunits to strengthen its binding process after its initial attachment process (Vetsch et al. 2004).

4.2 Type 1 pili

Type 1 pili are also referred to as mannose sensitive pili and they are commonly expressed in pathogenic and non pathogenic strains of E. coli. They are termed mannose sensitive as haemagglutination of erythrocytes is inhibited in the presence of mannose (Reid and Sobel 1987). Type 1 pili are composed of a helical rod with repeating Fim A subunits that are bound to a distal tip structure containing the Fim H adhesin (Jones et al. 1995). During the colonisation process Fim H adhesins bind to mannosylated receptors that are found on the host's uroepithelium. An inflammatory process occurs shortly after this binding process has been initiated. A number of studies have demonstrated that interactions between the Fim H adhesin and epithelial cells on the bladder's surface are essential for colonisation and infection of bladder epithelium with strains of uropathogenic E. coli (Sun 1996, Wu et al. 1996). This specific 'adhesin-epithelial cell' binding process occurs when type 1 pili bind to uroplakin 1a (UP1a) and uroplakin 1b (UP1b) (Malaviya and Abraham 1998). (Fig. 4) Uroplakins are membrane proteins that are found on umbrella cells which line the luminal surface of the urinary bladder. Initially adhesin binding mechanisms were investigated in a mouse cystitis model where numerous bacteria attached to the urothelial surface of the mouse urinary tract shortly after an inoculation period. Scanning electron microscopy of the urothelial layers demonstrated that Fim H containing pili bound to the central cavity of uroplakin hexameric rings and this binding process is responsible for the initial steps leading to active UTI (Mulvey et al. 1998).

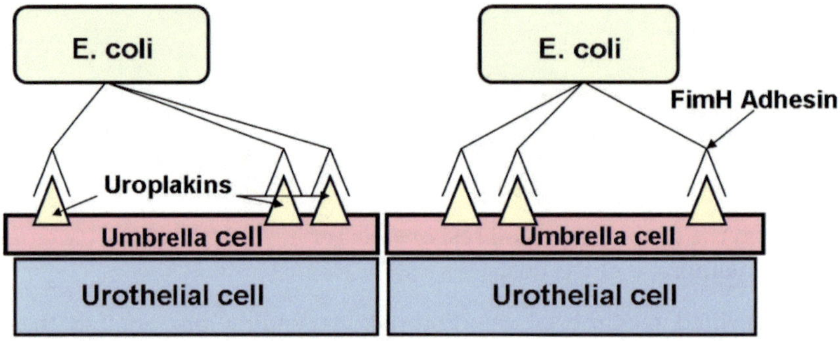

Fig. 4. During the colonisation period FimH adhesins bind to umbrella cells via uroplakin 1a and uroplakin 1b membrane receptors.

After binding to the epithelial surface the activated Fim H adhesins migrate towards deeper urothelial layers and penetrate the cell membrane (Mulvey et al. 2000). Once the uropathogen is intracellular the invasive process continues as bacteria proliferate within the cytosol to form clusters (Anderson et al. 2004b). Eight hours after inoculation the phenotypic appearance of the bacteria changes to an engulfing 'biofilm' like structure that protects against the host's immune response and shields the uropathogen from its surrounding environment (Justice et al. 2004) (Fig. 5). A decrease in the rate of bacterial proliferation will allow for effective production of a 'biofilm matrix'. This matrix can prevent the host's neutrophils from penetrating its surface. The 'biofilm' concept stems from the idea that bacteria co-operate with one another to remain viable and proliferate after attaching to a suitable substrate. Previously, it has been demonstrated that biofilms play an important role in a number of disease processes (Kau et al. 2005, Parsek and Singh 2003). Bacterial biofilms can form within infected urinary tract calculi, during Pseudomonas infections in patients with cystic fibrosis and in infective endocarditis. During the disease process biofilms form irreversible associations with their host by forming extracellular polysaccharides that have specialised functions (Justice et al. 2004).

Biofilms can form on many different types of bacteria however the sequence of events during the 'formation process' remains similar in all bacteria. Firstly, bacteria express extracellular polymeric substances that are initially reversible and subsequently become irreversible. Bacteria that have irreversibly attached to a surface will serve as a nidus for continued replication and recruitment of other bacteria. Irreversible attachment is usually established after 24 hours where the bacteria will develop into a complicated 'tower' like structure and become filamentous (up to 70 μm in length). Morphological changes allow the uropathogen to evade the host's immune response (Justice et al. 2004). Bacteria that have clustered will eventually detach from their group, become motile and flee the host cell. Bacterial adherence and replication will recur after the uropathogen escapes its intracellular environment and this effective replication process will allow bacterial invasion to persist (Anderson et al. 2004a) (Fig. 5).

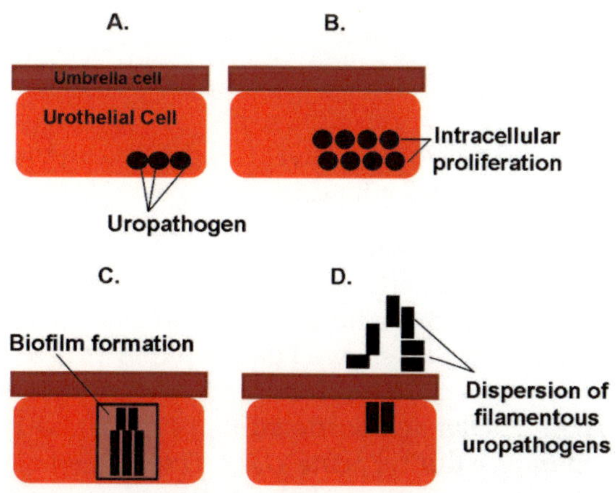

Fig. 5. After attaching to the epithelial surface the uropathogen will enter the cytosol (A). Intracellular bacteria rapidly proliferate within the first 24 hours (B). Subsequently, proliferation rate decreases and a protective biofilm matrix forms (C). Morphological changes allow the uropathogen to evade the host's immune response. Uropathogens that have clustered become motile and detach from the biofilm to disperse (D).

4.3 P Fimbriated pili

P fimbriated pili or mannose resistant strains of E. coli are associated with uncomplicated pyelonephritis as the receptor for P fimbriae is the major glycolipid component present on renal cell membranes (Mulvey 2002). They are termed mannose resistant as they are not affected by mannose during the haemagglutination process for human erythrocytes (Vaisanen et al. 1981). PapG is an adhesin found at the tip of the pilus and it recognizes the α-d-galctopyranosyl-(1-4)-β-d-galctopyranoside receptor which is found on P-blood group antigens on the host's uroepithelium (Kallenius et al. 1981) (Fig. 6). Mannose resistant adhesins that do not demonstrate digalactoside-binding affinity are referred to as 'X' adhesins. A correlation between severe UTIs and bacterial adherence was first identified in 1976 (Eden et al. 1976). Strains of uropathogenic E. coli in girls with established pyelonephritis had an adhesive ability of 70-80% compared to 10% in strains that caused asymptomatic bacteriuria. P pili were present in 91% of strains that caused pyelonephritis compared to a prevalence of 7% in bowel isolates from healthy children (Eden et al. 1976). Although mannose resistant haemagglutinins (MRHA) are associated with pyelonephritis it is important to note that no link exists between MRHA and renal scarring.

4.4 Phase variation

Interestingly, in vivo studies have shown that environmental factors are responsible for rapid changes in pili in E. coli isolates. This transformation process is known as known as

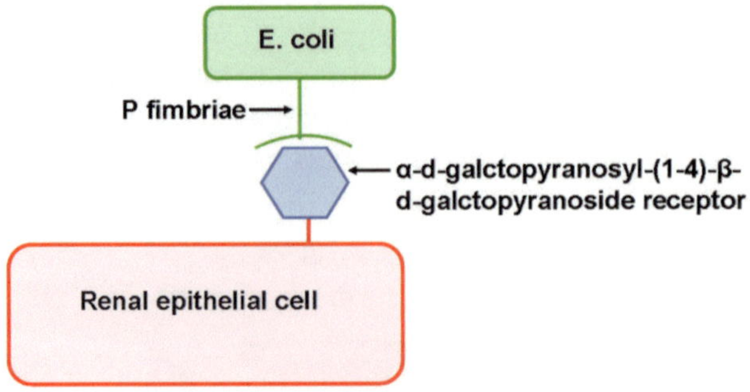

Fig. 6. P fimbiae bind to the α-d-galctopyranosyl-(1-4)-β-d-galctopyranoside receptor on the host's renal epithelial cell via the PapG adhesin.

phase variation and it involves alternating periods of piliated and nonpiliated adhesins during *in vivo* E. coli infection (Hultgren et al. 1986, Schaeffer et al. 1987). One study showed phase variation of pili using indirect immunofluorescense assays of voided urine in human patients. Analysis of the urine samples showed type 1 pili in 31 of 41 samples and P pili in 6 of 18 samples with piliation status varying from predominantly piliated to nonpiliated cells (Kisielius et al. 1989). These results demonstrated that type 1 and P pili are expressed and subject to phase variation *in vivo* during acute UTIs. The process of phase variation among adhesins has notable clinical implications. Importantly, the presence of type 1 pili may facilitate adherence and colonisation of the host's mucosa in the lower urinary tract. However, P pili may predominate as the infective process progresses and ascends. This transformation process occurs because primary mediators for the attachment of P pili to their glycolipid receptors are found within the kidney (Mulvey et al. 1998).

4.5 Cell receptivity

Epithelial cell receptivity also plays an important pathogenic role in female patients that are susceptible to recurrent UTI. The receptivity concept was established after vaginal epithelial cells were collected from patients susceptible to recurrent UTI with E. coli and compared with control samples that were resistant to UTI (Fowler and Stamey 1977). Results from this study demonstrated that strains of E. coli associated with cystitis ardently adhered to vaginal epithelial cells of susceptible females. Notably, buccal cell receptivity is also increased for different strains of E. coli in females with increased vaginal cell receptivity. These findings indicate a genotypic trait as the increase in receptor sites for strains of E. coli is not confined to the vagina in females with recurrent UTIs. Further analysis of this genetic concept by assessing human leukocyte antigens (HLAs) in females with recurrent UTIs has demonstrated that HLA-A3 may be a contributing factor. It has also been shown that a greater number of uropathogens attach to epithelial cell surface in females that are greater than 65 years of age compared to premenopausal females (i.e. age 18-40) (Schaeffer et al. 1983).

5. Predisposing factors for pathogenic adherence

5.1 Alterations to the host's natural defence mechanisms

Normal flora around the vaginal introitus, periurethral region and urethra include microorganisms such as lactobacilli, coagulase negative staphylococci and streptococci that form a barrier against pathogenic colonisation. Alterations in the vaginal mucosa and decreases in its pH are thought to play an important role for with coliforms (Hooton et al. 1996a). Acute disruptions to this mucosal barrier are frequently attributed to spermicidal and antimicrobial agents that alter normal flora and induce increased receptivity for uropathogens (Hooton et al. 1996a). Host factors that contribute to the disruption of this mucosal barrier are illustrated in table 2.

Comorbidities such as diabetes mellitus, sickle cell disease, hyperphosphataemia, gout and analgesics are also associated with altering the host's natural defence mechanisms (Freedman 1975). The incidence of pyelonephritis is up to fivefold higher in diabetics compared to non diabetic patients (Nicolle et al. 1996). Furthermore, female patients with diabetes mellitus are 3 times more likely to develop pyelonephritis compared to male patients with the condition (Nicolle et al. 1996). Diabetes also predisposes patients to more complicated UTIs with an inflammatory urothelial response occurring in the upper tracts of up to 80% of diabetic patients with UTIs (Forland et al. 1977, Stapleton 2002). In addition, UTIs in this patient cohort are often caused by atypical organisms and complications may progress to include papillary necrosis, perinephric abscesses or multisystemic infections (Stapleton 2002).

Urinary tract obstruction and stasis of urine flow can significantly alter the host's defence mechanisms and both factors strongly predispose to complicated UTIs (Hooton 2000). During the obstructive process local mucosal defence mechanisms are disturbed as the epithelial lining over-distends and pooled urine functions as a mean for bacterial growth and proliferation (Hooton et al. 2000). Urinary catheters, particularly in patients with high residual volumes, are also ideal media for uropathogens to colonise the urinary tract. Finally, fistulae can facilitate direct access into the genoitourinary tract via the gastrointestinal system.

Genetic	Biological	Behavioural	Others
Blood group antigen	Congenital abnormalities	Sexual intercourse	Decreased mental status
Non-secretor status	Urinary obstruction	Use of diaphragm	
Increased density of adhesion receptors	Calculi	Use of spermicides	
	Diabetes mellitus	Antimicrobial use	
	Anatomical		
	Residual urine		
	Atrophic vaginitis		
	Urinary incontinence		
	Prior history of UTI		
	Maternal history of UTI		
	Urinary catheters		
	Stents		
	Immunological deficiency (HIV)		
	Renal transplant		

Table 2. Host factors that contribute to the pathogenesis of UTIs in female patients.

5.2 Anatomical and physiological factors

It is widely acknowledged that a number of factors contribute to a greater prevalence in UTIs in females compared to males. In particular, female pelvic anatomy plays an important predisposing role for recurrent UTIs in female patients. One study investigated differences in perineal anatomical measurements and voiding characteristics in 100 females with a history of recurrent UTIs and in 113 females with no prior history of UTIs. Analysis of the results demonstrated that the urethra and anus were significantly closer together in cases of UTI (4.8 ± 0.6cm) compared to controls (5.0 ± 0.7cm, p= 0.03) (Hooton 2000). Other important physiological and anatomical factors that predispose to bacterial adherence in females (compared to males) include a drier urethral meatus, a shorter urethra and the absence of antibacterial properties provided by prostatic fluid (Lipsky 1989).

5.3 Spermicidal compounds

Nonoxynol-9 is a non-ionic surfactant that is the most active ingredient found in spermicidal compounds in the USA. Results from *in vitro* studies have shown that it is less active against uropathogenic bacteria compared to Lactobacillus (Hooton et al. 1991a, McGroarty et al. 1990) with hydrogen peroxide-producing strains being particularly susceptible (Hooton et al. 1991a). Therefore, it appears that vaginal colonisation with hydrogen peroxide vaginal strains of lactobacilli may play an important role in bacterial resistance (Eschenbach et al. 1989). This hypothesis has been tested in other studies where hydrogen peroxide-producing lactobacilli had a protective effect against bacterial vaginosis, symptomatic candidosis and vaginal colonisation with genital pathogens (Hawes et al. 1996, Hillier et al. 1992). In support of this hypothesis one case-control study has also demonstrated that vaginal colonisation with E. coli occurs more frequently in females without hydrogen peroxide-producing lactobacilli compared to females with these strains (odds ratio 4.0; p=0.01) (Gupta et al. 1998). In this study, spermicidal use among females correlated with an increased risk of vaginal colonisation with E. coli (odds ratio 12.5; p<0.001) and with the absence of hydrogen peroxide-producing lactobacilli. Another study also showed decreased vaginal lactobacilli and an increase in vaginal coliforms after nonoxynol-9 instillation in the absence of sexual activity and diaphragm use (Rosenstein et al. 1998).

Based on these studies, it seems likely that the antimicrobial activity of spermicides alters the vaginal ecosystem and provides a suitable environment for growth and proliferation of uropathogens. It is interesting to note that small amounts of nonoxynol-9 on condoms can increase the risk of UTI in females in the absence of sexual intercourse (Fihn et al. 1998, Fihn et al. 1996).

5.4 Premenopausal females

In premenopausal healthy females sexual intercourse and spermicide use are the most important factors predisposing to UTIs. One study demonstrated a 2.6 fold increased risk of UTI in females (age 24) that have sexual intercourse 3 times a week compared to females that do not have intercourse (Hooton et al. 1996a). It is hypothesised that an increased risk of UTI from sexual intercourse occurs from trauma at the introitus (Foxman et al. 1997, Hooton et al. 1991b) or through mechanical introduction of the uropathogen into the bladder (Hooton et al. 1991b). Other predisposing factors to UTI in premenopausal patients are a new sexual partner during the last year, having a first UTI less than 15 years of age and having a mother with a history of UTIs (Hooton et al. 1996a). Interestingly, the latter two are associated with a two- to four- fold increase in risk compared to normal females, perhaps suggesting a genetic predisposition. Finally, a previous history of UTI is a strong predictor of having a subsequent UTI. This may be attributable to a host's biological or behavioural features or from persistent colonisation of a particular bacterial strain.

5.5 Oestrogen

The role of oestrogen in the pathogenesis of UTIs is controversial. In vitro studies have demonstrated that oestrogen permits adherence of uropthogens to vaginal epithelial cells (Hooton et al. 1996b). However, other studies also suggest that oestrogen deficiency in postmenopausal females may increase the risk of UTI (Haspels et al. 1981, Thomas et al. 1980). In fact, one study showed that half of females aged 61 or older had genitourinary symptoms and 29% of this cohort also complained of urinary incontinence (Iosif and Bekassy 1984). Furthermore, the risk of UTI in postmenopausal females is decreased by topical application of oestrogen creams as demonstrated in one double-blinded-placebo controlled study (Raz and Stamm 1993). In this study results showed that vaginal colonization with E. coli was halved and lactobacillus colonization was re-established after topical application of oestrogen in postmenopausal females (Fig. 7). As a result vaginal pH was decreased along with colonisation with Enterobacteriaceae.

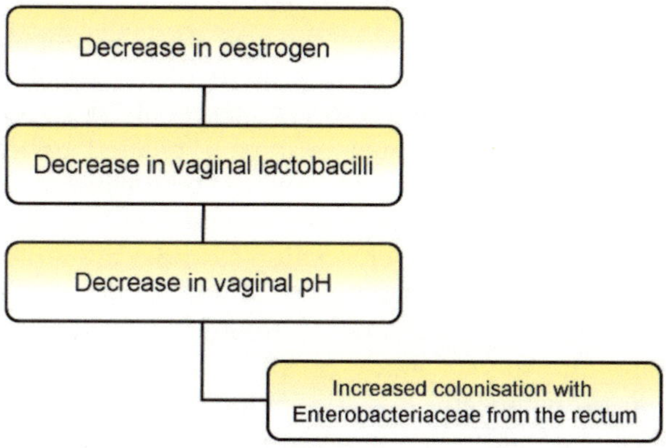

Fig. 7. Proposed pathophysiology of UTIs in patients with oestrogen deficiency (Raz 2001).

5.6 Genetic susceptibility

Interleukin-8 is an inflammatory cytokine that promotes neutrophil migration across infected urothelial cells (Godaly et al. 1998, Godaly et al. 1997). Absence of its receptor CXCR1 has recently been shown to promote bacteraemia within the urinary tract as demonstrated in one study in knockout mice that lacked CXCR1 (Frendeus et al. 2001). A genetic predisposition to UTIs has been suggested in paediatric patients where children with recurrent pyelonephritis demonstrated a defect in the CXCR1 receptor (Frendeus et al. 2000).

5.7 Antimicrobial agents

Animal and human studies suggest that antimicrobial agents predispose females to UTIs by altering their host's vaginal ecology (Herthelius-Elman et al. 1992, Winberg et al. 1993).

Colonisation with E. coli is increased after administering β-lactam antimicrobial agents in monkeys (Herthelius-Elman et al. 1992). Notably, trimethoprim and nirofuarantoin do not enhance vaginal colonisation with E.coli in similar trials on monkeys and these findings suggest that β-lactam antibiotics may be responsible for altering the genital flora of female patients. Less vaginal colonisation with uropathogens occurs after a course of co-trimoxazole or fluoroquinolones when compared to β-lactam antimicrobials. Finally, the timing of antimicrobial agents also appears to play a role for increasing the risk of UTI. One prospective study on premenopausal females demonstrated an increased risk for UTI in females that had been prescribed antimicrobial therapy during the preceding 15-28 days compared to the previous 3-14 days (Smith et al. 1997).

5.8 Urological factors

Several urological factors are associated with a predisposition to UTIs in female patients. Cystocele, high post-void residual volume and urinary incontinence are strongly associated with recurrent UTIs as demonstrated in one case control study (Raz et al. 2000). In addition, surgery of the genitourinary tract often precedes the onset of a UTI and urological surgery itself is also an independent risk factor for recurrent UTI (Raz et al. 2000).

6. Host response to pathogenic adherence

A series of defence pathways are activated by the host after the uropathogen adheres to the mucosal surface. Epithelial cells exfoliate within hours of the initial infection and infected urothelial cells are shed during this process (Mysorekar et al. 2002). Secretion and excretion of the infected urothelial cells is mediated by type 1 piliated bacteriae that induce cell apoptosis (Mulvey et al. 1998). In healthy patients the epithelium lining the surface of the bladder is quiescent as the umbrella cell layer is renewed every few months. However these normally repressed proliferation and differentiation cascades are rapidly activated after the infective process in the murine cystitis model. These proliferation cascades have the potential to induce effective regeneration of an umbrella cell layer within 24 hours of the exfoliation process (Fig. 8) Another study in mice has demonstrated that exfoliation of urothelial cells prevents uropathogenic E. coli from forming clusters (Anderson et al. 2004b). Notably, mice that elicited a mild exfoliation process in response to the uropathogen were more likely to form biofilms that migrated into deeper layers.

The host's innate immune response is primarily responsible for providing resistance to the invading uropathogen. Numerous cell types such as neutrophils, macrophages, eosinophils and natural killer cells are activated as the uropathogen invades. In addition, polymorphonuclear leukocytes synthesise nitric oxide by increasing the transcription of nitric oxide synthase and this process has a toxic effect on the invading pathogen (Poljakovic and Persson 2003, Poljakovic et al. 2001). During the initial inflammatory response period it is important to note that neutrophils play a key role as they migrate towards the infected site. The migratory process is mediated by pathogen-associated molecular pattern receptors (PAMPs) and Toll-like receptors (TLRs) (Anderson et al. 2004b). After lipopolysaccharides (LPS), peptidoglycans (PG) and other bacterial products are recognised TLRs activate signalling pathways that initiate immune and inflammatory responses to kill pathogens (Anderson et al. 2004a). TLR4 and its co-receptors (CD14 and MD2) recognise Gram-negative bacterial LPS and activate the innate immune response (Haraoka et al. 1999). In addition, TLR11 is released from the kidney and activated to prevent the infection from ascending towards the renal parenchyma (Zhang et al. 2004). Notably, more recent studies have demonstrated that uropathogens can suppress NFκB and consequentially decrease the host's inflammatory response. This tactic allows the uropathogen to invade into deeper tissues (Klumpp et al. 2001). After 7-10 days the adaptive immune response is activated where specific uropathogens are recognised by B and T lymphocytes with high affinity antibodies.

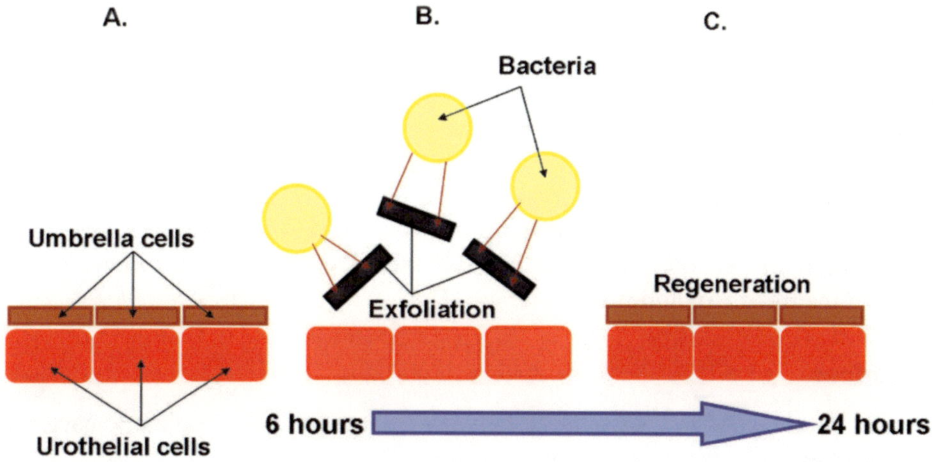

Fig. 8. In healthy patients the umbrella cell layer lining the lumen of the urinary bladder is renewed every few months (A). However, epithelial cells exfoliate within 6 hours after infection with an invasive uropathogen (B). This excretory process allows for effective excretion of infected urothelial cells. Within 24 hours of exfoliation proliferation cascades induce effective regeneration of a new umbrella cell layer.

Apart from triggering the initial inflammatory response, recruited neutrophils are also important for providing resistance to UTIs as demonstrated in one study on mice (Haraoka et al. 1999). Results from this study showed that UTIs are persistent in mice with specific genetic backgrounds and that UTIs will resolve spontaneously in mice with normal backgrounds. These findings suggest that specific host genes may be important for effective resolution of the UTI as demonstrated in another study on mice where TLR11 recognised uropathogenic E. coli and prevented its ascension into the kidneys (Hopkins et al. 1998). Interestingly, TLR11 is truncated in humans and susceptibility for pyelonephritis is increased. Furthermore, a study by Mysorekar *et al* demonstrated that females with recurrent UTIs had reduced levels of CD16 which led to decreased bacterial phagocytosis (Mysorekar et al. 2002).

The urinary tract is a component of the secretory immune system as it is the first defence system encountered by invading uropathogens. Infections of the kidneys are associated with serum and kidney immunoglobulin synthesis and type specific antibodies have been detected in the host's urine. Serum antibodies targeting type 1 and P pili have been detected after episodes of pyelonephritis with IgG and SIgA antibodies also detected in the urine (Rene et al. 1982). Synthesis of these specific antibodies occurs locally to enhance the opsonisation process in infected patients and to reduce adherence of E. coli (de Ree and van den Bosch 1987). The potential for modifying these immunological factors to decrease the incidence of UTIs in susceptible patients has been explored through immunisation techniques in animal models. Vaccination with P fimbria has been shown to decrease adherence of P-fimbriated E. coli to uroepithelial cells and prevent pyelonephritis in monkeys (Roberts and Phillips 1979). In addition, vaccination with FimH adhesin has been shown to prevent cystitis in mice (Langermann et al. 1997). It is therefore plausible that vaccination techniques may reduce colonisation and ascending infections in susceptible female patients (Uehling et al. 1994a, Uehling et al. 1994b).

7. Conclusions

A renewed interest in the pathogenesis of UTIs has developed over recent years. Pathogenic mechanisms are complicated and influenced by the biological and behavioural features of the host as well as adhesins from the invading uropathogen. Advances at a molecular level have led to a greater understanding in adherence mechanisms between bacterial virulence factors and the host's uroepithelial receptors. An improved understanding of these pathogenic mechanisms and associated host risk factors is important for developing novel strategies for the treatment and prevention of UTIs.

8. References

Abrutyn, E., Boscia, J. A. and Kaye, D. (1988) 'The treatment of asymptomatic bacteriuria in the elderly', *J Am Geriatr Soc,* 36(5), 473-5.

Anderson, G. G., Dodson, K. W., Hooton, T. M. and Hultgren, S. J. (2004a) 'Intracellular bacterial communities of uropathogenic Escherichia coli in urinary tract pathogenesis', *Trends Microbiol,* 12(9), 424-30.

Anderson, G. G., Martin, S. M. and Hultgren, S. J. (2004b) 'Host subversion by formation of intracellular bacterial communities in the urinary tract', *Microbes Infect,* 6(12), 1094-101.

Bonadio, M., Meini, M., Gigli, C., Longo, B. and Vigna, A. (1999) 'Urinary tract infection in diabetic patients', *Urol Int,* 63(4), 215-9.

Bronsema, D. A., Adams, J. R., Pallares, R. and Wenzel, R. P. (1993) 'Secular trends in rates and etiology of nosocomial urinary tract infections at a university hospital', *J Urol,* 150(2 Pt 1), 414-6.

Brooks, H. J., Benseman, B. A., Peck, J. and Bettelheim, K. A. (1981) 'Correlation between uropathogenic properties of Escherichia coli from urinary tract infections and the antibody-coated bacteria test and comparison with faecal strains', *J Hyg (Lond),* 87(1), 53-61.

Busch, R. and Huland, H. (1984) 'Correlation of symptoms and results of direct bacterial localization in patients with urinary tract infections', *J Urol,* 132(2), 282-5.

Coker, C., Poore, C. A., Li, X. and Mobley, H. L. (2000) 'Pathogenesis of Proteus mirabilis urinary tract infection', *Microbes Infect,* 2(12), 1497-505.

de Ree, J. M. and van den Bosch, J. F. (1987) 'Serological response to the P fimbriae of uropathogenic Escherichia coli in pyelonephritis', *Infect Immun,* 55(9), 2204-7.

Eden, C. S., Hanson, L. A., Jodal, U., Lindberg, U. and Akerlund, A. S. (1976) 'Variable adherence to normal human urinary-tract epithelial cells of Escherichia coli strains associated with various forms of urinary-tract infection', *Lancet,* 1(7984), 490-2.

Eschenbach, D. A., Davick, P. R., Williams, B. L., Klebanoff, S. J., Young-Smith, K., Critchlow, C. M. and Holmes, K. K. (1989) 'Prevalence of hydrogen peroxide-producing Lactobacillus species in normal women and women with bacterial vaginosis', *J Clin Microbiol,* 27(2), 251-6.

Fihn, S. D., Boyko, E. J., Chen, C. L., Normand, E. H., Yarbro, P. and Scholes, D. (1998) 'Use of spermicide-coated condoms and other risk factors for urinary tract infection caused by Staphylococcus saprophyticus', *Arch Intern Med,* 158(3), 281-7.

Fihn, S. D., Boyko, E. J., Normand, E. H., Chen, C. L., Grafton, J. R., Hunt, M., Yarbro, P., Scholes, D. and Stergachis, A. (1996) 'Association between use of spermicide-coated condoms and Escherichia coli urinary tract infection in young women', *Am J Epidemiol,* 144(5), 512-20.

Forland, M., Thomas, V. and Shelokov, A. (1977) 'Urinary tract infections in patients with diabetes mellitus. Studies on antibody coating of bacteria', *JAMA,* 238(18), 1924-6.

Fowler, J. E., Jr. and Stamey, T. A. (1977) 'Studies of introital colonization in women with recurrent urinary infections. VII. The role of bacterial adherence', *J Urol,* 117(4), 472-6.

Foxman, B. (2002) 'Epidemiology of urinary tract infections: incidence, morbidity, and economic costs', *Am J Med,* 113 Suppl 1A, 5S-13S.

Foxman, B., Marsh, J., Gillespie, B., Rubin, N., Koopman, J. S. and Spear, S. (1997) 'Condom use and first-time urinary tract infection', *Epidemiology,* 8(6), 637-41.

Freedman, L. R. (1975) 'Natural history of urinary infection in adults', *Kidney Int Suppl,* 4, S96-100.

Frendeus, B., Godaly, G., Hang, L., Karpman, D., Lundstedt, A. C. and Svanborg, C. (2000) 'Interleukin 8 receptor deficiency confers susceptibility to acute experimental pyelonephritis and may have a human counterpart', *J Exp Med,* 192(6), 881-90.

Frendeus, B., Godaly, G., Hang, L., Karpman, D. and Svanborg, C. (2001) 'Interleukin-8 receptor deficiency confers susceptibility to acute pyelonephritis', *J Infect Dis,* 183 Suppl 1, S56-60.

Godaly, G., Frendeus, B., Proudfoot, A., Svensson, M., Klemm, P. and Svanborg, C. (1998) 'Role of fimbriae-mediated adherence for neutrophil migration across Escherichia coli-infected epithelial cell layers', *Mol Microbiol,* 30(4), 725-35.

Godaly, G., Proudfoot, A. E., Offord, R. E., Svanborg, C. and Agace, W. W. (1997) 'Role of epithelial interleukin-8 (IL-8) and neutrophil IL-8 receptor A in Escherichia coli-induced transuroepithelial neutrophil migration', *Infect Immun,* 65(8), 3451-6.

Gruneberg, R. N. (1969) 'Relationship of infecting urinary organism to the faecal flora in patients with symptomatic urinary infection', *Lancet,* 2(7624), 766-8.

Gupta, K., Scholes, D. and Stamm, W. E. (1999) 'Increasing prevalence of antimicrobial resistance among uropathogens causing acute uncomplicated cystitis in women', *JAMA,* 281(8), 736-8.

Gupta, K., Stapleton, A. E., Hooton, T. M., Roberts, P. L., Fennell, C. L. and Stamm, W. E. (1998) 'Inverse association of H2O2-producing lactobacilli and vaginal Escherichia coli colonization in women with recurrent urinary tract infections', *J Infect Dis,* 178(2), 446-50.

Handley, M. A., Reingold, A. L., Shiboski, S. and Padian, N. S. (2002) 'Incidence of acute urinary tract infection in young women and use of male condoms with and without nonoxynol-9 spermicides', *Epidemiology,* 13(4), 431-6.

Haraoka, M., Hang, L., Frendeus, B., Godaly, G., Burdick, M., Strieter, R. and Svanborg, C. (1999) 'Neutrophil recruitment and resistance to urinary tract infection', *J Infect Dis,* 180(4), 1220-9.

Haspels, A. A., Luisi, M. and Kicovic, P. M. (1981) 'Endocrinological and clinical investigations in post-menopausal women following administration of vaginal cream containing oestriol', *Maturitas,* 3(3-4), 321-7.

Hawes, S. E., Hillier, S. L., Benedetti, J., Stevens, C. E., Koutsky, L. A., Wolner-Hanssen, P. and Holmes, K. K. (1996) 'Hydrogen peroxide-producing lactobacilli and acquisition of vaginal infections', *J Infect Dis,* 174(5), 1058-63.

Herthelius-Elman, M., Mollby, R., Nord, C. E. and Winberg, J. (1992) 'The effect of amoxycillin on vaginal colonization resistance and normal vaginal flora in monkeys', *J Antimicrob Chemother,* 29(3), 329-40.

Hillier, S. L., Krohn, M. A., Klebanoff, S. J. and Eschenbach, D. A. (1992) 'The relationship of hydrogen peroxide-producing lactobacilli to bacterial vaginosis and genital microflora in pregnant women', *Obstet Gynecol,* 79(3), 369-73.

Hooton, T. M. (2000) 'Pathogenesis of urinary tract infections: an update', *J Antimicrob Chemother,* 46 Suppl A, 1-7.

Hooton, T. M., Fennell, C. L., Clark, A. M. and Stamm, W. E. (1991a) 'Nonoxynol-9: differential antibacterial activity and enhancement of bacterial adherence to vaginal epithelial cells', *J Infect Dis,* 164(6), 1216-9.

Hooton, T. M., Hillier, S., Johnson, C., Roberts, P. L. and Stamm, W. E. (1991b) 'Escherichia coli bacteriuria and contraceptive method', *JAMA,* 265(1), 64-9.

Hooton, T. M., Scholes, D., Hughes, J. P., Winter, C., Roberts, P. L., Stapleton, A. E., Stergachis, A. and Stamm, W. E. (1996a) 'A prospective study of risk factors for symptomatic urinary tract infection in young women', *N Engl J Med,* 335(7), 468-74.

Hooton, T. M., Scholes, D., Stapleton, A. E., Roberts, P. L., Winter, C., Gupta, K., Samadpour, M. and Stamm, W. E. (2000) 'A prospective study of asymptomatic bacteriuria in sexually active young women', *N Engl J Med,* 343(14), 992-7.

Hooton, T. M. and Stamm, W. E. (1997) 'Diagnosis and treatment of uncomplicated urinary tract infection', *Infect Dis Clin North Am,* 11(3), 551-81.

Hooton, T. M., Winter, C., Tiu, F. and Stamm, W. E. (1996b) 'Association of acute cystitis with the stage of the menstrual cycle in young women', *Clin Infect Dis,* 23(3), 635-6.

Hopkins, W. J., Gendron-Fitzpatrick, A., Balish, E. and Uehling, D. T. (1998) 'Time course and host responses to Escherichia coli urinary tract infection in genetically distinct mouse strains', *Infect Immun,* 66(6), 2798-802.

Hultgren, S. J., Schwan, W. R., Schaeffer, A. J. and Duncan, J. L. (1986) 'Regulation of production of type 1 pili among urinary tract isolates of Escherichia coli', *Infect Immun,* 54(3), 613-20.

Iosif, C. S. and Bekassy, Z. (1984) 'Prevalence of genito-urinary symptoms in the late menopause', *Acta Obstet Gynecol Scand,* 63(3), 257-60.

Jones, C. H., Pinkner, J. S., Roth, R., Heuser, J., Nicholes, A. V., Abraham, S. N. and Hultgren, S. J. (1995) 'FimH adhesin of type 1 pili is assembled into a fibrillar tip structure in the Enterobacteriaceae', *Proc Natl Acad Sci U S A,* 92(6), 2081-5.

Justice, S. S., Hung, C., Theriot, J. A., Fletcher, D. A., Anderson, G. G., Footer, M. J. and Hultgren, S. J. (2004) 'Differentiation and developmental pathways of uropathogenic Escherichia coli in urinary tract pathogenesis', *Proc Natl Acad Sci U S A,* 101(5), 1333-8.

Kallenius, G., Mollby, R., Svenson, S. B. and Winberg, J. (1981) 'Microbial adhesion and the urinary tract', *Lancet,* 2(8251), 866.

Kau, A. L., Hunstad, D. A. and Hultgren, S. J. (2005) 'Interaction of uropathogenic Escherichia coli with host uroepithelium', *Curr Opin Microbiol,* 8(1), 54-9.

Kennedy, R. P., Plorde, J. J. and Petersdorf, R. G. (1965) 'Studies on the Epidemiology of Escherichia Coli Infections. Iv. Evidence for a Nosocomial Flora', *J Clin Invest,* 44, 193-201.

Khan, S. W. and Ahmed, A. (2001) 'Uropathogens and their susceptibility pattern: a retrospective analysis', *J Pak Med Assoc,* 51(2), 98-100.

Kisielius, P. V., Schwan, W. R., Amundsen, S. K., Duncan, J. L. and Schaeffer, A. J. (1989) 'In vivo expression and variation of Escherichia coli type 1 and P pili in the urine of adults with acute urinary tract infections', *Infect Immun,* 57(6), 1656-62.

Klemm, P. (1985) 'Fimbrial adhesions of Escherichia coli', *Rev Infect Dis,* 7(3), 321-40.

Klumpp, D. J., Weiser, A. C., Sengupta, S., Forrestal, S. G., Batler, R. A. and Schaeffer, A. J. (2001) 'Uropathogenic Escherichia coli potentiates type 1 pilus-induced apoptosis by suppressing NF-kappaB', *Infect Immun,* 69(11), 6689-95.

Kuehn, M. J., Ogg, D. J., Kihlberg, J., Slonim, L. N., Flemmer, K., Bergfors, T. and Hultgren, S. J. (1993) 'Structural basis of pilus subunit recognition by the PapD chaperone', *Science,* 262(5137), 1234-41.

Langermann, S., Palaszynski, S., Barnhart, M., Auguste, G., Pinkner, J. S., Burlein, J., Barren, P., Koenig, S., Leath, S., Jones, C. H. and Hultgren, S. J. (1997) 'Prevention of mucosal Escherichia coli infection by FimH-adhesin-based systemic vaccination', *Science,* 276(5312), 607-11.

Lau, Y. E., Rozek, A., Scott, M. G., Goosney, D. L., Davidson, D. J. and Hancock, R. E. (2005) 'Interaction and cellular localization of the human host defense peptide LL-37 with lung epithelial cells', *Infect Immun,* 73(1), 583-91.

Lipsky, B. A. (1989) 'Urinary tract infections in men. Epidemiology, pathophysiology, diagnosis, and treatment', *Ann Intern Med,* 110(2), 138-50.

Malaviya, R. and Abraham, S. N. (1998) 'Clinical implications of mast cell-bacteria interaction', *J Mol Med,* 76(9), 617-23.

McCarty, J. M., Richard, G., Huck, W., Tucker, R. M., Tosiello, R. L., Shan, M., Heyd, A. and Echols, R. M. (1999) 'A randomized trial of short-course ciprofloxacin, ofloxacin, or trimethoprim/sulfamethoxazole for the treatment of acute urinary tract infection in women. Ciprofloxacin Urinary Tract Infection Group', *Am J Med,* 106(3), 292-9.

McGroarty, J. A., Soboh, F., Bruce, A. W. and Reid, G. (1990) 'The spermicidal compound nonoxynol-9 increases adhesion of Candida species to human epithelial cells in vitro', *Infect Immun,* 58(6), 2005-7.

Mobley, H. L., Island, M. D. and Massad, G. (1994) 'Virulence determinants of uropathogenic Escherichia coli and Proteus mirabilis', *Kidney Int Suppl,* 47, S129-36.

Mulvey, M. A. (2002) 'Adhesion and entry of uropathogenic Escherichia coli', *Cell Microbiol,* 4(5), 257-71.

Mulvey, M. A., Lopez-Boado, Y. S., Wilson, C. L., Roth, R., Parks, W. C., Heuser, J. and Hultgren, S. J. (1998) 'Induction and evasion of host defenses by type 1-piliated uropathogenic Escherichia coli', *Science,* 282(5393), 1494-7.

Mulvey, M. A., Schilling, J. D., Martinez, J. J. and Hultgren, S. J. (2000) 'Bad bugs and beleaguered bladders: interplay between uropathogenic Escherichia coli and innate host defenses', *Proc Natl Acad Sci U S A,* 97(16), 8829-35.

Munoz, P., Llancaqueo, A., Rodriguez-Creixems, M., Pelaez, T., Martin, L. and Bouza, E. (1997) 'Group B streptococcus bacteremia in nonpregnant adults', *Arch Intern Med,* 157(2), 213-6.

Mysorekar, I. U., Mulvey, M. A., Hultgren, S. J. and Gordon, J. I. (2002) 'Molecular regulation of urothelial renewal and host defenses during infection with uropathogenic Escherichia coli', *J Biol Chem,* 277(9), 7412-9.

Nicolle, L. E., Friesen, D., Harding, G. K. and Roos, L. L. (1996) 'Hospitalization for acute pyelonephritis in Manitoba, Canada, during the period from 1989 to 1992; impact of diabetes, pregnancy, and aboriginal origin', *Clin Infect Dis,* 22(6), 1051-6.

Parsek, M. R. and Singh, P. K. (2003) 'Bacterial biofilms: an emerging link to disease pathogenesis', *Annu Rev Microbiol,* 57, 677-701.

Poljakovic, M. and Persson, K. (2003) 'Urinary tract infection in iNOS-deficient mice with focus on bacterial sensitivity to nitric oxide', *Am J Physiol Renal Physiol,* 284(1), F22-31.

Poljakovic, M., Svensson, M. L., Svanborg, C., Johansson, K., Larsson, B. and Persson, K. (2001) 'Escherichia coli-induced inducible nitric oxide synthase and cyclooxygenase expression in the mouse bladder and kidney', *Kidney Int,* 59(3), 893-904.

Raz, R. (2001) 'Postmenopausal women with recurrent UTI', *Int J Antimicrob Agents,* 17(4), 269-71.

Raz, R., Gennesin, Y., Wasser, J., Stoler, Z., Rosenfeld, S., Rottensterich, E. and Stamm, W. E. (2000) 'Recurrent urinary tract infections in postmenopausal women', *Clin Infect Dis,* 30(1), 152-6.

Raz, R. and Stamm, W. E. (1993) 'A controlled trial of intravaginal estriol in postmenopausal women with recurrent urinary tract infections', *N Engl J Med,* 329(11), 753-6.

Reid, G. and Sobel, J. D. (1987) 'Bacterial adherence in the pathogenesis of urinary tract infection: a review', *Rev Infect Dis,* 9(3), 470-87.

Rene, P., Dinolfo, M. and Silverblatt, F. J. (1982) 'Serum and urogenital antibody responses to Escherichia coli pili in cystitis', *Infect Immun,* 38(2), 542-7.

Roberts, A. P. and Phillips, R. (1979) 'Bacteria causing symptomatic urinary tract infection or asymptomatic bacteriuria', *J Clin Pathol,* 32(5), 492-6.

Ronald, A. (2003) 'The etiology of urinary tract infection: traditional and emerging pathogens', *Dis Mon,* 49(2), 71-82.

Ronald, A. and Ludwig, E. (2001) 'Urinary tract infections in adults with diabetes', *Int J Antimicrob Agents,* 17(4), 287-92.

Rosenstein, I. J., Stafford, M. K., Kitchen, V. S., Ward, H., Weber, J. N. and Taylor-Robinson, D. (1998) 'Effect on normal vaginal flora of three intravaginal microbicidal agents potentially active against human immunodeficiency virus type 1', *J Infect Dis,* 177(5), 1386-90.

Schaeffer, A. J., Jones, J. M. and Dunn, J. K. (1981) 'Association of vitro Escherichia coli adherence to vaginal and buccal epithelial cells with susceptibility of women to recurrent urinary-tract infections', *N Engl J Med,* 304(18), 1062-6.

Schaeffer, A. J., Radvany, R. M. and Chmiel, J. S. (1983) 'Human leukocyte antigens in women with recurrent urinary tract infections', *J Infect Dis,* 148(3), 604.

Schaeffer, A. J., Schwan, W. R., Hultgren, S. J. and Duncan, J. L. (1987) 'Relationship of type 1 pilus expression in Escherichia coli to ascending urinary tract infections in mice', *Infect Immun,* 55(2), 373-80.

Schlager, T. A. (2001) 'Urinary tract infections in children younger than 5 years of age: epidemiology, diagnosis, treatment, outcomes and prevention', *Paediatr Drugs,* 3(3), 219-27.

Schlager, T. A., Hendley, J. O., Bell, A. L. and Whittam, T. S. (2002) 'Clonal diversity of Escherichia coli colonizing stools and urinary tracts of young girls', *Infect Immun,* 70(3), 1225-9.

Smellie, J., Edwards, D., Hunter, N., Normand, I. C. and Prescod, N. (1975) 'Vesico-ureteric reflux and renal scarring', *Kidney Int Suppl,* 4, S65-72.

Smith, H. S., Hughes, J. P., Hooton, T. M., Roberts, P., Scholes, D., Stergachis, A., Stapleton, A. and Stamm, W. E. (1997) 'Antecedent antimicrobial use increases the risk of uncomplicated cystitis in young women', *Clin Infect Dis,* 25(1), 63-8.

Stamm, W. E. and Hooton, T. M. (1993) 'Management of urinary tract infections in adults', *N Engl J Med,* 329(18), 1328-34.

Stapleton, A. (2002) 'Urinary tract infections in patients with diabetes', *Am J Med,* 113 Suppl 1A, 80S-84S.

Sun, T. T. (1996) 'Epithelial growth and differentiation: an overview', *Mol Biol Rep,* 23(1), 1-2.

Talan, D. A., Stamm, W. E., Hooton, T. M., Moran, G. J., Burke, T., Iravani, A., Reuning-Scherer, J. and Church, D. A. (2000) 'Comparison of ciprofloxacin (7 days) and trimethoprim-sulfamethoxazole (14 days) for acute uncomplicated pyelonephritis pyelonephritis in women: a randomized trial', *JAMA,* 283(12), 1583-90.

Thomas, T. M., Plymat, K. R., Blannin, J. and Meade, T. W. (1980) 'Prevalence of urinary incontinence', *Br Med J,* 281(6250), 1243-5.

Uehling, D. T., Hopkins, W. J., Dahmer, L. A. and Balish, E. (1994a) 'Phase I clinical trial of vaginal mucosal immunization for recurrent urinary tract infection', *J Urol,* 152(6 Pt 2), 2308-11.

Uehling, D. T., Hopkins, W. J., James, L. J. and Balish, E. (1994b) 'Vaginal immunization of monkeys against urinary tract infection with a multi-strain vaccine', *J Urol,* 151(1), 214-6.

Vaisanen, V., Elo, J., Tallgren, L. G., Siitonen, A., Makela, P. H., Svanborg-Eden, C., Kallenius, G., Svenson, S. B., Hultberg, H. and Korhonen, T. (1981) 'Mannose-resistant haemagglutination and P antigen recognition are characteristic of Escherichia coli causing primary pyelonephritis', *Lancet,* 2(8260-61), 1366-9.

Vetsch, M., Puorger, C., Spirig, T., Grauschopf, U., Weber-Ban, E. U. and Glockshuber, R. (2004) 'Pilus chaperones represent a new type of protein-folding catalyst', *Nature,* 431(7006), 329-33.

Vosti, K. L., Goldberg, L. M., Monto, A. S. and Rantz, L. A. (1964) 'Host-Parasite Interaction in Patients with Infections Due to Escherichia Coli. I. The Serogrouping of E. Coli from Intestinal and Extraintestinal Sources', *J Clin Invest,* 43, 2377-85.

Winberg, J., Gezelius, L., Guldevall, L. and Mollby, R. (1993) 'Cephadroxil promotes vaginal colonization with Escherichia coli', *Infection,* 21(4), 201-5.

Wright, S. W., Wrenn, K. D. and Haynes, M. L. (1999) 'Trimethoprim-sulfamethoxazole resistance among urinary coliform isolates', *J Gen Intern Med,* 14(10), 606-9.

Wu, X. R., Sun, T. T. and Medina, J. J. (1996) 'In vitro binding of type 1-fimbriated Escherichia coli to uroplakins Ia and Ib: relation to urinary tract infections', *Proc Natl Acad Sci U S A,* 93(18), 9630-5.

Yamamoto, S., Tsukamoto, T., Terai, A., Kurazono, H., Takeda, Y. and Yoshida, O. (1997) 'Genetic evidence supporting the fecal-perineal-urethral hypothesis in cystitis caused by Escherichia coli', *J Urol,* 157(3), 1127-9.

Zhang, D., Zhang, G., Hayden, M. S., Greenblatt, M. B., Bussey, C., Flavell, R. A. and Ghosh, S. (2004) 'A toll-like receptor that prevents infection by uropathogenic bacteria', *Science,* 303(5663), 1522-6.

8

Urinary Tract Immunology

Kelesidis Theodoros
Department of Medicine, Division of Infectious Diseases,
David Geffen School of Medicine at UCLA,
Los Angeles, California,
USA

1. Introduction

Urinary tract infection (UTI) is one of the most common infections in humans. It is estimated that 40% of women and 12% of men will experience a symptomatic UTI, with incidences peaking in their early 20s or after age 85, respectively (1). Approximately 25% of these women will experience recurrence within 6 to 12 months (1). Uropathogenic *Escherichia coli* (UPEC) is the most common etiological agent responsible for uncomplicated UTI. In the United States alone, the estimated annual societal cost of UTI is more than 3 billion dollars (1).

Despite significant advances in the understanding of UPEC biology, mechanistic details regarding the host response to UTI and full comprehension of genetic loci that influence susceptibility require additional work. As new and intriguing details of how uropathogens initiate infections and persist within the urinary tract have emerged, so has important information regarding how the immune system functions within the urinary tract. The complex cross-linking for innate and adaptive immune response as well as humoral and cellular effectors is the key to the urinary tract immune system and to its defense against pathogenic microorganisms. As antibiotic therapy becomes increasingly ineffective, modulating the innate and adaptive immune system in the urinary tract using TLR4 ligands and other immunomodulators may become viable options to combat UTIs.

2. Innate responses to urinary tract infections

2.1 Host factors that prevent colonization of urinary tract with UPEC

Uroepithelial adherence is critical for establishment of UTI. The urinary tract, comprised of the urethra, bladder, ureters and the kidneys, represents a formidable mechanical barrier to infection. In addition to the relative impregnability of the epithelium lining the tract, potential pathogens have to contend with the powerful flushing action of urine and the aggregating actions of urinary mucins (2;3). UPEC strains possess an impressive repertoire of adhesins that enable them to aggregate and adhere to cellular surfaces (4). Consequently, the first line of host defense against UTI is concentrated on preventing UPEC adherence to the bladder mucosa. The luminal surface of the bladder is lined with highly sulfated and anionic glycosaminoglycans (GAGs) that contribute to bladder wall impermeability and afford an antimicrobial anti-adherence property. Intuitively, urine flow seems to be a convenient defense mechanism; however, FimH binds to mannose moieties using "catch-bonds," interactions that are actually strengthened by the sheer stress induced during urine flow (5). Thus, more active mechanisms, like umbrella cell exfoliation (6) that occurs by an apoptosis-like mechanism and is promoted by FimH (7) remove adherent UPEC. Tamm-Horsfall protein (THP) is a high-molecular-weight protein present in human urine (8) that binds E. coli fimbriae (9) by virtue of its mannose moieties, inhibiting fimbrial interaction with uroplakin receptors (10). This phenotype translated in vivo as thp−/− mice were unable to control lower-UTI (11). THP also appears to act as an innate-adaptive immunoregulatory molecule that can activate dendritic cells (12).

2.2 Host signaling in response to UPEC recognition

Of the various immune surveillance molecules the Toll-like receptor (TLR) family is the best characterized (13-16). Unlike the receptor for the FimH adhesin of UPEC, which promotes bacterial invasion and subsequent invasion of BECs (17), the TLRs function by detecting different PAMPs and then mobilizing appropriate immune defences. The common TLRs encountered in the urinary tract include TLR2 (recognizes bacterial lipoteichoic acid or lipoprotein), TLR3 (recognizes double stranded RNA), TLR4 [recognizes lipopolysaccharides (LPS)], TLR5 (recognizes flagellin), TLR9 (recognizes unmethylated CpG DNA of bacteria and viruses), and TLR11 (recognizes profiling of parasites). TLR5 and TLR11 are other TLRs shown in *in vivo* studies to contribute to immune defence in the urinary tract (13;16). TLR5 is predominantly expressed on bladder cells whereas TLR11 is primarily on kidney cells (13;16). Perhaps the best studied of these TLRs is TLR4, which is well expressed on epithelial cells of the kidney and bladder (14).

Toll-like receptor 4 (TLR4) is important for signalling of innate immunity in response to UTI

Upon successful adherence to the uroepithelium, Toll-like receptor (TLR) recognition of pathogen-associated molecular patterns generates signaling cascades to control infection and direct adaptive responses (18). Particular close attention has been given to the role of TLR4 in UTIs. LR4 mutation (TLR4-/-) mice failed to initiate an immune response against UTI, and they developed an asymptomatic carrier state resembling human asymptomatic bacteriuria (ABU) (19) . Interestingly, recent studies have shown that TLR4 has antimicrobial roles that appear to be specific to the urinary tract (20) (21). These include promotion of IL-6 and IL-8 secretion by activation of the MyD88- or cAMP-dependent signaling pathway, inhibition of bladder epithelial cell (BEC) invasion by bacteria, and expulsion of UPEC harboring in BECs (21-24). Clinical research found that children with UTI have lower TLR4 expression than age-matched controls without UTI. In relation to UTI history, children with low TLR4 expression on their neutrophils display an asymptomatic bacteriuria (ABU) carrier state lacking both inflammation and bacterial clearance (25). Meanwhile, adult patients with chronic UTI were found to have lower TLR4 expression than healthy controls without UTI (26). All these imply that enhanced TLR4 expression possibly contributes to increased mucosal immune response.

It has been known that C3H/HeJ mice, harboring a mutation in the Toll/interleukin-1 receptor (TIR) domain of TLR4, cannot resolve UTI as efficiently as LPS-responsive C3H/HeN counterparts (27). In accordance, tlr4−/− mice had significantly higher bacterial burdens in their bladders than similarly infected wild-type mice (28). This clearance defect is the result of insufficient downstream cytokine and chemokine production and neutrophil recruitment (29). Data from mouse chimeras disclosed that TLR4 on both stromal and hematopoietic cells is critical for normal inflammatory responses and clearance of UPEC in the bladder and kidney (30). Correspondingly, children with low TLR4 expression on their neutrophils display an asymptomatic bacteriuria (ABU) carrier state lacking both inflammation and bacterial clearance (25). A similar response is exhibited by C3N/HeJ mice following UPEC inoculation (31).

TLR4-mediated signaling is mainly LPS independent

TLR4-mediated signaling in the urinary tract does not appear to be the result of the archetypal interaction with LPS. Both the role of LPS in and the molecular trigger of TLR4 signaling by UPEC are topics of debate (32). Studies using the A498 human kidney cell line indicate that TLR4 signaling in response to UPEC requires P fimbriae and can be mediated independently of LPS (33). Mechanistic details regarding this phenomenon include P fimbriae binding to surface glycosphingolipids (GSLs) and subsequent release of the GSL membrane-anchoring domain, ceramide (34). Ceramide appears to act as a TLR4 agonist and the putative intermediate for TLR4 signaling initiated by P fimbriae (34). Lastly, the FimH tip adhesin of type 1 fimbriae was recently shown to directly interact with TLR4, an additional means for LPS-independent stimulation by UPEC fimbriae (35)

TLR4-mediated signaling is also LPS dependent

In contrast to LPS-independent signaling by P fimbriae, there appears to be a cooperative stimulation of TLR4 by LPS and type 1 fimbriae (36). This cooperative stimulation directly correlates with the level of cluster of differentiation 14 (CD14) expression on bladder cells (24). CD14 is an accessory molecule required for optimal TLR4 signaling in response to LPS (24). Immunohistochemical (IHC) analysis of human bladder biopsies revealed that CD14 expression is localized to the submucosa (37), suggesting that uroepithelial cells exposed to the lumen have little to no CD14 expression and therefore may not respond efficiently to LPS alone. These results support a role for both independent and cooperative TLR4 stimulation by UPEC fimbriae.

Downstream signalling pathways important for signalling of innate immunity in response to UTI

Infection of knockout mice has revealed critical roles for myeloid differentiation primary response protein 88 (MyD88), TIR domain-containing adaptor inducing beta interferon (TRIF), and TRIF-related adaptor molecule (TRAM) in signaling for UPEC clearance (38). It is also apparent that different fimbrial types influence the corresponding downstream signaling pathways (38). Regardless of the fimbria involved in stimulation, all pathways involving these adaptor molecules result in activation of NF-κB and proinflammatory gene expression. Song and colleagues identified an accompanying proinflammatory bladder cell signaling pathway that is also dependent on TLR4 but results in a spike in intracellular calcium levels (39). This calcium spike leads to adenylyl cyclase 3 (AC3)-mediated increase in cAMP, protein kinase A (PKA) activation, phosphorylation of the cAMP response element-binding protein transcription factor (CREB), and proinflammatory gene expression such as transcription of IL-6 and IL-8 (39). Using selective blockade of these signaling cascades, Song et al. determined that activation of epithelial IL-6 secretion by *E. coli* might even be faster via the CREB pathway than the canonical pathway and can also be activated by TLR2 and TLR3 ligands (39).

Other TLR pathways important for signalling of innate immunity in response to UTI

Other TLR pathways have been implicated in host defense during UTI. In a recent case-control study of adult women with a history of UTI in which TLR genes were examined, polymorphisms in TLR1, TLR4, and TLR5 were correlated with protection from, or susceptibility to, some UTI phenotypes (40). TLR2 is stimulated by peptidoglycan, as might be presented by gram-positive uropathogens, including *Enterococcus* and *Staphylococcus* species, as well as by lipoproteins and perhaps OmpA (41) of other extraintestinal pathogenic *E. coli*. Tlr2−/− mice appear to respond normally to acute UTI (31). TLR5 appears to play a UPEC recognition role in the bladder (13). TLR5 recognizes the structural subunit of flagella, which are essential for UPEC motility in the urinary tract induces inflammatory cytokines and chemokines (13). Mice lacking TLR5, which responds to bacterial flagellin, permit higher bacterial loads in the bladder and kidney following transurethral inoculation (13). In contrast to TLR5 which has a bladder-specific role during UTI, TLR11 has a kidney-specific role during UTI (16). The murine receptor TLR11, associated with a pseudogene in humans, also appears to respond to uropathogenic bacteria (16). Conversely, tlr11−/− mice are more susceptible than wild-type mice to UPEC kidney infection (16) a UPEC-encoded homolog has yet to be identified for TLR11 ligand. The fact that there is a stop codon in the open reading frame of human genomic and cell line tlr11 sequences may help explain acute and recurrent UTI susceptibility in humans (16).

Other Non-TLR pathways important for signalling of innate immunity in response to UTI

Surface molecules other than TLRs are also involved in host-UPEC interactions. Upon UPEC exposure, the cytoplasmic tail of uroplakin IIIa undergoes phosphorylation, and intracellular calcium levels increase, presumably important events for uroepithelial cell apoptosis and exfoliation(42) Although uroplakin Ia is thought to be the main receptor for UPEC FimH in vivo (167, 256, 286), type 1 fimbriae may bind to a number of host molecules, including uroplakin complexes (42) extracellular matrix proteins (43) CD molecules (44), and integrins (45). The CD44 ligand, hyaluronic acid (HA), accumulates in the urinary tract during UTI; UPEC can bind HA, thereby facilitating interaction with CD44 and tissue invasion (46). In accordance with this, cd44−/− mice are more resistant to UPEC kidney colonization and successive dissemination (46). Also, there are still unidentified players in inflammation and clearance of UPEC. For example, LPS-responder C3H/OuJ mice were found to be equally susceptible to UTI as non-LPS-responder C3H/HeJ mice yet demonstrated elevated levels of inflammation (47), revealing a susceptibility locus to map.

2.3 Metabolic host pathways against UPEC during UTI

Host factors against iron metabolism of UPEC

That E. coli strains causing UTI have several functionally redundant systems dedicated to iron uptake (48) suggests that the urinary tract, like other host niches, is an iron-limited environment (49). Siderophores are secreted iron-chelating molecules that allow bacteria to scavenge free and host protein-bound iron (50). Enterobactin, for instance, can bind free ferric ions with a higher affinity than transferrin (51) a host iron transport protein responsible for regulating the free iron concentration in serum(52). A transferrin family member, lactoferrin, evokes antimicrobial activity by sequestering iron over a range of pH. Lactoferrin is secreted by kidney cells and is found in neutrophil granules and thus could be involved in combating UTI (53). Both transferrin and lactoferrin have been shown to evoke direct antimicrobial activity by disrupting Gram-negative membranes (54).

In addition to iron sequestration, there are host factors that directly counter the action of siderophores. Early studies indicated that serum albumin, alone or in concert with other serum proteins, can impede bacterial siderophore function (55). In addition, the mammalian protein lipocalin 2 (Lcn2) can bind and sequester enterobactin and similar catecholate siderophores (56). Lcn2 inhibits enterobactin-dependent propagation of E. coli in vitro, and lcn2−/− mice are unable to control systemic E. coli burdens as well as wild-type mice (56) Production of Lcn2 is induced by TLR4, implicating iron regulation as a part of the immune response to infection(56). Murine GeneChip and quantitative PCR (qPCR) analyses confirmed that Lcn2 mRNA is upregulated by the uroepithelium of infected mice (57). Interestingly, these results were obtained in C3H/HeJ mice, indicating that a TLR4-independent signaling pathway can activate transcription of the lcn2 gene in response to UTI. Not surprisingly, UPEC has evolved a mechanism to counter Lcn2 siderophore sequestration. Encoded within the iroA gene cluster are glycosyltransferases that modify enterobactin in such a way that it cannot be bound by Lcn2 (58). Thus, both the host and UPEC have systems in place to manage their own iron stores and to inhibit iron acquisition by the other—a molecular arms race for an essential nutrient.

2.4 Metabolic host factors against UPEC

The role for bacterial central metabolism during infection has only been recently appreciated (59). Genes important for glucose import were upregulated by the uroepithelium of C3H/HeJ mice experiencing UTI, possibly for either nutrient sequestration or energy to combat infection(57). This fact, coupled with the knowledge that UPEC does not chemotax toward glucose in vitro (60) or utilize glucose as a primary carbon source in vivo (61) implies that UPEC may have evolved to use alternative carbon sources in the urinary tract. These results imply that nutrient acquisition is also a crucial aspect of bacterial pathogenesis and the host response that may influence the outcome of UTI.

2.5 Epithelial host pathways against UPEC during UTI

Life cycle of UPEC in urinary tract epithelium

There has been a growing body of literature revealing that UPEC appears to have three distinct intracellular lifestyle components within the urinary tract (62). The first is uptake by apical endocytosis of Rab27b+/CD63+ fusiform vesicles, which are subsequently recycled back to the cell surface and exocytosed (20). The other two pathways both begin with uptake into a membrane-bound compartment which can lead to either a quiescent nonreplicative existence (63) or escape from compartmental life to undergo a highly replicative phase in the cell cytoplasm. While internalization via the fusiform vesicle pathway may be a side effect of normal bladder epithelium function, cellular uptake by the other two pathways is perhaps intended by UPEC to establish a reservoir to persist in the urinary tract (63). Indeed, UPEC has been shown to exist in the urinary tract for weeks, even after antibiotic treatment (64). Infection of 10 genetically distinct mouse strains also revealed that some strains were more susceptible to persistence than others, indicating that host hereditary components may also contribute to the ability of UPEC to persevere in the urinary tract (65).

2.6 Epithelial host factors have important role against compartmental escape of UPEC

Infected mouse bladder explants monitored by time lapse fluorescence videomicroscopy generated a model for the intracellular UPEC life cycle instigated after uptake in a membrane-bound compartment (nonfusiform vesicle route)(66). While the mechanism of compartmental escape remains undefined, once contained in cytoplasmic "intracellular bacterial communities" (IBCs), UPEC can undergo several changes in morphology, categorized as early, middle, and late IBC stages (66). Late IBCs that escape exfoliation with umbrella cells contain filamentous UPEC that are not present in C3H/HeJ mice, indicating that this morphological change may be a bacterial stress response to TLR4-mediated immune activation (66). This murine background also experienced increased incidence and severity of IBCs compared to immunocompetent mice (66). Urothelial cells proximal to IBCs in C3H/HeJ mice upregulate transferrin receptor, Lcn2, complement system components (C3, factor B, and CD55), and lysozyme (57). Involucrin and suprabasin transcripts were also increased, indicating that, in addition to gene products that function to eradicate bacteria, proteins important for epithelial integrity may be an imperative host response during UTI (57).

Notably, TLR4 also plays a noninflammatory role in host defense against UPEC by modulating the activity of the observed secretory and vesicular internalization pathways. TLR4-mediated PKA activation suppresses the lipid raft endocytic pathway (21), a possible effort to prevent the establishment of persistence reservoirs. Also along these lines, UPEC exocytosis in fusiform vesicles was actually accelerated by TLR4-mediated recognition of LPS and dependent on the activities of cAMP, Rab27b, caveolin-1, and the scaffolding protein MyRIP (22).

The role of urothelial regeneration in response to UPEC infection

One of the consequences of UPEC infection is exfoliation of the superficial facet cell layer that lines the surface of the bladder lumen (67). Microarray analyses probing regenerative signals revealed that, in addition to genes involved in cell biological processes, inflammatory cytokines, chemokines, signaling molecules, and transcription factors are also upregulated in response to inoculation (68). While regeneration itself appears to be a function of basal stem/progenitor cells in the transitional epithelium (68) studies of the gut epithelium unveiled macrophages as "cellular transceivers" that relay MyD88-dependent inputs from the epithelium to colonic epithelial progenitors via direct contact (69). Whether or not macrophages play a similar role in the urinary tract remains unknown.

2.7 Antimicrobial peptides, cytokines and chemokines against UPEC during UTI

Antimicrobial peptides (AMPs) are short positively charged peptides secreted by both epithelial and hematopoietic cells that disrupt bacterial membranes and can be chemotactic for certain immune cells (70). Human β-defensin-1 mRNA and protein were found in kidney tissue, implicating this AMP in host defense against UPEC (71). More convincingly, mice deficient in defb1, a murine homolog of human β-defensin, have a significantly higher incidence of bacteriuria (72). Murine β-defensin is also a dendritic cell (DC) ligand that instigates upregulation of costimulatory molecules and maturation (73). The human cathelicidin, LL-37, and its murine homolog, cathelin-related antimicrobial peptide (CRAMP), are secreted in response to UPEC exposure (44). Studies using CRAMP-deficient mice revealed that epithelial-derived CRAMP is important during the early stages of UTI while leukocyte-derived CRAMP likely functions later when bacteria penetrate the kidney epithelium (46).

2.8 Cytokines and chemokines against UPEC during UTI

The role of IL-8-mediated neutrophil recruitment in phenotypic susceptibility to UTIs

Human C-X-C ligand 8 (hCXCL8; interleukin-8 [IL-8]) is the main chemoattractant for neutrophils in humans, and murine CXCL1 (mCXCL1) and mCXCL2 (also known as KC and MIP-2, respectively) are the functional mouse homologs of IL-8 (26). Bladder and kidney cell lines secrete IL-8 in response to UPEC (26). Human and murine studies both demonstrate that neutrophil migration to the UPEC-infected urinary tract is dependent on IL-8 (26). Additionally, mCXCL2 secretion is dependent on TLR4, as secretion was deficient in infected C3H/HeJ mice (100). hCXCR1 and hCXCR2 are receptors for a number of chemokines, including IL-8 (26). Both are expressed in bladder and kidney biopsies, and transmigration studies indicated that hCXCR1 plays a dominant role in IL-8-dependent neutrophil migration (74). Consistent with this, children prone to pyelonephritis tend to have low hCXCR1 expression and heterozygous hCXCR1 polymorphisms (74). Using a large cohort of families that included children with a history of recurrent UTIs, Svanborg and colleagues found that low CXCR1 (IL-8 receptor) expression levels correlated with the incidence of acute pyelonephritis (75). Subsequently, CXCR1 mutations and polymorphisms were identified in several patients with recurrent pyelonephritis (76). Although CXCR1 mutations were not correlated with pyelonephritis in a separate cohort of Italian children, IL-8 gene polymorphisms were found in this latter group (77). hCXCR1 deficiency results in impaired bacterial clearance but, unlike TLR4 deficiency, with intact inflammatory signaling that ultimately results in tissue damage(31).

Similarly, mice lacking mCXCR2 (the functional homolog for hCXCL1) experience subepithelial accumulation of neutrophils, increased bacterial titers, and renal scarring after UPEC inoculation (78) and increased susceptibility to experimental UTI and urinary tract-derived bacteremia (79;80). These data indicate that normal function of neutrophils, their chemotactic ligands, and their chemokine receptors are required for bacterial clearance without postinflammatory sequelae.

The role of other cytokines in phenotypic susceptibility to UTIs

Despite ample information on IL-8 in vitro and in vivo, a complete picture of the cytokine and chemokine dynamics during UTI was lacking. In response, a longitudinal assessment using a Bio-Plex format was conducted(81). Chemokine (C-C motif) ligand 2 (CCL2 or MCP-1), CCL4 (or MIP-1b), CCL5 (or RANTES), CXCL1, IL-1β, IL-6, IL-12p40, IL-17, tumor necrosis factor alpha (TNF-α), and granulocyte-colony stimulating factor (G-CSF) were all upregulated in bladder homogenates from UPEC-infected C57BL/6 mice (81). These results agreed with patient and cell line data regarding upregulation of IL-6 in response to UPEC (82). In mice, TNF-α expression was elevated at 1 h post-inoculation for rapid mobilization of acute responses (81); this waned at later time points, likely to prevent the deleterious effects of uncontrolled TNF-α signaling (16). Expression of most cytokines and chemokines peaked around 24 h post-inoculation, returning to near baseline at 2 weeks (81). These dynamics correlate well with the peak and resolution of bacterial burdens in C57BL/6 mice(81). One notable exception was IL-17, which was highly upregulated from 6 h to 1 week post-inoculation, remaining above baseline through the 2-week experimental duration(81). Importantly, IL-17A (the Th17 signature cytokine) contributes to innate clearance of UPEC through a mechanism involving cytokine and chemokine secretion and macrophage and neutrophil influx (26). Similar to TLR adaptor molecule usage (38) the type of fimbriae expressed also seems to influence the repertoire of chemokines secreted. Specifically, kidney cells exposed to type 1-fimbriated UPEC secrete neutrophil-associated chemokines, while P fimbriae-stimulated cells secrete chemokines targeting antigen-presenting cell (APC)- and Th1-specific cytokines, exemplified by CCL2 and CCL5 expression (83). In addition, IFN-γ and IL-4 (signature cytokines of the Th1 and Th2 lineages, respectively) and IL-10 (a T-regulatory [Treg] effector cytokine) knockout mice were tested for susceptibility to both acute cystitis and pyelonephritis (84). While il4−/− and il10−/− mice appear to experience infection dynamics similar to the wild type, ifnγ−/− mice had increased incidence and severity of UTI (84) implying a role for IFN-γ and Th1-mediated inflammatory responses during UTI.

2.9 The role of neutrophils in immune responses to UPEC-mediated UTI

Infected mouse bladders examined histologically display thickening of epithelium accompanied by robust infiltration of inflammatory cells and edema in the lamina propria (85). Neutrophils are the most rapid and abundant responders to the infected urinary tract (85). Efficient migration of neutrophils requires intracellular adhesion molecule 1 (ICAM-1) expression by epithelial cells and β2 integrin (CD11b/CD18) expression by neutrophils (30). G-CSF is also required for the neutrophil response, and unexpectedly, mice with neutralized G-CSF are more resistant to UTI(81). Although monocyte/macrophage numbers were similar in anti-G-CSF-treated mice, cytokines important for macrophage activation were upregulated, potentially leading to accelerated clearance by enhanced phagocytic killing (81). Despite counterintuitive phenotypes with respect to cytokine knock-down, antibody-mediated knockdown of the neutrophil population confirmed their crucial role in bacterial clearance, especially within the kidney (86). Lastly, the electrostatic properties of the UPEC P fimbrial tip adhesin may interfere with neutrophil binding, a potential host response evasion tactic specific to the kidney (86).

2.10 The role of APCs in immune responses to UPEC-mediated UTI

Compared to the neutrophil response, relatively little is known about APCs in the context of UTI. In mice, resident CD11c+ cells that express low to intermediate levels of F4/80 and CD11b macrophage markers were found in the kidney (87) while CD11c+ cells expressing the major histocompatibility class II activation marker were found in the bladder (30). In spite of macrophage marker expression, CD11c+ kidney cells had physical and functional characteristics of DCs (87). At 24 h post inoculation, CD11c+ cells that migrate to the bladder did not express CD8α, Gr-1, or B220 and thus were not plasmacytoid or lymphoid but appeared to be TNF-α- and inducible NOS (iNOS)-producing (Tip)-DCs (88) that express intermediate levels of CD11b. Infection studies in mice lacking Tip-DCs suggested that they are not necessary for the host response to acute UTI (88). Since Tip-DCs are necessary for the generation of mucosal IgA (89), their role may lie in mediating the humoral response to UPEC. Similar to what was observed for DCs, there appears to be a resident population of macrophages in bladder tissue that increases by several orders of magnitude in response to UTI (81). Monocytes expressing high levels of Gr-1, which can give rise to macrophages or DCs, are also recruited to the bladder in response to UPEC infection. Release of these cells from the bone marrow was dependent on CCR2 (90), and, correspondingly, CCL2 is upregulated in the bladder response to UTI(81).

2.11 The role of the antimicrobial compound nitric oxide (NO) in immune responses to UPEC-mediated UTI

Some of the factors utilized by neutrophils, macrophages, and DCs for pathogen uptake and destruction have been described during UTI. iNOS generates the antimicrobial compound nitric oxide (NO) from l-arginine and was originally reported to be secreted by macrophages

(91). Although iNOS is rapidly upregulated in the inoculated bladder(92) two independent groups reported that inos−/− mice are equally as susceptible to UTI as wild-type mice, suggesting that neuronal NOS, endothelial NOS, or myeloperoxidase may act as compensatory factors (93) Alternatively or in addition, inos−/− animals may lack a colonization phenotype because there are several factors (Hfq and Nsr-regulated genes, polyamines, and flavohemoglobin) expressed by UPEC that enhance tolerance to reactive nitrogen species in vitro (94) suggesting that NO production may be an ineffective host defense against UPEC.

2.12 The role of the complement in immune responses to UPEC-mediated UTI

With respect to the complement system, it appears that UPEC is able to bind C3 to enter host uroepithelial cells via the surface receptors Crry or CD46 (95). Correspondingly, c3−/− mice are more resistant to renal damage and infection (95). As C3 levels are significantly higher in the urine of UTI patients (96) UPEC may stimulate C3 production for pathogenic means or has evolved to exploit this host defense factor.

2.13 The role of innate-like lymphocytes (ILLs) in acute UTI host defense

Infection studies using severe combined immunodeficient (SCID) mice that lack functional B and T cells and nude mice that lack thymically derived T cells provide preliminary evidence of a role for innate-like lymphocytes (ILLs) in acute UTI host defense (97). Epithelial γδ T cells, B-1 cells, and natural killer T (NKT) cells are ILLs: cellular subsets that have relatively invariant receptors and reside in specific locations of the body (26). After a 2-day primary infection, SCID mice had significantly higher bacterial counts in their bladder and kidneys, while nude mice were colonized similarly to wild-type animals (97). The lack of a colonization phenotype in nude mice suggests that either antibody responses independent of thymus-derived T-cell help or extrathymically produced T cells may play a role in innate clearance of UPEC. The latter suggestion has some experimental support.

The role of γδ T cells

γδ T cells can be produced extrathymically and rapidly secrete cytokines in response to stimulation (98). Resident γδ T cells found in the bladder increase in response to UTI (26), and TCR δ−/− mice are more susceptible to UTI than isogenic controls (84). As γδ TCR+ cells express IL-17A during UPEC-mediated UTI (26) this rapid-response cell population may function in concert with other innate factors to mediate neutrophil influx for clearance of UPEC.

The role of B-1 cells

B-1 cells spontaneously secrete large quantities of polyspecific IgM against bacterial and self-antigens, and in contrast to conventional (B-2) B cells, do not require T-cell help (99). While IgM secreted by B-1 cells might play a role in innate clearance of UPEC, current evidence suggests otherwise. JHD mice, lacking both B-1 and B-2 cells (100) infected and monitored over a 14-day time period exhibited no significant increase in incidence or severity of cystitis (84).

The role of NK T cells

On a final note regarding ILLs, administration of α-galactosylceramide (α-GalCer), a ligand for CD1d-restricted NKT cells, alleviates renal UPEC infection (101). Consistent with this, a resident population of NK1.1+ cells (potentially NK or NKT cells) in the bladder of C57BL/6 mice that increases in response to UTI has been reported (26). Studies using a systemic E. coli infection model suggested that, similar to γδ T cells, NKT cells may act as early amplifiers of the innate immune response to UTI by rapid cytokine secretion (102).

3. Genetic factors that contribute to innate immunity

Although susceptibility to UTI thus far appears to be related primarily to function of the innate immune system, additional determinants are likely important in this polygenic phenotype. For example, the increased susceptibility of C3H/HeJ mice was recently suggested to be due to at least two other loci in addition to *Tlr4 (103)* Accelerating progress in genomic sequencing methodology might facilitate the elucidation of other contributing genes, but these efforts may be hampered somewhat by the continuous, rather than discrete, nature of UTI susceptibility phenotypes in human populations.

The individual's response to UTI is variable and the susceptibility to the infection is inheritable. Lundstedt et al. found in a family study, 15% of the relatives of pyelonephritis-prone children had UTI history, whereas the value was 3% in the controls(75). A evaluation of a familal predisposition about women with recurrent UTI described that 65.5% of mothers, 60.7% of daughters, and 48.6% of sisters of the women had a similar history (104). Many studies discovered that genitic variations of TLR4 and CXCR1 are association with susceptibility to different type of UTIs. And TLR4(896)AG genotype and TLR4(896)G alleles could increase the risk for UTI in childhood (76;105), CXCR1 G (2608) C gene polymorphism and expression are strong linked to acute pyelonephritis in children (77). Reduced expression levels of CXCR1 and TLR4 in neutrophils are associated with pyelonephritis, recurrent cystitis, and asymptomatic bacteriuria in children and premenopausal women (25)(78;106). Although these studies suggest the association of gene polymorphisms and expression of TLR4 and CXCR1 to UTIs, whether the variants are associated with UTI in adults is still unknown.

3.1 Other host factors that contribute to innate immunity

Other mediators also shape the extent of the polymorphonuclear leukocyte (PMN) response to infection. Perpetuation of the PMN response might be controlled by cytokines such as IL-17, which has an emerging role in bridging innate to adaptive immunity(107) and is present at high levels in the bladder at later time points. Plasminogen activator inhibitor type 1 (PAI-1) influences cell migration through its effects on integrin binding; upon UPEC infection of mice lacking PAI-1, kidneys bore significantly higher bacterial burdens and fewer PMN infiltrates than wild-type counterparts did (108). UPEC infection was recently demonstrated to induce the secretion of granulocyte colony-stimulating factor (gCSF) in the bladder, and antibody-mediated depletion of this cytokine reduced PMN influx following UPEC infection (81).

Finally, the secretion of a number of soluble antibacterial compounds into the urinary tract is induced by UPEC infection. UPEC infection also elicits the production of nitric oxide in association with upregulation of the iNOS gene (92). However, UPEC may employ strategies to resist the antibacterial effect of nitric oxide, as mice deficient in iNOS generally have shown no increased susceptibility to UTI (93;109). Among short antibacterial peptides, the human cathelicidin LL-37 is detectable in the urine during human cystitis, and mice deficient in its ortholog (CRAMP) demonstrate increased susceptibility to UTI (110).

4. Cellular and humoral adaptive immune responses to UPEC-mediated UTI

Existing data regarding adaptive immune responses to UPEC are relatively limited. In a seminal study, Thumbikat and colleagues engineered a strain of UPEC to express ovalbumin to examine mechanisms behind antigen-specific adaptive immune responses in experimental UTI (111). In response to reinfection, CD4+ and CD8+ cells infiltrated the bladder and expressed the CD69 activation marker in the spleen (111), extending the findings of early IHC studies probing T- and B-cell populations in infected bladders (109). Furthermore, splenocytes, enriched splenic T cells, or serum antibodies from previously infected donor mice each protected wild-type naïve recipient mice against UPEC challenge (111). This result suggests that protection derived from natural infection is antibody mediated, as UPEC-specific antibody-secreting plasma cells could be present in both splenocyte and enriched T-cell preparations. As expected, transfers from naïve donor mice did not facilitate enhanced protection to recipients (111). This result is in contrast to a previous murine adoptive transfer study where SCID recipients receiving splenocytes from either naïve or vaccinated wild-type donors exhibited equal levels of enhanced clearance, despite the presence of antigen-specific plasma cells in the vaccinated donor cells (97). This result suggests that simply reconstituting immunosuppressed mice with lymphoid cells provides the means (likely stimulatory cytokines for phagocytic cells) for enhanced clearance. Conversely, wild-type recipient mice used in the former study only exhibited enhanced clearance when given cells or serum from antigen-educated, vaccinated donors (111), indicating that enhanced protection in individuals with intact immune systems will be provided only by stimulation of an effective adaptive immune response.

4.1 The role of T cells in adaptive immune responses to UPEC-mediated UTI

T-cell subsets are characterized by transcription factors and cytokines involved in their differentiation and the particular effector cytokines they secrete. To date, studies have not implicated a skew toward Th1- or Th2-mediated UTI immunity (111). DC phagocytosis of infected apoptotic cells is the key event required for DCs to secrete the cytokine milieu necessary for Th17 development (112), and both DCs and infected apoptotic cells are present in the bladder during UTI. Despite this connection, IL-17A is dispensable for the generation of a protective response in a murine reinfection model, suggesting that Th17 cells may not play a role in adaptive responses to UPEC infection (26). Similar to APCs and other lymphocytes, there are resident CD8+ cells in the bladder that increase in response to infection (26;111). It has been suggested that the observed CD8+ cells are either classical cytotoxic T cells or intraepithelial lymphocytes that exert cytotoxic effects on UPEC- or virus-infected cells or rapidly secrete cytokines to mobilize innate immune responses (26). Lastly, the role of Treg subsets in UTI host defense has not been formally examined.

4.2 The role of antibody-mediated clearance in adaptive immune responses to UPEC-mediated UTI

Despite the lack of detail regarding T-cell responses to UTI, there is ample evidence for antibody-mediated clearance of UPEC. The genitourinary tract has been recognized as part of the secretory immune system (113). UPEC-specific antibodies are detected in the urine of infected patients and in the urine or serum of animals exposed to UPEC antigens (111). Urinary IgG and IgA from UTI patients are capable of inhibiting UPEC adherence (114). Patient studies have also suggested that antibody responses to pyelonephritis are, in general, stronger and last longer than humoral responses to cystitis (115). Analysis of murine urine and serum samples collected before and after vaccination with OMP iron receptors allowed identification of immunological correlates of vaccine-induced protection against UTI (116). Specifically, levels of either urinary IgA or serum IgG (relative to serum IgM; denoted the class switch index) inversely correlated with bladder colonization in vaccinated mice (116). Presumably, urinary IgA plays a direct role in UPEC clearance from the bladder mucosa, while IgG may be a marker for class switching by B cells or also play a direct role in mucosal bacterial clearance. As mentioned earlier, infected JHD mice had wild-type levels of colonization in response to primary infection, suggesting that B cells have no role in innate clearance of UPEC (84). However, this result is not unexpected since both antigen presentation and antibody-mediated protection provided by B cells would likely play a role in adaptive responses, indicating a need for reevaluation of these mice in UPEC reinfection and vaccination challenge models.

5. Immunomodulation as therapeutic option for UTI

There are several practiced and proposed therapeutics for UTI management. Prophylactic treatments include estrogen in postmenopausal women (117) or cranberry juice (118) although the efficacy of the former remains controversial. Immunomodation strategies are emerging therapies for UTIs especially in the setting of increasing antimicrobial resistance.

5.1 Non-vaccine strategies

Since the lining of the urinary tract is highly enriched in TLR4 molecules, administering TLR4 specific ligands directly to the urinary tract could trigger TLR4 mediated innate immune responses thereby enhancing local reactivity and resistance to infection. Treatment of UPEC-infected mice with forskolin, a drug that increases intracellular cyclic AMP (cAMP) levels, expels UPEC from intracellular vesicles into the extracellular milieu, rendering the bacteria susceptible to immune responses and antibiotics (20). Similarly, exposing the bladder to protamine sulfate, a highly cationic protein, removes bound and intracellular UPEC by causing umbrella cells to exfoliate (63)), unfortunately with a significant level of discomfort, as reported by study volunteers (119). In addition to a number of nonspecific chemical treatments (120)), both small-molecule inhibitors (121) and specific antibody directed against FimH (122) demonstrated some utility in preventing bacterial adherence. While antibiotic therapy remains the standard treatment for UTI, overuse leads to deleterious alterations of the normal host microbiota (123) and selection for resistant strains (124), prompting the need for vaccine-mediated prevention of UTI.

Astragalus is a Chinese herbal medicine, and Astragalus polysaccharide (APS) is its main components. Previous studies have demonstrated that APS could induce enhancement of expression of TLR4 on bladder epithelial cells (125) and astragalus also increases the TLR4 expression on monocytes in UTI patients. These suggest that similar to LPS, APS can activate pre-inflammatory factor secretion during the early stages of infection similar to LPS, promote TLR4 expression, and involve mucosal innate immunity of the urinary tract. However it remains to be seen whether this herbal medicine can be a therapeutic option for UTI.

These observations suggest that activators of the TLR4 signalling pathway in the urinary tract can be effective therapeutic agents against infections. Furthermore, it is not necessary to use TLR4 ligands for activation of the pathway. Inducers of downstream substrates of the pathway are also effective activators of the innate immune response. Even if TLR4 ligands are employed for therapeutic use, it is unlikely that LPS will be the ligand of choice since LPS has intrinsic toxicity. A TLR4 ligand with greatly improved safety profiles, such as monophosphoryl lipid (MPL), could be used in its place (126).

5.2 Vaccines

The involvement of TLRs in the immune response to UTI and current knowledge of their ability to incite innate and direct adaptive responses make them attractive adjuvant candidates for UTI vaccines (127). These and other mucosal adjuvants and variations in vaccination routes and schedules must be tested in an effort to generate UPEC-specific local and systemic antibodies(128) and optimize production of immunological memory, not tolerance . A more detailed knowledge of adaptive immune responses to UPEC is a prerequisite for the development of next-generation candidate vaccines for the prevention of UTI. More recently, a variety of experimental approaches have been applied to search for immunodominant epitopes, revealing an array of new candidate targets, and thus a number of vaccine antigens have been explored (26).

Lipopolysaccharide (LPS) and side chain (O) antigen as vaccine targets

Early vaccine studies focused on the lipopolysaccharide (LPS) side chain (O) antigen (129). There are trends regarding the frequencies of particular O antigens among UTI isolates(130) and O-antigen-specific antibodies demonstrate an anti-adhesive effect (130). Nonetheless, significant structural heterogeneity may represent an insurmountable obstacle for development of an O-antigen-based vaccine. Furthermore, a study evaluating antibody responses in mice intranasally vaccinated with a killed *E. coli* lacking capsule and O antigen demonstrated that these surface features actually obstruct optimal humoral responses (131)

P fimbriae as vaccine targets

Later studies involved vaccines directed against particular virulence factors. The pore-forming toxin alpha-hemolysin (HlyA) and P fimbriae are proposed minimal factors required for colonization of and dissemination from the kidney (132). P fimbriae are adherence organelles that play a role in kidney colonization in mice and humans (133). There are convincing data using both murine (132) and primate models (134) that vaccination against P fimbriae or HlyA prevents renal colonization and damage. Additionally, to overcome P fimbrial allelic variability, linear peptide sequences that generated cross-reactive antibodies were evaluated as protective antigens (135). Despite these successes, vaccines targeting P fimbriae may not be effective because of their limited role during bladder colonization. Type 1 fimbria is a *bona fide* virulence factor of UPEC and, in contrast to P fimbria, is critical for bladder colonization (136). Animals vaccinated with various components of type 1 fimbriae had increased levels of antigen-specific antibodies and decreased levels of colonization upon challenge (137). Unfortunately, expression of type 1 fimbria is subject to phase variation, allowing UPEC to evade humoral responses targeting this organelle(138). Additionally, since nonpathogenic isolates also express type 1 fimbriae (139), targeting this population may result in detrimental disruption of the host microbiota. Also of note, both P and type 1 fimbriae were not necessary for colonization of the human neurogenic bladder, indicating the need for alternative targets in certain high-risk patient groups (140). Although vaccines based on P or type 1 pilus components have generated substantial mucosal antibody responses, protection from subsequent infections has been incomplete, perhaps because of phase variation in the expression of these antigens during infection.

Iron pathway as target for vaccine

Iron is essential for nearly all organisms (141) and UPEC strains encode a battery of genes involved in iron acquisition. Vaccination with UPEC outer membrane protein (OMP) fractions enriched for iron receptors protects against experimental sepsis (142). Additionally, mice vaccinated subcutaneously with denatured IroN, an OMP siderophore receptor and urovirulence factor (143), had both increased levels of antigen-specific serum IgG and reduced kidney colonization upon challenge (144). Undetectable levels of IgA in the bladder mucosa after this vaccination may explain why these animals were not protected from cystitis (144). Recently, a broad functional vaccinology initiative was conducted using an "omics" approach to identify vaccine candidates: UPEC proteins that are pathogen-specific, antigenic, surface-exposed, and *in vivo* expressed (26). Strikingly, the top targets identified by this approach were all OMPs functioning in iron uptake. Intranasal vaccination with three of six candidates afforded protection from cystitis and pyelonephritis, suggesting that combining antigenic motifs found in these proteins may be an effective multivalent vaccine for UTI (26).

Other vaccine targets

Vaccines consisting of bacterial components or whole cells have also been assessed. Transurethral immunization of mice with a live-attenuated UPEC strain lacking the ability to persist in the urinary tract engendered heterologous protection (145) a potential platform for further development. SolcoUrovac, a vaginal suppository containing 10 heat-killed uropathogenic strains, has been tested in mice , in nonhuman primates , and in clinical trials (26). While safe, SolcoUrovac vaccination did not result in appreciable increases in local specific antibody, nor did it afford protection without periodic readministration (146).

Vaccine strategies to combat UTIs

Since B and T cells, which mediate adaptive immunity are critically dependent on signals derived from the innate immune system, modulators that boost innate immune responses may be of value in boosting adaptive immune responses (147-150). Thus, immunomodulators used to boost innate immune responses in the urinary tract may be also employed to boost adaptive immune responses. One of the reasons for administering vaccine antigens against UTIs in the genitourinary tract, as in the case of the vaginal mucosal vaccine mentioned above, is to evoke secretory IgA (sIgA) antibodies in the mucosal surfaces of the urinary tract. Whereas subcutaneous, intramuscular, or intravenous immunization evokes strong systemic IgG responses to the vaccine antigens, they fail to evoke IgA antibodies in the mucosal surfaces of the urinary tract where infections are initiated and where antibodies are most needed (111).

However, administering vaccines directly to the urinary tract is neither easy nor practical. A much more accessible mucosal site for the delivery of vaccines is the nasal passages. Delivery of proteus antigens into the nasal passages of mice have been shown to evoke high levels of sIgA in the urine and this was accompanied by impressive protection against *Proteus mirabilis* induced UTI (151). Immunization at nasal sites has been shown to be highly effective in evoking antigen specific serum IgG as well as sIgA responses in various mucosal sites presumably due to activation of the nasal associated lymphoid tissue (NALT) found in the nasal passage. Since the NALT is a potent immunologically inductive and sampling site, it can respond vigorously to vaccine antigens and if TLR ligands or other adjuvants are present, this response may be even more magnified (152). Taken together, an alternate or complementary approach for the management of UTIs in the future could be targeted administration of modulators of the TLR signalling pathway to boost both innate and adaptive responses in the urinary tract.

Cumulatively, all the indications suggest that the urinary tract is able to mount an appreciable and protective adaptive immune response and that this property can be harnessed for vaccination purposes. An important and as yet unanswered question is the duration of protection in the urinary tract following infection or vaccination. Since up to 25% of women with UTIs that have no underlying immune competency issues have recurrences (153) it is conceivable that the immunity generated in the urinary tract could be relatively short lived and therefore frequent vaccinations may be required.

6. Conclusion

The over use of broad spectrum antibiotics has led to the emergence of antibiotic resistant bacteria many of which have been implicated in UTIs. As a consequence, management of these infections constitutes a serious and growing medical challenge. Modulating or co-opting the powerful innate and adaptive immune systems of the urinary tract could potentially have important therapeutic and prophylactic implications for the treatment of UTIs, particularly where conventional approaches are ineffective.

There is considerable work to be done to better understand the mechanisms of protective immunity against UPEC in the bladder. Specifically, available knockout mouse strains could be used to systematically evaluate the role of various receptors, signaling molecules, cytokines and chemokines, and cell types in controlling UPEC-mediated UTI and eliciting potent adaptive and memory immune responses. Ideally, the field can acquire insights on UTI immunity at a level suitable to rationally develop a much-needed vaccine that elicits sterilizing immunity against UPEC in the human urinary tract.

Unlike antibiotic treatment, immunomodulation will not be broadly applicable. Instead, it will have to be tailored to each patient and must take into consideration, among other factors, the virulence and antibiotic resistance profile of the infecting bacteria as well as the age, immune competence and genetic make-up of the patient. For example, employing TLR4 ligands to boost immunity in patients with defective TLR4 genes will not be productive but the use of activators of downstream components of the pathway could be useful. Thus, for these proposed emerging strategies to be completely effective, comprehensive information regarding relevant traits of the pathogen and the host will become necessary.

7. References

[1] Foxman B. Epidemiology of urinary tract infections: incidence, morbidity, and economic costs. Am J Med 2002; 113 Suppl 1A:5S-13S.

[2] Denman SJ, Burton JR. Fluid intake and urinary tract infection in the elderly. JAMA 1992; 267(16):2245, 2249.

[3] Eckford SD, Keane DP, Lamond E, Jackson SR, Abrams P. Hydration monitoring in the prevention of recurrent idiopathic urinary tract infections in pre-menopausal women. Br J Urol 1995; 76(1):90-93.

[4] Pizarro-Cerda J, Cossart P. Bacterial adhesion and entry into host cells. Cell 2006; 124(4):715-727.

[5] Shrom SH, Parsons CL, Mulholland SG. Role of urothelial surface mucoprotein in intrinsic bladder defense. Urology 1977; 9(5):526-533.

[6] Mulvey MA, Schilling JD, Hultgren SJ. Establishment of a persistent Escherichia coli reservoir during the acute phase of a bladder infection. Infect Immun 2001; 69(7):4572-4579.

[7] Mulvey MA, Lopez-Boado YS, Wilson CL, Roth R, Parks WC, Heuser J et al. Induction and evasion of host defenses by type 1-piliated uropathogenic Escherichia coli. Science 1998; 282(5393):1494-1497.

[8] Tamm I, HORSFALL FL, Jr. A mucoprotein derived from human urine which reacts with influenza, mumps, and Newcastle disease viruses. J Exp Med 1952; 95(1):71-97.

[9] Parkkinen J, Virkola R, Korhonen TK. Identification of factors in human urine that inhibit the binding of Escherichia coli adhesins. Infect Immun 1988; 56(10):2623-2630.

[10] Pak J, Pu Y, Zhang ZT, Hasty DL, Wu XR. Tamm-Horsfall protein binds to type 1 fimbriated Escherichia coli and prevents E. coli from binding to uroplakin Ia and Ib receptors. J Biol Chem 2001; 276(13):9924-9930.

[11] Bates JM, Raffi HM, Prasadan K, Mascarenhas R, Laszik Z, Maeda N et al. Tamm-Horsfall protein knockout mice are more prone to urinary tract infection: rapid communication. Kidney Int 2004; 65(3):791-797.

[12] Saemann MD, Weichhart T, Zeyda M, Staffler G, Schunn M, Stuhlmeier KM et al. Tamm-Horsfall glycoprotein links innate immune cell activation with adaptive immunity via a Toll-like receptor-4-dependent mechanism. J Clin Invest 2005; 115(2):468-475.

[13] Andersen-Nissen E, Hawn TR, Smith KD, Nachman A, Lampano AE, Uematsu S et al. Cutting edge: Tlr5-/- mice are more susceptible to Escherichia coli urinary tract infection. J Immunol 2007; 178(8):4717-4720.

[14] Samuelsson P, Hang L, Wullt B, Irjala H, Svanborg C. Toll-like receptor 4 expression and cytokine responses in the human urinary tract mucosa. Infect Immun 2004; 72(6):3179-3186.

[15] Schilling JD, Mulvey MA, Vincent CD, Lorenz RG, Hultgren SJ. Bacterial invasion augments epithelial cytokine responses to Escherichia coli through a lipopolysaccharide-dependent mechanism. J Immunol 2001; 166(2):1148-1155.

[16] Zhang D, Zhang G, Hayden MS, Greenblatt MB, Bussey C, Flavell RA et al. A toll-like receptor that prevents infection by uropathogenic bacteria. Science 2004; 303(5663):1522-1526.

[17] Martinez JJ, Mulvey MA, Schilling JD, Pinkner JS, Hultgren SJ. Type 1 pilus-mediated bacterial invasion of bladder epithelial cells. EMBO J 2000; 19(12):2803-2812.

[18] Medzhitov R, Janeway CA, Jr. Innate immunity: the virtues of a nonclonal system of recognition. Cell 1997; 91(3):295-298.

[19] Hagberg L, Hull R, Hull S, McGhee JR, Michalek SM, Svanborg EC. Difference in susceptibility to gram-negative urinary tract infection between C3H/HeJ and C3H/HeN mice. Infect Immun 1984; 46(3):839-844.

[20] Bishop BL, Duncan MJ, Song J, Li G, Zaas D, Abraham SN. Cyclic AMP-regulated exocytosis of Escherichia coli from infected bladder epithelial cells. Nat Med 2007; 13(5):625-630.
[21] Song J, Bishop BL, Li G, Duncan MJ, Abraham SN. TLR4-initiated and cAMP-mediated abrogation of bacterial invasion of the bladder. Cell Host Microbe 2007; 1(4):287-298.
[22] Song J, Bishop BL, Li G, Grady R, Stapleton A, Abraham SN. TLR4-mediated expulsion of bacteria from infected bladder epithelial cells. Proc Natl Acad Sci U S A 2009; 106(35):14966-14971.
[23] Miyazaki J, Kawai K, Oikawa T, Johraku A, Hattori K, Shimazui T et al. Uroepithelial cells can directly respond to Mycobacterium bovis bacillus Calmette-Guerin through Toll-like receptor signalling. BJU Int 2006; 97(4):860-864.
[24] Schilling JD, Martin SM, Hunstad DA, Patel KP, Mulvey MA, Justice SS et al. CD14- and Toll-like receptor-dependent activation of bladder epithelial cells by lipopolysaccharide and type 1 piliated Escherichia coli. Infect Immun 2003; 71(3):1470-1480.
[25] Ragnarsdottir B, Samuelsson M, Gustafsson MC, Leijonhufvud I, Karpman D, Svanborg C. Reduced toll-like receptor 4 expression in children with asymptomatic bacteriuria. J Infect Dis 2007; 196(3):475-484.
[26] Sivick KE, Mobley HL. Waging war against uropathogenic Escherichia coli: winning back the urinary tract. Infect Immun 2010; 78(2):568-585.
[27] Svanborg EC, Briles D, Hagberg L, McGhee J, Michalec S. Genetic factors in host resistance to urinary tract infection. Infection 1985; 13 Suppl 2:S171-S176.
[28] Ashkar AA, Mossman KL, Coombes BK, Gyles CL, Mackenzie R. FimH adhesin of type 1 fimbriae is a potent inducer of innate antimicrobial responses which requires TLR4 and type 1 interferon signalling. PLoS Pathog 2008; 4(12):e1000233.
[29] Shahin RD, Engberg I, Hagberg L, Svanborg EC. Neutrophil recruitment and bacterial clearance correlated with LPS responsiveness in local gram-negative infection. J Immunol 1987; 138(10):3475-3480.
[30] Schilling JD, Martin SM, Hung CS, Lorenz RG, Hultgren SJ. Toll-like receptor 4 on stromal and hematopoietic cells mediates innate resistance to uropathogenic Escherichia coli. Proc Natl Acad Sci U S A 2003; 100(7):4203-4208.
[31] Ragnarsdottir B, Fischer H, Godaly G, Gronberg-Hernandez J, Gustafsson M, Karpman D et al. TLR- and CXCR1-dependent innate immunity: insights into the genetics of urinary tract infections. Eur J Clin Invest 2008; 38 Suppl 2:12-20.
[32] Poltorak A, He X, Smirnova I, Liu MY, Van HC, Du X et al. Defective LPS signaling in C3H/HeJ and C57BL/10ScCr mice: mutations in Tlr4 gene. Science 1998; 282(5396):2085-2088.
[33] Hedges S, Svensson M, Svanborg C. Interleukin-6 response of epithelial cell lines to bacterial stimulation in vitro. Infect Immun 1992; 60(4):1295-1301.
[34] Fischer H, Ellstrom P, Ekstrom K, Gustafsson L, Gustafsson M, Svanborg C. Ceramide as a TLR4 agonist; a putative signalling intermediate between sphingolipid receptors for microbial ligands and TLR4. Cell Microbiol 2007; 9(5):1239-1251.
[35] Mossman KL, Mian MF, Lauzon NM, Gyles CL, Lichty B, Mackenzie R et al. Cutting edge: FimH adhesin of type 1 fimbriae is a novel TLR4 ligand. J Immunol 2008; 181(10):6702-6706.
[36] Hedlund M, Frendeus B, Wachtler C, Hang L, Fischer H, Svanborg C. Type 1 fimbriae deliver an LPS- and TLR4-dependent activation signal to CD14-negative cells. Mol Microbiol 2001; 39(3):542-552.

[37] Hedlund M, Wachtler C, Johansson E, Hang L, Somerville JE, Darveau RP et al. P fimbriae-dependent, lipopolysaccharide-independent activation of epithelial cytokine responses. Mol Microbiol 1999; 33(4):693-703.

[38] Fischer H, Yamamoto M, Akira S, Beutler B, Svanborg C. Mechanism of pathogen-specific TLR4 activation in the mucosa: fimbriae, recognition receptors and adaptor protein selection. Eur J Immunol 2006; 36(2):267-277.

[39] Song J, Duncan MJ, Li G, Chan C, Grady R, Stapleton A et al. A novel TLR4-mediated signaling pathway leading to IL-6 responses in human bladder epithelial cells. PLoS Pathog 2007; 3(4):e60.

[40] Hawn TR, Scholes D, Li SS, Wang H, Yang Y, Roberts PL et al. Toll-like receptor polymorphisms and susceptibility to urinary tract infections in adult women. PLoS One 2009; 4(6):e5990.

[41] Jeannin P, Magistrelli G, Goetsch L, Haeuw JF, Thieblemont N, Bonnefoy JY et al. Outer membrane protein A (OmpA): a new pathogen-associated molecular pattern that interacts with antigen presenting cells-impact on vaccine strategies. Vaccine 2002; 20 Suppl 4:A23-A27.

[42] Thumbikat P, Berry RE, Zhou G, Billips BK, Yaggie RE, Zaichuk T et al. Bacteria-induced uroplakin signaling mediates bladder response to infection. PLoS Pathog 2009; 5(5):e1000415.

[43] Wu XR, Sun TT, Medina JJ. In vitro binding of type 1-fimbriated Escherichia coli to uroplakins Ia and Ib: relation to urinary tract infections. Proc Natl Acad Sci U S A 1996; 93(18):9630-9635.

[44] Khan NA, Kim Y, Shin S, Kim KS. FimH-mediated Escherichia coli K1 invasion of human brain microvascular endothelial cells. Cell Microbiol 2007; 9(1):169-178.

[45] Eto DS, Jones TA, Sundsbak JL, Mulvey MA. Integrin-mediated host cell invasion by type 1-piliated uropathogenic Escherichia coli. PLoS Pathog 2007; 3(7):e100.

[46] Rouschop KM, Sylva M, Teske GJ, Hoedemaeker I, Pals ST, Weening JJ et al. Urothelial CD44 facilitates Escherichia coli infection of the murine urinary tract. J Immunol 2006; 177(10):7225-7232.

[47] Hopkins W, Gendron-Fitzpatrick A, McCarthy DO, Haine JE, Uehling DT. Lipopolysaccharide-responder and nonresponder C3H mouse strains are equally susceptible to an induced Escherichia coli urinary tract infection. Infect Immun 1996; 64(4):1369-1372.

[48] Welch RA, Burland V, Plunkett G, III, Redford P, Roesch P, Rasko D et al. Extensive mosaic structure revealed by the complete genome sequence of uropathogenic Escherichia coli. Proc Natl Acad Sci U S A 2002; 99(26):17020-17024.

[49] Barasch J, Mori K. Cell biology: iron thievery. Nature 2004; 432(7019):811-813.

[50] Neilands JB. Siderophores: structure and function of microbial iron transport compounds. J Biol Chem 1995; 270(45):26723-26726.

[51] Fischbach MA, Lin H, Liu DR, Walsh CT. How pathogenic bacteria evade mammalian sabotage in the battle for iron. Nat Chem Biol 2006; 2(3):132-138.

[52] Raymond KN, Dertz EA, Kim SS. Enterobactin: an archetype for microbial iron transport. Proc Natl Acad Sci U S A 2003; 100(7):3584-3588.

[53] Abrink M, Larsson E, Gobl A, Hellman L. Expression of lactoferrin in the kidney: implications for innate immunity and iron metabolism. Kidney Int 2000; 57(5):2004-2010.

[54] Ellison RT, III, Giehl TJ, LaForce FM. Damage of the outer membrane of enteric gram-negative bacteria by lactoferrin and transferrin. Infect Immun 1988; 56(11):2774-2781.

[55] Konopka K, Neilands JB. Effect of serum albumin on siderophore-mediated utilization of transferrin iron. Biochemistry 1984; 23(10):2122-2127.

[56] Flo TH, Smith KD, Sato S, Rodriguez DJ, Holmes MA, Strong RK et al. Lipocalin 2 mediates an innate immune response to bacterial infection by sequestrating iron. Nature 2004; 432(7019):917-921.

[57] Reigstad CS, Hultgren SJ, Gordon JI. Functional genomic studies of uropathogenic Escherichia coli and host urothelial cells when intracellular bacterial communities are assembled. J Biol Chem 2007; 282(29):21259-21267.

[58] Smith KD. Iron metabolism at the host pathogen interface: lipocalin 2 and the pathogen-associated iroA gene cluster. Int J Biochem Cell Biol 2007; 39(10):1776-1780.

[59] Fabich AJ, Jones SA, Chowdhury FZ, Cernosek A, Anderson A, Smalley D et al. Comparison of carbon nutrition for pathogenic and commensal Escherichia coli strains in the mouse intestine. Infect Immun 2008; 76(3):1143-1152.

[60] Lane MC, Lloyd AL, Markyvech TA, Hagan EC, Mobley HL. Uropathogenic Escherichia coli strains generally lack functional Trg and Tap chemoreceptors found in the majority of E. coli strains strictly residing in the gut. J Bacteriol 2006; 188(15):5618-5625.

[61] Alteri CJ, Smith SN, Mobley HL. Fitness of Escherichia coli during urinary tract infection requires gluconeogenesis and the TCA cycle. PLoS Pathog 2009; 5(5):e1000448.

[62] Eto DS, Mulvey MA. Flushing bacteria out of the bladder. Nat Med 2007; 13(5):531-532.

[63] Mysorekar IU, Hultgren SJ. Mechanisms of uropathogenic Escherichia coli persistence and eradication from the urinary tract. Proc Natl Acad Sci U S A 2006; 103(38):14170-14175.

[64] Kerrn MB, Struve C, Blom J, Frimodt-Moller N, Krogfelt KA. Intracellular persistence of Escherichia coli in urinary bladders from mecillinam-treated mice. J Antimicrob Chemother 2005; 55(3):383-386.

[65] Hopkins WJ, Gendron-Fitzpatrick A, Balish E, Uehling DT. Time course and host responses to Escherichia coli urinary tract infection in genetically distinct mouse strains. Infect Immun 1998; 66(6):2798-2802.

[66] Justice SS, Hung C, Theriot JA, Fletcher DA, Anderson GG, Footer MJ et al. Differentiation and developmental pathways of uropathogenic Escherichia coli in urinary tract pathogenesis. Proc Natl Acad Sci U S A 2004; 101(5):1333-1338.

[67] Mulvey MA, Schilling JD, Hultgren SJ. Establishment of a persistent Escherichia coli reservoir during the acute phase of a bladder infection. Infect Immun 2001; 69(7):4572-4579.

[68] Mysorekar IU, Isaacson-Schmid M, Walker JN, Mills JC, Hultgren SJ. Bone morphogenetic protein 4 signaling regulates epithelial renewal in the urinary tract in response to uropathogenic infection. Cell Host Microbe 2009; 5(5):463-475.

[69] Pull SL, Doherty JM, Mills JC, Gordon JI, Stappenbeck TS. Activated macrophages are an adaptive element of the colonic epithelial progenitor niche necessary for regenerative responses to injury. Proc Natl Acad Sci U S A 2005; 102(1):99-104.

[70] Zasloff M. Antimicrobial peptides, innate immunity, and the normally sterile urinary tract. J Am Soc Nephrol 2007; 18(11):2810-2816.

[71] Valore EV, Park CH, Quayle AJ, Wiles KR, McCray PB, Jr., Ganz T. Human beta-defensin-1: an antimicrobial peptide of urogenital tissues. J Clin Invest 1998; 101(8):1633-1642.

[72] Morrison G, Kilanowski F, Davidson D, Dorin J. Characterization of the mouse beta defensin 1, Defb1, mutant mouse model. Infect Immun 2002; 70(6):3053-3060.
[73] Biragyn A, Ruffini PA, Leifer CA, Klyushnenkova E, Shakhov A, Chertov O et al. Toll-like receptor 4-dependent activation of dendritic cells by beta-defensin 2. Science 2002; 298(5595):1025-1029.
[74] Godaly G, Hang L, Frendeus B, Svanborg C. Transepithelial neutrophil migration is CXCR1 dependent in vitro and is defective in IL-8 receptor knockout mice. J Immunol 2000; 165(9):5287-5294.
[75] Lundstedt AC, Leijonhufvud I, Ragnarsdottir B, Karpman D, Andersson B, Svanborg C. Inherited susceptibility to acute pyelonephritis: a family study of urinary tract infection. J Infect Dis 2007; 195(8):1227-1234.
[76] Lundstedt AC, McCarthy S, Gustafsson MC, Godaly G, Jodal U, Karpman D et al. A genetic basis of susceptibility to acute pyelonephritis. PLoS One 2007; 2(9):e825.
[77] Artifoni L, Negrisolo S, Montini G, Zucchetta P, Molinari PP, Cassar W et al. Interleukin-8 and CXCR1 receptor functional polymorphisms and susceptibility to acute pyelonephritis. J Urol 2007; 177(3):1102-1106.
[78] Frendeus B, Godaly G, Hang L, Karpman D, Lundstedt AC, Svanborg C. Interleukin 8 receptor deficiency confers susceptibility to acute experimental pyelonephritis and may have a human counterpart. J Exp Med 2000; 192(6):881-890.
[79] Svensson M, Irjala H, Alm P, Holmqvist B, Lundstedt AC, Svanborg C. Natural history of renal scarring in susceptible mIL-8Rh-/- mice. Kidney Int 2005; 67(1):103-110.
[80] Svensson M, Irjala H, Svanborg C, Godaly G. Effects of epithelial and neutrophil CXCR2 on innate immunity and resistance to kidney infection. Kidney Int 2008; 74(1):81-90.
[81] Ingersoll MA, Kline KA, Nielsen HV, Hultgren SJ. G-CSF induction early in uropathogenic Escherichia coli infection of the urinary tract modulates host immunity. Cell Microbiol 2008; 10(12):2568-2578.
[82] Hedges S, Anderson P, Lidin-Janson G, de MP, Svanborg C. Interleukin-6 response to deliberate colonization of the human urinary tract with gram-negative bacteria. Infect Immun 1991; 59(1):421-427.
[83] Godaly G, Otto G, Burdick MD, Strieter RM, Svanborg C. Fimbrial lectins influence the chemokine repertoire in the urinary tract mucosa. Kidney Int 2007; 71(8):778-786.
[84] Jones-Carson J, Balish E, Uehling DT. Susceptibility of immunodeficient gene-knockout mice to urinary tract infection. J Urol 1999; 161(1):338-341.
[85] Johnson DE, Lockatell CV, Russell RG, Hebel JR, Island MD, Stapleton A et al. Comparison of Escherichia coli strains recovered from human cystitis and pyelonephritis infections in transurethrally challenged mice. Infect Immun 1998; 66(7):3059-3065.
[86] Tewari R, Ikeda T, Malaviya R, MacGregor JI, Little JR, Hultgren SJ et al. The PapG tip adhesin of P fimbriae protects Escherichia coli from neutrophil bactericidal activity. Infect Immun 1994; 62(12):5296-5304.
[87] Kruger T, Benke D, Eitner F, Lang A, Wirtz M, Hamilton-Williams EE et al. Identification and functional characterization of dendritic cells in the healthy murine kidney and in experimental glomerulonephritis. J Am Soc Nephrol 2004; 15(3):613-621.
[88] Engel D, Dobrindt U, Tittel A, Peters P, Maurer J, Gutgemann I et al. Tumor necrosis factor alpha- and inducible nitric oxide synthase-producing dendritic cells are rapidly recruited to the bladder in urinary tract infection but are dispensable for bacterial clearance. Infect Immun 2006; 74(11):6100-6107.

[89] Tezuka H, Abe Y, Iwata M, Takeuchi H, Ishikawa H, Matsushita M et al. Regulation of IgA production by naturally occurring TNF/iNOS-producing dendritic cells. Nature 2007; 448(7156):929-933.

[90] Engel DR, Maurer J, Tittel AP, Weisheit C, Cavlar T, Schumak B et al. CCR2 mediates homeostatic and inflammatory release of Gr1(high) monocytes from the bone marrow, but is dispensable for bladder infiltration in bacterial urinary tract infection. J Immunol 2008; 181(8):5579-5586.

[91] Stuehr DJ, Gross SS, Sakuma I, Levi R, Nathan CF. Activated murine macrophages secrete a metabolite of arginine with the bioactivity of endothelium-derived relaxing factor and the chemical reactivity of nitric oxide. J Exp Med 1989; 169(3):1011-1020.

[92] Mysorekar IU, Mulvey MA, Hultgren SJ, Gordon JI. Molecular regulation of urothelial renewal and host defenses during infection with uropathogenic Escherichia coli. J Biol Chem 2002; 277(9):7412-7419.

[93] Poljakovic M, Persson K. Urinary tract infection in iNOS-deficient mice with focus on bacterial sensitivity to nitric oxide. Am J Physiol Renal Physiol 2003; 284(1):F22-F31.

[94] Svensson L, Marklund BI, Poljakovic M, Persson K. Uropathogenic Escherichia coli and tolerance to nitric oxide: the role of flavohemoglobin. J Urol 2006; 175(2):749-753.

[95] Springall T, Sheerin NS, Abe K, Holers VM, Wan H, Sacks SH. Epithelial secretion of C3 promotes colonization of the upper urinary tract by Escherichia coli. Nat Med 2001; 7(7):801-806.

[96] Li K, Feito MJ, Sacks SH, Sheerin NS. CD46 (membrane cofactor protein) acts as a human epithelial cell receptor for internalization of opsonized uropathogenic Escherichia coli. J Immunol 2006; 177(4):2543-2551.

[97] Hopkins WJ, James LJ, Balish E, Uehling DT. Congenital immunodeficiencies in mice increase susceptibility to urinary tract infection. J Urol 1993; 149(4):922-925.

[98] Chien YH, Jores R, Crowley MP. Recognition by gamma/delta T cells. Annu Rev Immunol 1996; 14:511-532.

[99] Berland R, Wortis HH. Origins and functions of B-1 cells with notes on the role of CD5. Annu Rev Immunol 2002; 20:253-300.

[100] Chen J, Trounstine M, Alt FW, Young F, Kurahara C, Loring JF et al. Immunoglobulin gene rearrangement in B cell deficient mice generated by targeted deletion of the JH locus. Int Immunol 1993; 5(6):647-656.

[101] Minagawa S, Ohyama C, Hatakeyama S, Tsuchiya N, Kato T, Habuchi T. Activation of natural killer T cells by alpha-galactosylceramide mediates clearance of bacteria in murine urinary tract infection. J Urol 2005; 173(6):2171-2174.

[102] Nagarajan NA, Kronenberg M. Invariant NKT cells amplify the innate immune response to lipopolysaccharide. J Immunol 2007; 178(5):2706-2713.

[103] Hopkins WJ, Elkahwaji J, Kendziorski C, Moser AR, Briggs PM, Suhs KA. Quantitative trait loci associated with susceptibility to bladder and kidney infections induced by Escherichia coli in female C3H/HeJ mice. J Infect Dis 2009; 199(3):355-361.

[104] Hopkins WJ, Uehling DT, Wargowski DS. Evaluation of a familial predisposition to recurrent urinary tract infections in women. Am J Med Genet 1999; 83(5):422-424.

[105] Karoly E, Fekete A, Banki NF, Szebeni B, Vannay A, Szabo AJ et al. Heat shock protein 72 (HSPA1B) gene polymorphism and Toll-like receptor (TLR) 4 mutation are associated with increased risk of urinary tract infection in children. Pediatr Res 2007; 61(3):371-374.

[106] Smithson A, Sarrias MR, Barcelo J, Suarez B, Horcajada JP, Soto SM et al. Expression of interleukin-8 receptors (CXCR1 and CXCR2) in premenopausal women with recurrent urinary tract infections. Clin Diagn Lab Immunol 2005; 12(12):1358-1363.

[107] Peck A, Mellins ED. Precarious balance: Th17 cells in host defense. Infect Immun 2010; 78(1):32-38.

[108] Roelofs JJ, Teske GJ, Bonta PI, de Vries CJ, Meijers JC, Weening JJ et al. Plasminogen activator inhibitor-1 regulates neutrophil influx during acute pyelonephritis. Kidney Int 2009; 75(1):52-59.

[109] Kang WS, Tamarkin FJ, Wheeler MA, Weiss RM. Rapid up-regulation of endothelial nitric-oxide synthase in a mouse model of Escherichia coli lipopolysaccharide-induced bladder inflammation. J Pharmacol Exp Ther 2004; 310(2):452-458.

[110] Chromek M, Slamova Z, Bergman P, Kovacs L, Podracka L, Ehren I et al. The antimicrobial peptide cathelicidin protects the urinary tract against invasive bacterial infection. Nat Med 2006; 12(6):636-641.

[111] Thumbikat P, Waltenbaugh C, Schaeffer AJ, Klumpp DJ. Antigen-specific responses accelerate bacterial clearance in the bladder. J Immunol 2006; 176(5):3080-3086.

[112] Torchinsky MB, Garaude J, Martin AP, Blander JM. Innate immune recognition of infected apoptotic cells directs T(H)17 cell differentiation. Nature 2009; 458(7234):78-82.

[113] Tomasi TB, Jr., Larson L, Challacombe S, McNabb P. Mucosal immunity: The origin and migration patterns of cells in the secretory system. J Allergy Clin Immunol 1980; 65(1):12-19.

[114] Trinchieri A, Braceschi L, Tiranti D, Dell'Acqua S, Mandressi A, Pisani E. Secretory immunoglobulin A and inhibitory activity of bacterial adherence to epithelial cells in urine from patients with urinary tract infections. Urol Res 1990; 18(5):305-308.

[115] Kantele A, Papunen R, Virtanen E, Mottonen T, Rasanen L, Ala-Kaila K et al. Antibody-secreting cells in acute urinary tract infection as indicators of local immune response. J Infect Dis 1994; 169(5):1023-1028.

[116] Alteri CJ, Hagan EC, Sivick KE, Smith SN, Mobley HL. Mucosal immunization with iron receptor antigens protects against urinary tract infection. PLoS Pathog 2009; 5(9):e1000586.

[117] Raz R, Stamm WE. A controlled trial of intravaginal estriol in postmenopausal women with recurrent urinary tract infections. N Engl J Med 1993; 329(11):753-756.

[118] Avorn J, Monane M, Gurwitz JH, Glynn RJ, Choodnovskiy I, Lipsitz LA. Reduction of bacteriuria and pyuria after ingestion of cranberry juice. JAMA 1994; 271(10):751-754.

[119] Lilly JD, Parsons CL. Bladder surface glycosaminoglycans is a human epithelial permeability barrier. Surg Gynecol Obstet 1990; 171(6):493-496.

[120] Uehling DT, Mizutani K, Balish E. Inhibitors of bacterial adherence to urothelium. Invest Urol 1980; 18(1):40-42.

[121] Bister B, Bischoff D, Nicholson GJ, Valdebenito M, Schneider K, Winkelmann G et al. The structure of salmochelins: C-glucosylated enterobactins of Salmonella enterica. Biometals 2004; 17(4):471-481.

[122] Thankavel K, Madison B, Ikeda T, Malaviya R, Shah AH, Arumugam PM et al. Localization of a domain in the FimH adhesin of Escherichia coli type 1 fimbriae capable of receptor recognition and use of a domain-specific antibody to confer protection against experimental urinary tract infection. J Clin Invest 1997; 100(5):1123-1136.

[123] Dethlefsen L, Huse S, Sogin ML, Relman DA. The pervasive effects of an antibiotic on the human gut microbiota, as revealed by deep 16S rRNA sequencing. PLoS Biol 2008; 6(11):e280.

[124] Czaja CA, Scholes D, Hooton TM, Stamm WE. Population-based epidemiologic analysis of acute pyelonephritis. Clin Infect Dis 2007; 45(3):273-280.

[125] Yin X, Chen L, Liu Y, Yang J, Ma C, Yao Z et al. Enhancement of the innate immune response of bladder epithelial cells by Astragalus polysaccharides through upregulation of TLR4 expression. Biochem Biophys Res Commun 2010; 397(2):232-238.

[126] Nurkkala M, Nordstrom I, Telemo E, Eriksson K. MHC expression and chemokine production in the murine vagina following intra-vaginal administration of ligands to toll-like receptors 3, 7 and 9. J Reprod Immunol 2007; 73(2):148-157.

[127] Lahiri A, Das P, Chakravortty D. Engagement of TLR signaling as adjuvant: towards smarter vaccine and beyond. Vaccine 2008; 26(52):6777-6783.

[128] Layton GT, Smithyman AM. The effects of oral and combined parenteral/oral immunization against an experimental Escherichia coli urinary tract infection in mice. Clin Exp Immunol 1983; 54(2):305-312.

[129] Uehling DT, Wolf L. Enhancement of the bladder defense mechanism by immunization. Invest Urol 1969; 6(5):520-526.

[130] Svanborg-Eden C, Svennerholm AM. Secretory immunoglobulin A and G antibodies prevent adhesion of Escherichia coli to human urinary tract epithelial cells. Infect Immun 1978; 22(3):790-797.

[131] Russo TA, Beanan JM, Olson R, Genagon SA, MacDonald U, Cope JJ et al. A killed, genetically engineered derivative of a wild-type extraintestinal pathogenic E. coli strain is a vaccine candidate. Vaccine 2007; 25(19):3859-3870.

[132] O'Hanley P, Lalonde G, Ji G. Alpha-hemolysin contributes to the pathogenicity of piliated digalactoside-binding Escherichia coli in the kidney: efficacy of an alpha-hemolysin vaccine in preventing renal injury in the BALB/c mouse model of pyelonephritis. Infect Immun 1991; 59(3):1153-1161.

[133] O'Hanley P, Low D, Romero I, Lark D, Vosti K, Falkow S et al. Gal-Gal binding and hemolysin phenotypes and genotypes associated with uropathogenic Escherichia coli. N Engl J Med 1985; 313(7):414-420.

[134] Roberts JA, Hardaway K, Kaack B, Fussell EN, Baskin G. Prevention of pyelonephritis by immunization with P-fimbriae. J Urol 1984; 131(3):602-607.

[135] Schmidt MA, O'Hanley P, Lark D, Schoolnik GK. Synthetic peptides corresponding to protective epitopes of Escherichia coli digalactoside-binding pilin prevent infection in a murine pyelonephritis model. Proc Natl Acad Sci U S A 1988; 85(4):1247-1251.

[136] Connell I, Agace W, Klemm P, Schembri M, Marild S, Svanborg C. Type 1 fimbrial expression enhances Escherichia coli virulence for the urinary tract. Proc Natl Acad Sci U S A 1996; 93(18):9827-9832.

[137] Langermann S, Palaszynski S, Barnhart M, Auguste G, Pinkner JS, Burlein J et al. Prevention of mucosal Escherichia coli infection by FimH-adhesin-based systemic vaccination. Science 1997; 276(5312):607-611.

[138] Eisenstein BI. Phase variation of type 1 fimbriae in Escherichia coli is under transcriptional control. Science 1981; 214(4518):337-339.

[139] Johnson JR. Virulence factors in Escherichia coli urinary tract infection. Clin Microbiol Rev 1991; 4(1):80-128.

[140] Hull RA, Donovan WH, Del TM, Stewart C, Rogers M, Darouiche RO. Role of type 1 fimbria- and P fimbria-specific adherence in colonization of the neurogenic human bladder by Escherichia coli. Infect Immun 2002; 70(11):6481-6484.
[141] Ganz T. Iron in innate immunity: starve the invaders. Curr Opin Immunol 2009; 21(1):63-67.
[142] Durant L, Metais A, Soulama-Mouze C, Genevard JM, Nassif X, Escaich S. Identification of candidates for a subunit vaccine against extraintestinal pathogenic Escherichia coli. Infect Immun 2007; 75(4):1916-1925.
[143] Russo TA, McFadden CD, Carlino-MacDonald UB, Beanan JM, Barnard TJ, Johnson JR. IroN functions as a siderophore receptor and is a urovirulence factor in an extraintestinal pathogenic isolate of Escherichia coli. Infect Immun 2002; 70(12):7156-7160.
[144] Russo TA, McFadden CD, Carlino-MacDonald UB, Beanan JM, Olson R, Wilding GE. The Siderophore receptor IroN of extraintestinal pathogenic Escherichia coli is a potential vaccine candidate. Infect Immun 2003; 71(12):7164-7169.
[145] Billips BK, Yaggie RE, Cashy JP, Schaeffer AJ, Klumpp DJ. A live-attenuated vaccine for the treatment of urinary tract infection by uropathogenic Escherichia coli. J Infect Dis 2009; 200(2):263-272.
[146] Uehling DT, Hopkins WJ, Elkahwaji JE, Schmidt DM, Leverson GE. Phase 2 clinical trial of a vaginal mucosal vaccine for urinary tract infections. J Urol 2003; 170(3):867-869.
[147] Pasare C, Medzhitov R. Toll-like receptors: linking innate and adaptive immunity. Adv Exp Med Biol 2005; 560:11-18.
[148] Iwasaki A, Medzhitov R. Toll-like receptor control of the adaptive immune responses. Nat Immunol 2004; 5(10):987-995.
[149] van DD, Medzhitov R, Shaw AC. Triggering TLR signaling in vaccination. Trends Immunol 2006; 27(1):49-55.
[150] Parker LC, Prince LR, Sabroe I. Translational mini-review series on Toll-like receptors: networks regulated by Toll-like receptors mediate innate and adaptive immunity. Clin Exp Immunol 2007; 147(2):199-207.
[151] Li X, Lockatell CV, Johnson DE, Lane MC, Warren JW, Mobley HL. Development of an intranasal vaccine to prevent urinary tract infection by Proteus mirabilis. Infect Immun 2004; 72(1):66-75.
[152] Davis SS. Nasal vaccines. Adv Drug Deliv Rev 2001; 51(1-3):21-42.
[153] Stapleton A. Host factors in susceptibility to urinary tract infections. Adv Exp Med Biol 1999; 462:351-358.
[154] Song J, Abraham SN. Innate and adaptive immune responses in the urinary tract. Eur J Clin Invest 2008; 38 Suppl 2:21-28.

9

Biofilm and Urogenital Infections

Peter Tenke[1], Bela Koves[1], Karoly Nagy[1], Shinya Uehara[2], Hiromi Kumon[2], Scott J. Hultgren[3], Chia Hung[3] and Werner Mendling[4]
[1]*Dep. of Urology, South-Pest Hospital, Budapest,*
[2]*Dep. of Urology, Okayama University, Okayama city,*
[3]*Dep. of Molecular Microbiology, Washington Uni. Medical School, St. Louis, MO*
[4]*Vivantes Clinic for Obstetrics and Gynecology, Klinikum Am Urban,*
[1]*Hungary*
[2]*Japan*
[3]*USA*
[4]*Berlin*

1. Introduction

Bacterial adherence and the growth of bacteria on solid surfaces as biofilm are both naturally occurring phenomena. Biofilms can be defined as an accumulation of microorganisms and their extracellular products forming structured communities attached to a surface. Biofilms are able to build up under natural circumstances, for instance on the urothelium or prostate stones and they can also colonize the surfaces of implanted medical devices. Biofilm infections have a major role on temporary and permanent implants or devices placed in the human body. In the process of endourological development a great variety of foreign bodies have been invented besides urethral catheters like ureter, prostatic stents, percutan nephrostomy, penile, testicular implants and artificial urinary sphincters. Many biofilms are quite harmful but others can have a positive impact, namely lining healthy intestine and female genito-urinary tract. Biofilms have significant implications for clinical pharmacology, particularly related to antibiotic resistance, drug adsorption onto and off of devices, and minimum inhibitory concentrations of drugs required for effective therapy.

2. Biofilm formation and growth

A biofilm is an aggregate of microorganisms in which cells adhere to each other and/or to a surface. These adherent cells are frequently embedded within a self-produced matrix of extracellular polymeric substance (EPS). Formation of a biofilm begins with the attachment of free-floating microorganisms to a surface. The first step of biofilm formation is always the deposition of a conditioning film produced by the host to the foreign body. It is followed by the attachment of microorganisms. The microbial adhesion and anchorage to the surface are made by exopolymer production. After this process their growth, multiplication and dissemination can be observed [1,2,3,4,5].

After insertion of the device into the body the material surface enters into contact with body fluids around the implant. In case of the urinary tract Tamm-Horsfall glycoprotein, various ions, polysaccharides and other components diffuse toward the implant surface from the urine within minutes [6]. Macromolecular components (serum albumin, fibrinogen, collagen, fibronectin) from these body fluids adsorb extremely fast onto the material surfaces to form a conditioning film, prior to the arrival of the first organisms [7]. The creation of a conditioning film alters the surface characteristics of implants. The role of the conditioning film is vital as many pathogens do not have mechanisms allowing them to adhere directly or strongly onto bare implant surfaces [8].

The next step in the development of a biofilm is the approach and attachment of microorganisms. The ability of microorganisms to adhere to surfaces is influenced by electrostatic and hydrophobic interactions, ionic strength, osmolality and urinary pH [9,10].

In order for bacteria to react to a surface or an interface like an air-water interface, these cells must be able to 'sense' their proximity to these surfaces. The planktonic 'free-floating' bacterial cells release both protons and signaling molecules as they move through the bulk fluid. These protons and signaling molecules must diffuse radially away from the floating cell, if not adjacent to any surface or interface. But a significantly higher concentration of either protons or signaling molecules can develop on the side of the bacterial cell close to any surface. This allows the cell to sense that it is near a surface because diffusion is limited on this side [4]. After the planktonic bacterial cell has sensed the surface, it may commit to the active process of adhesion and biofilm formation.

There is no single process or theory, which can completely describe microbial adhesion. The initial adhesion is reversible and involves hydrophobic and electrostatic forces. It is followed by irreversible attachment provided by bacterial polysaccharides which anchor the organisms to the surface. Subsequently, colonization takes by species factors, such as slow migration and spreading, rolling, packing and adhesion of the progress. A developed biofilm consists of groups of microorganisms, sometimes in mushroom-like forms, separated by interstitial spaces that are filled with the surrounding fluid [11]. The growth rates of organisms on a surface as well as the strategies used by microorganisms to spread over a surface are important for colonization. These strategies are species specific which can influence the distribution of a biofilm on a surface [12].

The final stage of microbial colonization of a surface is the formation of a biofilm structure. At this point, the microorganisms have created a microenvironment protective against many antimicrobial agents and host immune defense mechanisms. Biofilm has been described as having a heterogeneous structure with a rough surface [13]. The microcolony is actually the basic structural unit of the biofilm, similar to the tissue which is the basic unit of growth of more complex organisms. Depending on the species involved, the microcolony may be composed of 10-25% cells and 75-90% exopolysaccharide (EPS) matrix. The biofilm contains 'water channels' which allow transporting of essential nutrients and oxygen for the growth of the cells [14]. Microorganisms within the biofilm also secrete chemical signals that mediate population density-dependent gene expression, which has an important role in biofilm development [15]. In summary, the biofilm is usually built up of three layers [16]:

1. the linking film which attaches to the surface of tissue or biomaterials
2. the base film of compact microorganisms
3. the surface film as an outer layer, where planktonic organisms can be released free-floating and spreading over the surface.

3. Antimicrobial susceptibility of bacteria in biofilm

Infections caused as a result of biofilm formation are characterized by particularly strong antibiotic and immune resistance patterns. Bacteria within the biofilms differ in behaviour and in phenotypic form from the planktonic bacteria. Antimicrobial agents are effective against planktonic bacteria and appear to clear mucosal surfaces of adherent bacterial microcolonies but frequently fail to eradicate bacterial biofilms on urological devices. The use of antibiotics is currently one of the possibilities of the prevention of biofilm formation. However, even in the presence of antibiotics bacteria can adhere, colonize and survive on implanted medical devices as has been shown for urinary catheters and ureteral stent surfaces in vitro and in vivo [17,18,19]. The problem in conventional clinical microbiology is how to treat patients in the best way when choosing antibiotics is based on bacterial cultures derived from planktonic bacterial cells which differ very much from bacteria in the biofilm mode. This can stand behind the clinical failure rate of treating chronic bacterial infection.

The failure of antimicrobial agents to treat biofilms has been associated with a variety of mechanisms (4) [18,19,20,21,22,23,24]. One mechanism of biofilm resistance to antimicrobial agents is the failure of an agent to penetrate the full depth of the biofilm (extrinsic resistance). The extracellular matrix for instance may block the penetration at the very beginning.

- One mechanism is the failure of an agent to penetrate the full depth of the biofilm (*extrinsic resistance*). The extracellular matrix may block the penetration at the very beginning.
- The organisms growing at a slower rate within the biofilm are more resistant to the effects of antimicrobial agents, which require active growth.
- Bacteria within biofilm are phenotypically so different from their planktonic counterparts that antimicrobial agents developed against the latter often fail to eradicate organisms in the biofilm. Bacteria within a biofilm activate many genes which alter the cell envelope, the molecular targets and the susceptibility to antimicrobial agents (intrinsic resistance). Current opinion is that phenotypic changes caused by a genetic switch, when approximately 65-80 proteins change, play a more important role in the protection from antimicrobial agents than the external resistance provided by the exopolysaccharide matrix.
- Bacteria within a biofilm can sense the external environment, communicate with each other and transfer genetic information and plasmids within biofilm.
- Bacteria in a biofilm can usually survive the presence of antimicrobial agents at a concentration 1000-1500 times higher than the concentration that kills planktonic cells of the same species.

According to in vitro and in vivo studies aminoglycosides and beta-lactam antibiotics can prevent the formation of 'young' biofilms, while fluoroquinolones are effective in case of both 'young' and 'older' biofilms because of their good penetrative qualities. They are present in biofilms even one or two weeks after the end of the antibiotic treatment [25-28].

Most researchers believe that antibiotics can only slow down the progress of biofilm formation by eliminating unprotected planktonic bacteria and reducing the metabolic activity of bacteria on the biofilm surface [23, 29-30]. However, during an acute febrile phase of a biofilm infection.

4. Indwelling urethral catheters

Due to the urinary catheter the development of bacteriuria and biofilm formation is inevitable. Urinary catheters are readily targets of biofilm development on their inner and outer surfaces once they are inserted. The long-term use of them leads to infection in most of the cases. The surface of a catheter (depending on its material) provides sufficient circumstances for bacteria to adhere and spread along in two ways. One route is when organisms ascend the catheter extraluminally by direct inoculation at the time of the catheter insertion or migrate in the mucous sheath that surrounds the external aspect of the catheter. Extraluminal organisms are primarily endogenous, originating from the gastrointestinal tract. These organisms colonize the patient's perineum and ascend the urethra after catheter insertion [13,31,32,33,34] Approximately 70% of bacteriuria in catheterized women is believed to occur through the extraluminal entry.
Bacteria can ascend the catheter also by an *intraluminal route,* which occurs when organisms gain access to the internal lumen of the catheter. These organisms are usually introduced from exogenous sources, for instance with cross transmission from the hands of health care personnel [13,32,33,35]. Adhesion of microorganisms to catheter materials depends on the hydrophobicity of the organism and catheter surface.

5. The biofilms and the encrustation and blockage of catheters

An additional problem in use of medical biomaterials in the urinary tract environment is the development of encrustation and consecutive obstruction. When the drained urinary tract becomes infected by urease producing bacteria such as *Proteus mirabilis,* the bacterial urease generates ammonia from urea and elevates the pH of the urine. Under these alkaline conditions, crystals of calcium phosphate (hydroxyapatite) and magnesium ammonium phosphate (struvite) are formed and trapped in the organic matrix surrounding the cells [20, 21, 36,37]. Progression of these encrustations eventually blocks the catheter lumen.

6. Ureteral stents

In vitro and in vivo studies confirmed the difficulty in detecting biofilm formation by using conventional laboratory procedures [38, 39]. Reid at al found that 90% of indwelling silicone double J stents were colonized by adherent bacteria, however the incidence of urinary infection detected clinically was only 27% [38]. The difficulty in detecting biofilm formation by using conventional laboratory procedures was confirmed in a large study where 237 ureteral stents were tested. It was shown that 68% of stents were actually colonized but only 30% of patients were found to have bacteriuria [39]. Therefore, a negative urine culture does not rule out the possibility of stent colonization. The study testified correlation between the length of the indwelling time and the development of infection.

7. Penile prostheses

The prosthesis-associated chronic pain due to subclinical infection is more common than clinically apparent infection (3). Staphylococcus species, especially Staphylococcus epidermidis are the most common pathogens found in penile prostheses infection (35-56%) [40], while Gram-negative enteric bacteria are liable for 20 % of infections [41,42]. S.

epidermidis was cultured in 40% of penile prosthesis removed for malfunction with no clinical evidence of infection [43]. Staphylococcal species were also found to enhance biofilm formation. These cases can be 'silent' for many years before becoming clinically evident [44] in contrast to Gram-negative bacterial infection (*Pseudomonas aeruginosa, E.coli, Serratia marcescens, and Proteus mirabilis*) being responsible for 20% of infections, which usually become manifest in a month after implantation [43].
To reduce the risk of device associated infections many modifications have been developed such as antibiotic and hydrophilic coated devices.Hydrophilic penile prosthesis coating was has been shown to decrease bacterial adherence in vitro and in animal models [45]. Antibiotic prophylaxis is desirable for the above-mentioned facts. Since the most common pathogen is the Staphylococcus epidermidis, first-generation cephalosporins, broad-spectrum penicillin should be used [46]. In cases of chronic pain, long-term administration of quinolones eased 60% of symptoms. Lack of success involves the necessity of implant removal.

8. Artificial urinary sphincters (AUS)

Around 3% of the AUS become infected and symptoms are mainly associated with the control pump device. Avoiding the risk factors as infected urine, prolonged urinary retention and large bladder residual can reduce this high occurrence [43,46]. Since the parts of the sphincter device form one continuous surface, the AUS is suggested to be removed entirely as the first step to eliminate the infection. The reimplantation must be preceded by the complete treatment of the infected area. This is not always achievable as many of these patients are paraplegic or have a neurogenic bladder with recurrent UTIs [43,46].

9. Infected urinary calculi

In case of urease-producing bacteriuria the infection can be conjoined with the formation of struvite and calcium phosphate calculi as described above. The infected calculi grow rapidly and provide safe environment for the bacteria adhered to the biofilm [47]. The complete removal of all stone fragments during stone operation (PCNL, URS, ±combined with ESWL), prolonged administration of antibiotics (8-10 weeks for destroying urease-producing bacteria) and metaphylaxis are the features of the most effective treatment strategy.

10. Chronic bacterial prostatitis

Although the diagnosis and classification of chronic prostatitis have been standardized, the differentiation of chronic non-bacterial from bacterial inflammation is still challenging. Being out of the sweeping effect of streaming urine the prostatic ducts and acini provides safe circumstances to planktonic bacteria to multiply rapidly and induce a host response with infiltration of acute inflammatory cells into the ducts. The ducts become engorged with infiltrate composed of dead and living bacteria as well as living and dying acute inflammatory cells, desquamated epithelial cells and cellular debris. At this point it is relatively easy to eradicate all the offending organisms which are in a 'planktonic state' with appropriate antibiotic therapy. If the bacteria persist from either clinically acute or more likely, subacute inflammation, they can form sporadic bacterial microcolonies or biofilms adherent to the epithelium of the ductal system (2b) [48,49]. These bacteria also produce an exopolysaccharide slime or glycocalyx that envelops these adherent microcolonies. The bacteria persisting in the prostate gland within these focal biofilms can provoke persistent immunological stimulation and subsequent chronic inflammation [48]. The diagnosis of chronic bacterial prostatitis can be difficult as colonized bacteria will not get into the prostatic secretion or urine sample. Antimicrobial therapy eradicates the planktonic bacteria but not the adherent bacterial biofilms deep within the prostate gland. Another cause of unsuccessful treatment may be the fact that the bacteria within biofilms differ significantly from their planktonic counterparts in metabolic rate, molecular targets and expression of antimicrobial binding proteins [3,19]. There is a need in development of diagnostic tools which would be able to recognize small adherent bacterial biofilms which exist deep within the prostate gland in chronic bacterial prostatitis. New treatment regimens should be carried out in order to be able to deliver much higher antibiotic concentrations to the biofilm within the prostatic duct.

11. Intracellular bacterial biofilm-like pods in the recurrent cystitis

Entry of E. coli into the urinary tract is not well understood, although sexual intercourse is the most clearly defined predisposing factor. Presumably, a small number of E. coli from the vaginal or enteric flora are introduced into the bladder during an average incident, and it seems plausible that in most cases the innate defenses in the bladder would be able to prevent infection. However, sometimes Uropathogenic E.Coli (UPEC) clearly possess mechanisms to overcome these defenses and establish a foothold in the bladder. UPEC pathogenesis initiates with bacterial binding of superficial bladder epithelial cells. Initial colonization events activate inflammatory and apoptotic cascades in the epithelium, which is normally inert and only turns over every 6 to 12 months. Bladder epithelial cells respond to invading bacteria in part by recognizing bacterial lipopolysaccharide (LPS) via the Toll-like receptor pathway, which results in strong neutrophil influx into the bladder. In addition, interactions mediated by adhesin FimH at the tips of type 1 pili with the bladder epithelium stimulate exfoliation of superficial epithelial cells, causing many of the pathogens to be shed into the urine. Genetic programs are activated that lead to differentiation and proliferation of the underlying transitional cells in an effort to renew the exfoliated superficial epithelium. Despite the robust inflammatory response and epithelial exfoliation, UPEC are able to maintain high titers in the bladder for several days.

A bacterial mechanism of FimH-mediated invasion into the superficial cells apparently allows evasion of these innate defenses. Initially, bacteria replicate rapidly inside superficial cells as disorganized clusters. Subsequently, bacteria in the clusters divide without much growth in cell size, resulting in coccoid-shaped bacteria, presumably due to changes in genetic programs. Furthermore, the bacterial clusters became highly compact and organized into biofilm-like structures, termed intracellular bacterial communities (IBCs), inside bladder superficial cells [50]. The IBCs push the bladder superficial cell membranes outward to give a "pod" like appearance by scanning electron microscopy. Bacteria in the IBCs are held together by exopolymeric matrices, reminiscent of biofilm structures [51]. At some point during this IBC developmental process, bacteria on the edges of IBCs become elongated again, become motile and start to move away from IBCs. Bacteria can exit out of infected bladder cells, probably due to compromised membrane integrity. UPEC undergo such IBC cascade to increase in numbers, resulting in high bacterial titers in the bladder. In addition, bacteria in these intracellular niches can create a chronic quiescent reservoir in the bladder, which can persist undetected for several months without bacteria shedding in the urine [52,53,54]. Bacteria in IBCs are completely resistant to 3- and 10-day courses of antibiotics [55].

12. Biofilm and pyelonephritis

Once bacteria reach the kidney either by ascending infection or vesicoureteral reflux they are able to adhere to the urothelium and papillae. Nickel et al showed that bacteria could adhere in thin biofilms to the urothelium before invading the renal tissue with resultant pyelonephritis [47]. These bacterial biofilms are more easily eradicated by antimicrobial agents, in contrast to the biofilms on catheter surfaces [51], which may be ascribed to the effective synergistic actions of antimicrobial agents and host defenses against the biofilms on urothelium [56].

13. Biofilm in bacterial vaginosis

Bacterial vaginosis (BV) is the most common vaginal disorder in adult women [57]. Although it is a non-fatal disease, BV presents an increased risk for other more severe clinical outcomes, such as preterm birth and HIV infections [58,59]. As defined by Amsel clinical criteria, BV exhibits at least 3 of the following 4 clinical symptoms: 1) elevation of vaginal fluid pH to above 4.5; 2) detectable "fishy odor" of vaginal fluid upon addition of 10% potassium hydroxide; 3) presence of clue cells, vaginal epithelial cells covered with bacteria, in vaginal fluid; and 4) milky vaginal discharge. The vaginal flora of healthy women consists predominantly of Gram-positive lactobacilli, especially *Lactobacillus cripatus* and *Lactobacillus jensenii* [60-62]. Productions of antimicrobial proteins as well as the maintenance of acidic pH and hydrogen peroxide (H_2O_2) in the vaginal fluid by these bacteria contribute critically to the establishment of a healthy ecosystem in the vagina [61-63]. On the other hand, the vaginal microbiota of women with BV showed a loss of *Lactobacillus* species and an increase in microbial diversity dominated by *Gardnerella vaginalis* and to a lesser extend, many other bacterial organisms, including *Porphyromonas, Mobiluncus,* and *Prevotella* species [64-66].

The attempts to demonstrate *G. vaginalis* as the causative pathogen of BV have failed [67], many studies have demonstrated unequivocally that *G. vaginalis* is present in the majority of BV vaginal cultures in high numbers [64, 68, 69]. One additional complication with BV is the high recurrent rate of infection, despite of efficient resolution of infection by antibiotic treatments [70]. The recurrence nature of this disease prompted the speculation that bacterial biofilms are involved in BV. *G. vaginalis* poses the intrinsic ability to form biofilm *in vitro* [71-73]. Similar to other bacterial biofilm phenotypes, *G. vaginalis* biofilm is more resistant to antibiotic treatments compared to it planktonic counterparts [73].

Swidsinski and co-workers demonstrated the presence of bacterial biofilms on the vaginal epithelium of biopsies from women with BV [68]. These biofilm showed characteristics of dense surface bacterial biofilm and were comprised predominantly of *G. vaginalis*. Although *G. vaginalis* was also detected in biopsies from healthy women, they were present in very small numbers and infrequent. The sensitivity and specificity of FISH technique also allowed the researchers to identify the presence of Gram-positive (*Streptococcus* spp.,

Enterococcus spp. and *Staphylococcus* spp.) and Gram-negative (*Escherichia coli* and *Proteus* spp.) bacteria embedded within the *G. vaginalis* biofilms. Furthermore, in a subsequent publication, Swidsinski and colleagues reported the resurgence of dense bacterial biofilms at 1-week post-cessation of metronidazole treatment [74]. These biofilms were comprised principally of *G. vaginalis* and *Atopobium vaginae*. These clinical data strongly support the presence and involvement of bacterial biofilm in BV. It is interesting to note, however, that Saunders et al. [72] demonstrated that incubation of preformed *G. vaginalis* biofilm with certain strains of *L. reuteri* or *L. iners* resulted in the disruption of biofilm and decreased viability of *G. vaginalis*.

14. Prevention of biofilm formation in the urinary tract

The harsh and potentially fatal consequences of microbial biofilm infections generated efforts to prevent their formation, particularly on indwelling medical devices using chemical and mechanical approaches. Catheters coated with hydrogel, silver salts, and antimicrobials have been evaluated; however, they provide minimal reduction in infection incidence (75).

Antibiotic (minocycline, rifampicin, nitrofurantoin) impregnated catheters lowered the rate of asymptomatic bacteriuria compared to catheters without impregnation at less than one week but difference was not statistically significant at greater than one week, and the authors concluded that the data were too few to draw conclusions about long-term catheterization. [76]

Silver alloy catheters significantly reduced the incidence of asymptomatic bacteriuria at less than one week of catheterization [76]. Beyond one week the estimated effect was smaller but the risk of asymptomatic bacteriuria was still less in the silver alloy group. There are no available clinical trials with appropriate setting about the effect of silver alloy coated catheters on bacteriuria or biofilm formation in case of long-term catheterisation.

De Ridder et al found that fewer patients using hydrophilic-coated catheter (64%) for CIC experienced UTIs compared to the uncoated catheter group (82%)[77]. However, in a randomised controlled study the authors did not find significant difference between hydrophilic-coated and uncoated indwelling urethral catheters in place for 6 weeks with respect to symptomatic urinary tract infection and microbiological analysis of urine culture [78].

Heparin coated ureteral stents did not show any organic (biofilms) or anorganic (crystals) deposits after being in situ for up to 6 weeks whereas significant biofilms were demonstrated in 33% of uncoated stents [79].

15. Use of low-energy surface acoustic waves (SAW)

Biofilm formation can be prevented- or delayed- by applying low intensity nanowaves along the surfaces of an indwelling catheter. This approach opens new options for pharmacological prevention of urinary tract infections (80,81).The concept of using low-energy SAW is based on the hypothesis that these acoustic waves are able to disrupt the formation of biofilms if transmitted directly to indwelling medical devices by inhibiting the adhesion of planktonic bacteria to their surface. Hazan et al. demonstrated the the effectiveness of Low-Energy Surface Acoustic Waves in the prevention of biofilm formation in an animal model in vivo. They found that SAW treatment reduced biofilm formation in vitro, leaving catheters virtually clean of adherent microorganisms, irrespective of the types

of bacteria that were examined. In the animal model SAW treated catheters showed strong inhibition of bacterial biofilm compared to controls [82].
In a double blind sham controlled randomized study related to short term catheterization, applying SAW releasing device to catheters prevented biofilm formation in all of the catheters whereas biofilm was present in 63% of the control group [83].
A workgroup of the authors of the present article performed a prospective parallel group comparative study on the efficacy of the SAW treatment in case of long-term catheterisation (8 weeks). SAW treatment lowered the rate of significant bacteriuria (33% vs. 81%) and the rate of biofilm formation was also significantly lower in the SAW group compared to the controls[84].

16. Conclusion

The number of biomaterial devices used in urology has been increasing permanently. Biofilm infections have a major impact on implants or devices placed in the human body. The mechanism and the different bacterial and host factors taking part in the formation of biofilms have been extensively researched in the last decades, such ideal method has not been developed yet. Antimicrobial agents are effective against planktonic bacteria and appear to clear mucosal surfaces of adherent bacterial microcolonies but frequently fail to eradicate bacterial biofilms on urological devices. Several different approaches to disease prevention are being investigated and some promising results have been obtained.

17. References

[1] Mardis HK, Kroeger RM (1988) Ureteral stents. Urol Clin North Am 15:471-479

[2] Biering-Sorensen F (2002) Urinary tract infection in individuals with spinal cord lesion. Current Opinion in Urology 12: 45-49

[3] Choong S, Whitfield H (2000) Biofilms and their role in infections in urology Brit J Urology 86: 935-941

[4] Costerton JW (1999) Introduction to biofilm. Int J Antimicrob Agents 11: 217-221

[5] Habash M, Reid G (1999) Microbial Biofilms: Their development and significance for medical device-related infections. J Clin Pharmacology 39: 887-898

[6] Fletcher M (ed.) (1996) Bacterial Adhesion: Molecular and Ecological Diversity. New York: Wiley-Liss

[7] Busscher HJ, Stokoos I, Schakenraad JM (1991) Two-dimensional spatial arrangement of fibronectin adsorbed to biomaterials with different wettabilities. Cells Mater 1: 49-57

[8] Busscher HJ, Weerkamp AH (1987) Specific and non-specific interactions in bacterial adhesion to solid substrata. FEMS Microbiol Rev 46:165-173

[9] Van Loosdrecht MCM, Lyklema J, Norde W, Schraa G, Zehnder AJB (1987) The role of bacterial cell hydrophobicity in adhesion. Appl Environ Microbiol 53:1893-1897

[10] Van Loosdrecht MCM, Lyklema J, Norde W, Schraa G, Zehnder AJB (1987) Electrophoretic mobility and hydrophobicity as a measure to predict the initial steps of bacterial adhesion. Appl Environ Microbiol 53:1989-1901

[11] Denstedt J.D., Wollin T.A., Reid G (1998) Biomaterials used in urology: Current issues of biocompatibility, infection and encrustation. J of Endourology 12:493-500

[12] Lawrence JR, Caldwell DE (1987) Behaviour of bacterial stream populations within the hydrodynamic boundary layers of surface microenvironments. Microbial Ecol 14:15-27

[13] Reid G, Habash MB (1998) Urogenital microflora and urinary tract infections. In, Tannock GW (ed.): Medical Importance of the Normal Microflora. London: Chapman & Hall 423-440

[14] Densted J.D., G. Reid, Sofer M (2000) Advances in ureteral stent tecnology. World J Urol 18: 237-242

[15] Costerton J, Lewandowski Z, Caldwell D, Korber D, Lappin-Scott H (1995) Microbial biofilms. Annu. Rev. Microbiol 49:711-745

[16] Busscher GJ, Bos R, van der Mei HC (1995) Initial microbial adhesion is a determinant for strength of biofilm adhesion. FEMS Microbiol Lett 128:229-234

[17] Caldwell DE. Cultivation and study of biofilm communities. In Lappin Scott HM, Costerton JW eds Microbial Biofilms Cambridge: Cambridge University Press, 1195: 4-69

[18] Brown MRW, Collier PJ, Gilbert P (1990) Influence of growth rate on susceptibility to antimicrobial agents: modification of the cell envelope and batch and continuous culture studies. Antimicrob Agents Chemother 34:1623-1628

[19] Brown MW, Allison DG, Gilbert P (1988) Resistance of bacterial biofilms to antibiotics: a growth-related effect J Antimicrob Chemother 22:777-783

[20] Goto T, Nakame Y, Nishida M (1999) Bacterial biofilms and catheters in experimental urinary tract infection. Int. J of Antimicrob. Agents 11: 227-231

[21] Choong S, Wood S, Whitfield HF (2001) Catheter-associated urinary tract infection and encrustation. Int J of Antimicrobial Agents 17: 305-310

[22] Nickel JC, Wright JB, Ruseska I, Marrie TJ, Whitfield C, Costerton JW (1985) Antibiotic resistance of Pseudomonas aeruginosa colonising a urinary catheter in vitro. Eur J Clin Microbiol 4:213-218

[23] Goto T, Nakame Y, Nishida M, Oh Y (1999) In vitro bactericidal activities of beta-lactamases, amikacin and fluoroquinolones against Pseudomonas aeruginosa biofilm in artificial urine. Urology 53: 1058-1062

[24] Tsukamoto T, Matsukawa M, Sano M, et al (1999) Biofilm in complicated urinary tract infection. Int. J.of Antimicrob. Agents 11: 233-236

[25] Kumon H (1996) Pathogenesis and management of bacterial biofilms in the urinary tract. J Infect Chemother 2:18-28

[26] Reid G, Habash M (2001) Oral fluoroquinolone therapy results in drug adsorption on ureteral stents and prevention of biofilm formation. Int J of Antimicrob Agents 17:317-332

[27] Reid G, Potter P, Dalenay G, Hsieh J, Nicoshia S, Hayes K (2000) Ofloxacin for treatment of urinary tract infections and biofilms in spinal cord injury. Int J Antimicrob. Agents 4:305-307.

[28] Shigeta M, Komatsuzawa H, Sugai M, Suginaka H, Usui T (1997) Effect of the growth rate of Pseudomonas aeruginosa biofilms on the susceptibility to antimicrobial agents. Chemotherapy 43 :137-141

[29] Reid G (1999) Biofilms in infectious diseases and on medical devices. Int. J. of Antimicrob.l Agents 11: 223-226

[30] Nickel JC, Downey J (1992) Movement of pseudomonas aeruginosa along catheter surfaces. Urology39: 93-98

[31] Warren J, Bakke A, Desgranchamps F, Johnson JR, Kumon H, Shah J, Tambyah P (2000) Catheter-Associated Bacteriuria and the Role of Biomaterial in Prevention. Nosocomial and Health Care Associated Infections In Urology 153-177

[32] Warren J (2001) Catheter-associated urinary tract infections. Int J Antimicrob Agents 17: 299-303

[33] Liedl B (2001) Catheter-associated urinary tract infections. Current Opinion in Urology 11: 75-79

[34] Nickel JC (1991) Catheter-associated urinary tract infection: new perspectives on old problems. Can J Infect Contrl 6:38-42

[35] Ganderton L, Chawla J, Winters C, Wimpenny J, Stickler D (1992) Scanning electron microscopy of bacterial biofilms on indwelling bladder catheters. Eur J Clin Microbiol Infect Dis 11:789-797

[36] Stickler DJ, Williams T, Jarman C, Howe N, Winters C (1995) The encrustation of urethral catheters. In: Wimpenny J, Handley P, Gilbert P. Lappin-Scott H, eds. The life and death of biofilm. Cardiff: Bioline 119-125

[37] Kunin CM, Chin QF, Chambers S (1987) Formation of encrustations on indwelling catheters in the elderly: a comparison of different types of catheter material in „blockers" and „non-blockers". J Urol 138:899-902

[38] Reid G, Denstedt JD, Kang YS, Lam D, Naus C (1992) Microbial adhesion and biofilm formation on ureteral stents in vitro and in vivo. J Urol 148:1592-1594

[39] Farsi HMA, Mosli HA, Al-Zemaity (1995) Bacteriuria and colonisation of double pigtail ureteral stents: long-term experience with 237 patients. J Endourol 9: 469-472

[40] Carson CC (1999) Management of prosthesis infections in urologic surgery. Urol Clin North Am 26: 829-839

[41] Abouassaly, R., D.K. Montague, and K.W. Angermeier, Antibiotic-coated medical devices: with an emphasis on inflatable penile prosthesis. Asian J Androl, 2004. 6(3): p. 249-57.

[42] Carson, C.C., Diagnosis, treatment and prevention of penile prosthesis infection. Int J Impot Res, 2003. 15 Suppl 5: p. S139-46.

[43] Licht MR, Montague DK, Angermeier KW et al (1995) Cultures from genitourinary prostheses at re-operation: Questioning the role of Staphylococcus epidermidis in periprosthetic infection. J Urol 154: 387-390

[44] Fishman IJ, Scott FB, Selam IN (1987) Rescue procedure: an alternative to complete removal for treatment of infected penile prosthesis J Urol 137: 202A

[45] Rajpurkar, A., et al., Antibiotic soaked hydrophilic coated bioflex: a new strategy in the prevention of penile prosthesis infection. J Sex Med, 2004. 1(2): p. 215-20

[46] Carson CC. (1989) Infections in genitourinary prostheses. Ural Clin North Am 16: 139-147

[47] Nickel JC, Olson ME, Mclean RJ, Grant SK, Costerton JW (1987) An ecological study of infected urinary stone genesis in an animal model. Br J Urol 59: 21-3145

[48] Nickel JC, Olson ME, Barabas A, Benediktsson H, Dasgupta MK, Costerton JW (1990) Pathogenesis of chronic bacterial prostatitis in an animal model. B.J of U rol 66, 47-54

[49] Nickel JC, Olson ME, Ceri H (1993) Experimental prostatitis. In Prostatitis (Weidner W, Madson P.O.P., Schiefer H.G, Eds). Springer-Verlag, Berlin
[50] Justice SS, Hung C, Theriot JA, Fletcher DA, Anderson GG, Footer MJ, Hultgren SJ. Differentiation and developmental pathways of uropathogenic Escherichia coli in urinary tract pathogenesis. Proc Natl Acad Sci U S A. 2004 Feb 3;101(5):1333-8.
[51] Nickel C, Costerton W, McLean RJC, Olson M (1994) Bacterial biofilms: influence on the pathogenesis, diagnosis and treatment of urinary tract infections. Antimicrobial Chemotherapy 33 (Suppl. A): 31-41
[52] Mysorekar IU and Hultgren SJ. Mechanisms of uropathogenic Escherichia coli persistence and eradication from the urinary tract. Proc Natl Acad Sci U S A. 2006 Sep 19;103(38):14170-5.
[53] Mulvey MA, Schilling JD, Hultgren SJ. Establishment of a persistent Escherichia coli reservoir during the acute phase of a bladder infection. Infect Immun. 2001 Jul;69(7):4572-9.
[54] Anderson GG, Palermo JJ, Schilling JD, Roth R, et al. Intracellular bacterial biofilm-like pods in urinary tract infections Science. Washington: Jul 4, 2003. Vol. 301, Iss. 5629; p. 105.
[55] Schilling JD, Lorenz RG, Hultgren SJ. Effect of trimethoprim-sulfamethoxazole on recurrent bacteriuria and bacterial persistence in mice infected with uropathogenic Escherichia coli. Infect Immun. 2002 Dec;70(12):7042-9.
[56] Nickel JC (1990) The bottle of the bladder: the pathogenesis and treatment of uncomplicated cystitis Int Urogynecol J 1: 218-222.
[57] Sobel, J.D., *What's new in bacterial vaginosis and trichomoniasis?* Infect Dis Clin North Am, 2005. 19(2): p. 387-406.
[58] Hillier, S.L., et al., *Association between bacterial vaginosis and preterm delivery of a low-birth-weight infant. The Vaginal Infections and Prematurity Study Group.* N Engl J Med, 1995. 333(26): p. 1737-42.
[59] Taha, T.E., et al., *Bacterial vaginosis and disturbances of vaginal flora: association with increased acquisition of HIV.* AIDS, 1998. 12(13): p. 1699-706.
[60] Vasquez, A., et al., *Vaginal lactobacillus flora of healthy Swedish women.* J Clin Microbiol, 2002. 40(8): p. 2746-9.
[61] Vallor, A.C., et al., *Factors associated with acquisition of, or persistent colonization by, vaginal lactobacilli: role of hydrogen peroxide production.* J Infect Dis, 2001. 184(11): p. 1431-6.
[62] Hillier, S.L., et al., *Characteristics of three vaginal flora patterns assessed by gram stain among pregnant women. Vaginal Infections and Prematurity Study Group.* Am J Obstet Gynecol, 1992. 166(3): p. 938-44.
[63] Aroutcheva, A.A., J.A. Simoes, and S. Faro, *Antimicrobial protein produced by vaginal Lactobacillus acidophilus that inhibits Gardnerella vaginalis.* Infect Dis Obstet Gynecol, 2001. 9(1): p. 33-9.
[64] Fredricks, D.N., T.L. Fiedler, and J.M. Marrazzo, *Molecular identification of bacteria associated with bacterial vaginosis.* N Engl J Med, 2005. 353(18): p. 1899-911.
[65] Sobel, J.D., *Bacterial vaginosis.* Annu Rev Med, 2000. 51: p. 349-56.
[66] Nugent, R.P., M.A. Krohn, and S.L. Hillier, *Reliability of diagnosing bacterial vaginosis is improved by a standardized method of gram stain interpretation.* J Clin Microbiol, 1991. 29(2): p. 297-301.

[67] Srinivasan, S. and D.N. Fredricks, *The human vaginal bacterial biota and bacterial vaginosis.* Interdiscip Perspect Infect Dis, 2008. 2008: p. 750479.

[68] Swidsinski, A., et al., *Adherent biofilms in bacterial vaginosis.* Obstet Gynecol, 2005. 106(5 Pt 1): p. 1013-23.

[69] Gardner, H.L. and C.D. Dukes, *Haemophilus vaginalis vaginitis: a newly defined specific infection previously classified non-specific vaginitis.* Am J Obstet Gynecol, 1955. 69(5): p. 962-76.

[70] Wilson, J., *Managing recurrent bacterial vaginosis.* Sex Transm Infect, 2004. 80(1): p. 8-11.

[71] Patterson, J.L., et al., *Effect of biofilm phenotype on resistance of Gardnerella vaginalis to hydrogen peroxide and lactic acid.* Am J Obstet Gynecol, 2007. 197(2): p. 170 e1-7.

[72] Saunders, S., et al., *Effect of Lactobacillus challenge on Gardnerella vaginalis biofilms.* Colloids Surf B Biointerfaces, 2007. 55(2): p. 138-42.

[73] Muli, F. and J.K. Struthers, *Use of a continuous-culture biofilm system to study the antimicrobial susceptibilities of Gardnerella vaginalis and Lactobacillus acidophilus.* Antimicrob Agents Chemother, 1998. 42(6): p. 1428-32.

[74] Swidsinski, A., et al., *An adherent Gardnerella vaginalis biofilm persists on the vaginal epithelium after standard therapy with oral metronidazole.* Am J Obstet Gynecol, 2008. 198(1): p. 97 e1-6.

[75] Thibon, P., X. Le Coutour, R. Leroyer, and J. Fabry. 2000. Randomized multi-centre trial of the effects of a catheter coated with hydrogel and silver salts on the incidence of hospital-acquired urinary tract infections. J. Hosp. Infect. 45:117–1124

[76] Schumm, K. and T.B. Lam, Types of urethral catheters for management of short-term voiding problems in hospitalised adults. Cochrane Database Syst Rev, 2008(2): p. CD004013.

[77] De Ridder, D.J., et al., Intermittent catheterisation with hydrophilic-coated catheters (SpeediCath) reduces the risk of clinical urinary tract infection in spinal cord injured patients: a prospective randomised parallel comparative trial. Eur Urol, 2005. 48(6): p. 991-5.

[78] Sarica, S., et al., Comparison of the use of conventional, hydrophilic and gel-lubricated catheters with regard to urethral micro trauma, urinary system infection, and patient satisfaction in patients with spinal cord injury: a randomized controlled study. Eur J Phys Rehabil Med, 2010. 46(4): p. 473-9.

[79] Riedl, C.R., et al., Heparin coating reduces encrustation of ureteral stents: a preliminary report. Int J Antimicrob Agents, 2002. 19(6): p. 507-10.

[80] Hazan Z, Zumeris J, Jacob H, Raskin H, Kratysh G, Vishnia M, Dror N, Barliya T, Mandel M, Lavie G. 2006. Effective Prevention of Microbial Biofilm Formation on Medical Devices by Low-Energy Surface Acoustic Waves. Antimicrob Agents Chemother. 2006 Dec;50(12):4144-52. Epub 2006 Aug 28.

[81] Ikinger U., Zillich S., Weber C. 2007. Biofilm Prevention by Surface Acoustic Nanowaves: A New Approach to Urinary Tract Infections? 25th World Congress of Endourology and SWL Cancun, Mexico, October 2007

[82] Hazan, Z., et al., Effective prevention of microbial biofilm formation on medical devices by low-energy surface acoustic waves. Antimicrob Agents Chemother, 2006. 50(12): p. 4144-52.

[83] Ikinger, U., S. Zillich, and C. Weber, Biofilm Prevention by Surface Acoustic Nanowaves: A New Approach to Urinary Tract Infections? . Poster presented at: 25th World Congress of Endourology and SWL; 2007; Cancun, Mexico.
[84] Nagy, K., B. Koves, and P. Tenke, The effectiveness of acoustic energy induced by UroShield device in the prevention of bacteriuria and the reduction of patients' complaints related to long-term indwelling urinary catheters. Poster accepted to: 26th Annual EAU Congress; 2011 March 18-22; Vienna, Austria

10

Biofilm Formation in Uropathogenic *Escherichia coli* Strains: Relationship with Urovirulence Factors and Antimicrobial Resistance

Sara M. Soto, Francesc Marco,
Elisabet Guiral and Jordi Vila
Department of Clinical Microbiology, Hospital Clinic,
School of Medicine, University of Barcelona
Spain

1. Introduction

1.1 *Escherichia coli* virulence and urinary tract infections

Urinary tract infections are a major public health concern in developed countries and also represent one of the most common hospital-acquired infections. Most uncomplicated UTIs are caused by *E. coli*, accounting for up to 90% of community-acquired and approximately 50% of nosocomial UTIs (Vila et al., 2002). The origin of these strains is frequently the patient's own intestinal flora. In comparison to commensal strains, UPEC present several virulence factors that allow them to colonize host mucosal uro-epithelium, injure and invade host tissues, overcome host defence mechanisms, incite a host inflammatory response and eventually proceed from the lower urinary tract to the renal cavities and tissues. The virulence factors involved in UTIs include surface virulence factors such as type 1 fimbriae, P, S and F1C fimbriae; exported virulence factors such as α-haemolysin, cytotoxic necrotising factor 1 (CNF1), secreted autotransporter toxin (SAT), cytolethal distending toxin (CDT) and cytolysin A (Caprioli et al., 1987; Lai et al., 2000; Smith et al., 1963; Tóth et al., 2000).

A common problem in UTI is recurrence, even in patients without anatomic abnormalities or indwelling bladder catheters. It is estimated that 40 to 50% of adult healthy women have experienced at least one UTI in their lifetime, and there is a tendency for these infections to become chronic due to a high rate of recurrence (Ulett et al., 2007). The persistence of the same *E. coli* strain in the urinary tract may be the cause of recurrent prostatitis. In fact, it has been shown that after an episode of acute prostatitis, cultures of expressed prostatic secretions are still positive three months after the end of a six-week course of therapy in one third of men (Kravchick et al., 2004). This may be related to the capacity of bacteria to form biofilm structures. Biofilm can promote persistence in the urinary tract and on biomaterial surfaces by protecting bacteria from the clearing out effect of hydrodynamic forces and the killing activity of host defence mechanisms and antibiotics (Hanna et al., 2003).

1.2 Biofilm and factors involved in its formation

Biofilm is defined as a structured community of bacterial cells enclosed in a self-produced polymeric matrix and adherent to an inert or living surface (Costerton et al., 1999). Biofilm formation is carried out in four steps: adhesion or attachment, early development of biofilm structure, maturation and dispersion of cells from the biofilm into the surrounding environment and return to the planktonic state.
Several surface determinants are involved in biofilm formation such as:

1.2.1 Flagella and motility

Motile *E. coli* generally present multiple peritrichous flagella. Motility is involved in colonization of host organisms or target organs and promotes initial cell-to-surface contact.

1.2.2 Fimbriae

Fimbriae are one of the virulent factors associated with host tissue adhesion of pathogenic *E. coli* strains (Finlay et al., 1997). Among these, type 1 fimbriae are the most common among *E. coli* and have an important role in the initial attachment to abiotic surface in biofilm formation (Pratt et al., 1998).

1.2.3 Autotransporter proteins

These secretory proteins present all the requirements for secretion across the cytoplasmic and the outer membrane to the bacterial cell surface (Desvaux et al., 2004). Among these proteins Ag43, AIDA (adhesin involved in diffuse adherence) and TibA are involved in adhesion. Antigen 43 promotes aggregation of cells through Ag43-Ag43 interactions by an intercellular handshake mechanism (Hasman et al., 1999). Ag43 and type 1 fimbriae are expressed co-ordinately in the cells which normally produce only one type of adherence structure at a time (Schembri et al., 2001). AIDA and TibA are autotransporters with homology to Ag43.

1.2.4 Curli

Curli fimbriae aggregate at the cell surface to form 6- to 12-nm-diameter structures whose length varies between 0.5 and 1 μm. Curli adhesive fibres also promote biofilm formation to abiotic surfaces both by facilitating initial cell–surface interactions and subsequent cell–cell interactions (Cookson et al., 2002; Uhlich et al., 2006; Vidal et al., 1998).

1.2.5 F conjugative pilus

The F-pilus promotes both initial adhesion and biofilm maturation through nonspecific attachment to abiotic surfaces and subsequent cell-to-cell contacts which stabilize the structure of the biofilm (Ghigo et al., 2001; Molin & Tolker-Nielsen, 2003; Reisner et al., 2003).

1.2.6 Exopolysaccharide production

The biofilm matrix is composed by exopolysaccharide. This matrix forms a hydrated viscous layer which protects embedded bacteria from desiccation and from host defences because bacteria forming this structure may not be recognised by the immune system. The matrix

may also be involved in the protection of the bacteria against toxic molecules such as antimicrobials, hydroxyl radicals, and superoxide anions). The biofilm matrix could also inhibit wash-out of enzymes, nutrients, or even signalling molecules that could then accumulate locally and create more favourable microenvironments within the biofilm (Redfield et al., 2002; Starkey et al., 2004; Welch et al., 2002). All these aspects of the matrix could contribute to development of phenotypic resistance of pathogenic *E. coli* biofilms and lead to persistent infections (Anderson et al. 2003; Justice et al. 2004). In addition, the exopolysaccharide interactions with other components of the matrix favour the three-dimensional growth of the biofilm (White et al., 2003). The exopolysaccharides most frequently found in the matrix are poly-β-1,6-N-acetyl-glucosamine, cellulose, colanic acid, lipopolysaccharides and capsules.
In this chapter, the role of biofilm in urinary tract infections and its relation with virulence factors and antimicrobial resistance is explained.

2. Evolution of antimicrobial resistance in uropathogenic *Escherichia coli* (UPEC)

Several studies have demonstrated an increase in antibiotic resistance levels in *E. coli* causing community-acquired urinary tract infection (UTI) (Barret et al., 1999; Daza et al., 2001; Goettsch et al., 2000; Goldstein, 2000; Gupta et al., 2001a). Some authors have suggested that most of these studies are likely to reflect a selection bias because few UTIs are being cultured routinely and culture results are available from patients with complications, recent treatment, and recurrence of infection or suspected resistance (Gupta et al., 2001b). However, taking into account the worldwide increase in antibiotic resistance, this factor can be a major problem in complicated and uncomplicated community-acquired UTIs. Hence, as suggested by the Infectious Diseases Society of America (IDSA), knowledge of local resistance rates and surveillance studies to monitor changes in the susceptibility of *E. coli* is highly recommended. (Warren et al., 1999)
Cotrimoxazole has been the drug of choice for empiric therapy of uncomplicated UTI in women during several years. However, resistance to this compound is higher than 20% in many countries. In Spain, a multicentre study performed in 2006 found a resistance level of 32%, (Andreu et al., 2008) quite similar to the result of 33.9 %found in a previous study completed four years beforehand (Andreu et al., 2005), making the differences found between regions noteworthy (range 23% to 37.3%). Results from a single centre also in Spain found a resistance rate of 25%, with isolates from complicated UTIs (28%) being more resistant than those than from uncomplicated UTIs (22%) (Alós et al., 2005). In the USA, resistance to cotrimoxazole has risen from 15% in 1998 to 21.3% in 2003-2004 (Gupta et al., 2001b)). Again, geographic variations were observed in another study among states (15% to 40%) in the USA and in Canada (10.2 to 48.5%) (Zhanel et al., 2006).
Betalactam antibiotics are widely used in the treatment of UTIs. Among them, ampicillin or amoxicillin are not recommended as first line drugs due to high levels of resistance. In the multicentre study from Spain (Andreu et al., 2008) the rate of resistance was 60.7% with clear differences between regions, the lowest value being 36.8%. Despite ampicillin not having been used to treat uncomplicated cystitis for a long time, resistance to this compound has increased along the years. Amoxicillin plus clavulanic acid shows a high

level of activity compared to ampicillin. Resistance to this drug was only found in 8.1% of isolates with a variation according to geographic zones of 3% to 18.3% (Andreu et al., 2008). Other oral betalactams like cefuroxime (8.9% of resistance) or cefixime (6.9% of resistance) show good activity against *E. coli* urinary isolates, but resistance to both drugs was higher in elderly patients (>60 years)(Andreu et al., 2008). An *E. coli* producer of extended spectrum betalactamases should always be considered as an aetiological agent of UTIs. In the Spanish multicentre study (Andreu et al., 2008) this agent represented 5.2% of *E. coli* isolates with most (79.1%) being recovered from patients over the age of 60 years. These isolates are also frequently resistant to fluorquinolones and cotrimoxazole.

Fluorquinolones can be an option to treat UTIs, but their utility is hampered by resistance rates. In Europe, resistance to ciprofloxacin in UPEC was low in the period from 1999-2000, with the highest values found in Portugal (5.8%) and Spain (14.7%) (Kahlmeter, 2003). The multicentre study published by Zhanel et al. (2006) reported a rate resistance in UPEC of only 1.1% in Canada and 6.8% in the USA, with great differences between regions (2.9% to 20.3%). In the Spanish multicentre study (Andreu et al., 2008) resistance to ciprofloxacin was found in 23.9% of all UPEC isolates and, again, significant geographical differences were found (12.5% to 37.3%). Interestingly, the study by Alós et al., (2005) showed that resistance to ciprofloxacin was higher in UPEC recovered in complicated UTIs (19.5%) than in UPEC isolated in uncomplicated UTIs (8.5%). Both studies found that elderly patients showed higher levels of resistance to fluorquinolones.

Nitrofurantoin shows a good activity against UPEC isolates with only 3.8% resistant isolates (Andreu et al., 2008). However, dosage and potential pulmonary toxicity limits their usefulness. Fosfomycin remains as the most active oral antibiotic against UPEC isolates. Resistance to this drug was of 1.7% in the multicentre study published by Andreu et al., (2008) and the compound usually maintains its activity against ESBL producers.

3. Relationship between virulence factors and antimicrobial resistance in UPEC

The level of quinolone-resistance in *E. coli* clinical isolates has steadily increased in most European countries. When the analysis is stratified according to the different UTIs it is found that the percentage of quinolone-resistant *E. coli* isolates causing pyelonephritis is lower that those causing cystitis (Velasco et al., 2001). This data suggested that the quinolone-resistant *E. coli* lost the ability to colonize the kidney epithelia. In order, to prove this hypothesis a study investigating some urovirulence factors in nalidixic acid resistant *E. coli* clinical isolates compared with a group of quinolone-susceptible clinical isolates was carried out. Haemolysin, cytotoxic necrotizing factor-1 (CNF-1) and the autotransporter toxin (sat) were less prevalent in nalidixic acid-resistant than in nalidixic acid susceptible strains. These results suggested that resistance to quinolones may be associated with a decrease in the presence of some virulence factors in uropathogenic *E. coli* (Vila et al., 2002). A study related quinolone resistance and low virulence with phylogenetic origin, mainly in phylogenetic group A, which show a high level of resistance to quinolones and has a low number of urovirulence factors (Johnson JR, et al., 2003). Among the four phylogenetic groups (A, B1, B2 and D), B2 is considered the most virulent. Therefore in a subsequent study, 31 virulence factors were analyzed among nalidixic acid-susceptible and –resistant *E.*

coli clinical isolates from phylogenetic group B2 and again haemolysin and CNF-1 were less prevalent among nalidixic acid-resistant *E. coli* strains (Horcajada JP, et al. 2005). All three genes (*hly*, encoding haemolysin; *cnf*, encoding the cytotoxic necrotizing factor and *sat*, encoding the autotransporter toxin) have their localization in pathogenicity islands in common. Therefore, we thought that the link between the acquisition of resistance to quinolone and lower prevalence of some virulence factors could be explained by the fact that quinolones have been shown to induce the SOS system (Phillips I. et al., 1987) and this induction can favour the release of a genome phage integrated in the bacterial chromosome. Since the structure of the genome phage and the pathogenicity islands is genetically similar it can be hypothesized that the induction of the SOS system by quinolones would favour the release and loss of the pathogenicity island. Indeed, this hypothesis was proven incubating haemolysin-positive, quinolone-susceptible *E. coli* strains with subinhibitory concentrations of ciprofloxacin and searching for haemolysin-negative *E. coli* mutants. It was shown that these mutants can suffer a partial or total loss of the pathogenicity island, carrying the *hly* and *cnf* genes through a dependent and independent SOS pathway, respectively (Soto et al., 2006). All the abovementioned results suggest that the acquisition of quinolone resistance may generate *E. coli* strains with lower virulence.

4. Relationship between biofilm formation, urovirulence factors and antimicrobial resistance

Biofilm formation may be considered as another pathogenic determinant which allows the strains to persist a long time in the genito-urinary tract and interfere with bacterial eradication. Biofilm endows bacteria with several advantages, such as the acquisition of antibiotic tolerance, expression of several virulence factors and an increased resistance against phagocytosis and other host defence mechanisms. Actually, biofilms are probably the usual living condition of bacteria in natural environments and they are, indeed, regularly involved in infections associated with biomaterials such as catheters or prostheses. In these clinical processes, biofilm formation is the main culprit of the characteristic persistence of the infection, despite appropriate antibiotic therapy and hydrodynamic forces (Hanna et al., 2003). More than 50% of all bacteria infections reported involve biofilm formation (Costerton et al., 1999).

Acute UTI caused by UPEC can lead to recurrent infection, which is denominated "relapse" when it is caused by the same strain as that involved in the original UTI or as "re-infection" when it involves different strains. Approximately 25% of women with an episode of acute cystitis later develop recurrent UTI being an important burden to the health system. A study of women with recurrent UTI showed that 74% of strains causing relapse were biofilm formers (Soto et al., 2007). It had been demonstrated that uropathogens can persist within the bladder tissue in underlying epithelial cells or creating pod-like bulges on the bladder surface being a source of recurrent UTI (Mulvey et al., 2000; Anderson et al., 2003). Two virulence factors related to iron-uptake system, yersiniabactin and aerobactin, have also been associated with relapse (Johnson et al., 2001; Soto et al., 2006) due to the need of the bacteria to capture iron for growth in a stressful environment such as the vagina. However, biofilm production may be the key determinant for the persistence of UPEC in the vaginal reservoir, the bladder epithelial cells or both.

The study of the factors contributing to biofilm formation may be important to conceive new therapeutic solutions for the treatment of these infections. On comparing UPEC collected from patients with cystitis, pyelonephritis or prostatitis it had been observed that strains causing prostatitis presented a higher capacity to form "in vitro" biofilm than those causing cystitis and pyelonephritis (Soto et al., 2007). The increased capacity to form biofilm of these strains could be a possible explanation for the persistence of such strains in the prostatic secretory system.

Wu and colleagues (Wu et al., 1996) suggested that the inhibition of bacterial attachment to an uroepithelial surface, a crucial initial event involving precise interactions between groups of bacterial adhesive molecules called adhesins and their cognate urinary tract receptors, could be interesting to avoid biofilm formation. One of the virulence factors involved in the initial steps of biofilm is type 1 fimbriae which play an important role in the adhesion to the host epithelial cells (Prüss et al., 2006) and confer binding to α-D-mannosylated proteins, such as uroplakins, which are abundant in the bladder (Wu et al., 1996). It had been found that biofilm-producing *E. coli* strains showed a significantly greater type 1 fimbriae expression than non-biofilm producing strains (Soto et al., 2007).

Another mechanism by which UPEC promotes the formation of biofilms is via expression of proteins that mediate cell-cell aggregation (Ulett et al., 2007). Of these, Ag43 is also associated with the early stages of biofilm development (Schembri et al., 2003), although it has been demonstrated that the Ag43 can be dispensable for biofilm formation being replaced by alternative factors, such as conjugative pili (Guigo et al., 2001; Reisner et al., 2003). Ag43 is expressed on the surface of UPEC cells located within intracellular biofilm-like bacterial pods in the bladder epithelium, indicating that it may contribute to survival and persistence during prolonged infection (Anderson et al., 2003).

On the other hand, among of the virulence factors studied, only haemolysin seems to present an association with biofilm production. In fact, haemolysin-positive UPEC strains were strongly linked to prostatitis also shown to have a higher frequency of "in vitro" biofilm formation (Andreu et al., 1997; Johnson et al., 2005; Mitsumori et al., 1999; Ruiz et al., 2002; Soto et al., 2007; Terai et al., 1997). These data confirm that the tropism and invasiveness of *E. coli* strains for the prostate rely mainly on haemolysin but also provide a possible explanation for the persistence of such strains in the prostatic secretory system by means of their increased ability to form biofilm.

It has been previously reported that most *E. coli* isolates collected from faeces belong to phylogenetic groups A and B1, with phylogenetic groups B2 and D being the most frequently isolated in urine and considered as virulent. The differences in the phylogenetic background of these two groups of isolates from urine and faeces indicate that the prostate was not, in most of the cases, colonized by commensal bacteria from the intestinal tract. Strains belonging to phylogenetic group B2 presented a higher capacity to form biofilm than those belonging to phylogenetic groups A, B1 and D (Soto et al., 2007).

A relationship between nalidixic acid susceptibility and "in vitro" biofilm formation seems to exist. Studies comparing biofilm positive UPEC strains versus biofilm negative UPEC strains showed that the percentage of nalidixic acid resistant strains was higher among those non-biofilm formers than among biofilm-formers (Soto et al., 2007). In fact, acquisition of quinolone resistance causes a decrease in the "in vitro" production of biofilm by a decrease in the expression of type 1 fimbriae, avoiding the first step of biofilm formation, the adhesion to the surfaces (unpublished data).

5. Conclusion

Biofilm formation is an important feature related to relapsed UTI, and likely plays an important role in prostatitis caused by *E. coli.* In addition, a link between acquisition of quinolone resistance acquisition and decrease in biofilm formation and loss of some virulence factors has been suggested.

6. Acknowledgements

This work was supported by the Spanish Network for Research in Infectious Diseases (REIPI RE06/0008), SGR091256 of the Department d'Universitats, Recerca I Societat de la Informació de la Generalitat de Catalunya, Fondo de Investigaciones Sanitarias (PI10/01579) of Spain, and by funding from the European Community (TROCAR contract HEALTH-F3-2008-223031). Sara M. Soto is a recipient of a contract "Miguel Servet" (CP05/00140) from "Fondo de Investigaciones Sanitarias" of the Spanish Ministry of Health.

7. References

Alós, I.; Serrano, M. G.; Gómez Garcés, J. L.; Perianes, J. (2005). Antibiotic resistance of *Escherichia coli* from community-acquired urinary tract infections in relation to demographic and clinical data. Clinical Microbiology and Infection, Vol. 11, No. 3, pp. 199–203, ISSN 1198-743X.

Anderson, G. G.; Palermo, J.J.; Schilling, J.D.; Roth, R.; Heuser, J.; Hultgren, S.J. (2003). Intracellular bacterial biofilm-like pods in urinary tract infections. *Science,* Vol. 301, No.5629, pp. 105-107, ISSN 1095-9203.

Andreu, A.; Stapleton, A.E.; Fennel, C.; Lockman, H.A.; Xercavins, M.; Fernandez, F.; Stamm, W.E. (1997). Urovirulence determinants in *Escherichia coli* strains causing prostatitis. *Journal of Infectious Diseases,* Vol. 176, No. 2, pp. 464, ISSN 0022-1899.

Andreu, A.; Alós, I.; Gobernado, M.; Marco, F.; de la Rosa , M.; García-Rodríguez, J. A. (2005). Etiology and antimicrobial susceptibility among uropathogens causing community-acquired lower urinary tract infections: a nationwide surveillance study. *Enfermedades Infecciosas y Microbiol ogia Clinica,* Vol. 23, No. 1, pp. 4-9, ISSN 0213-005X.

Andreu, A.; Planells, I.; Grupo cooperativo Español para el estudio de la sensibilidad antimicrobiana a los patógenos urinarios. (2008). Etiology of community-acquired lower urinary infections and antimicrobial resistance of *Escherichia coli*: a national surveillance study. *Medicina Clinica* (Barcelona). Vol. 130, No. 13, pp. 481-486, ISSN 0025-7753.

Barrett, S. P.; Savage, M. A.; Rebec, M. P.; Guyot, A.; Andrews, N.; Shrimpton, S. B. (1999). Antibiotic sensitivity of bacteria associated with community-acquired urinary tract infection in Britain. *Journal of Antimicrobial Chemotherapy*, Vol. 44, No. 3, pp. 359–365, ISSN 0305-7453.

Caprioli, A.; Falbo, V.; Ruggeri, F.M.; Baldassarri, L.; Bisicchia, R.; Ippolito, G.; Romoli, E.; Donelli, G. (1987). Cytotoxic necrotizing factor production by hemolytic strains of *Escherichia coli* causing extraintestinal infections. *Journal of Clinical Microbiology*, Vol. 25, No. 1, pp. 146-149, ISSN 0095-1137.

Cookson, A. L.; Cooley, W.A; Woodward, M.J. (2002). The role of type 1 and curli fimbriae of Shiga toxin-producing *Escherichia coli* in adherence to abiotic surfaces. *International Journal of Medical Microbiology*, Vol. 292, No. 3-4, pp. 195-205, ISSN 1438-4221.

Costerton, J.W.; Lewandowski, Z.; Caldurell, D.E.; Korber, D.R.; Lappin-Scott, H.M. (1995). Microbial biofilms. *Annual Reviews in Microbiology*, Vol. 49, pp. 711-745, ISSN 0066-4227.

Costerton, J. W. (1999a). Introduction to biofilm. *International Journal of Antimicrobial Agents*, Vol. 11, No. 3-4, pp. 217-221, ISSN 0924-8579.

Costerton, J. W.; Stewart P.S.; Greenberg, E.P. (1999b). Bacterial biofilms: a common cause of persistent infections. *Science*, Vol. 284, No. 5418, pp. 1318-1322, ISSN 1095-9203.

Daza, R.; Gutierrez, J.; Piedrola, G. (2001). Antibiotic susceptibility of bacterial strains isolated from patients with community-acquired urinary tract infections. *International Journal of Antimicrobial Agents*, Vol. 18, No. 3, pp. 211–215, ISSN 0924-8579.

Desvaux, M.; Parham, N.J.; et al. (2004). The autotransporter secretion system. *Research in Microbiology*, Vol. 155, No. 2, pp. 53-60, ISSN 0923-2508.

Finlay, B. B. (1997). Interactions of enteric pathogens with human epithelial cells. Bacterial exploitation of host processes. *Advances in Experimental and Medical Biology*, Vol. 412, pp. 289-293, ISSN 0065-2598.

Ghigo, J. M. (2001). Natural conjugative plasmids induce bacterial biofilm development. *Nature* Vol. 412, No. 6845, pp. 442-445, ISSN 0028-0836.

Goettsch, W.; van Pelt, W.; Nagelkerke, N.; Hendrix, M. G.; Buiting, A. G.; et al. (2000). Increasing resistance to fluoroquinolones in *Escherichia coli* from urinary tract infections in the Netherlands. *Journal of Antimicrobial Chemotherapy*, Vol. 46, No. 2, pp. 223–228, ISSN 0305-7453.

Goldstein, F. W. (2000). Antibiotic susceptibility of bacterial strains isolated from patients with community-acquired urinary tract infections in France. Multicentre Study Group. *European Journal of Clinical Microbioloy and Infectious Diseases*, Vol. 19, No. 2, pp. 112–117, ISSN 0934-9723.

Gupta, K.; Hooton, T. M.; Stamm, W. E. (2001a). Increasing antimicrobial resistance and the management of uncomplicated community-acquired urinary tract infections. *Annual of International Medicine*, Vol. 135, No. 1, pp. 41–50, ISSN 0003-4819.

Gupta, K.; Sahm, D. F.; Mayfield, D.; Stamm, W. E. (2001b). Antimicrobial resistance among uropathogens that cause community-acquired urinary tract infections in women: a nationwide analysis. *Clinical Infectious Diseases*, Vol. 33, No. 1, pp. 89-94, ISSN 1058-4838.

Hanna, A.; Berg, M.; Stout, V.; Razatos, A. (2003). Role of capsular colanic acid in adhesion of uropathogenic *Escherichia coli*. *Applied Environmental Microbiology*, Vol. 69, No. 8, pp. 4474-4481, ISSN 0099-2240.

Hasman, H.; Chakraborty, T.; Klemm, P. (1999). Antigen-43-mediated autoaggregation of *Escherichia coli* is blocked by fimbriation. *Journal of Bacteriology*, Vol. 181, No. 16, pp. 4834-4841, ISSN 0021-9193.

Horcajada, J.P.; Soto, S.M.; Gajewski, A.; Jiménez de Anta, M.T.; Mensa, J.; Vila, J.; Johnson, J.R. (2005). Quinolone resistant uropathogenic *Escherichia coli* from phylogeneticgroup B2 have fewer virulence factors than their susceptible counterparts. *Journal of Clinical Microbiology*, Vol. 43, No. 6, pp. 2962-2964, ISSN 0095-1137.

Johnson, J.R.; O'Bryan, T.T.; Delavari, P.; Kuskowski, M.; Stapleton, A.; Carlino, U.; et al. (2001). Clonal relationships and extended virulence genotypes among *Escherichia coli* isolates from women with a first or recurrent episode of cystitis. *Journal of Infectious Diseases*, Vol. 183, pp. 1508-1517, ISSN 0022-1899.

Johnson, J.R.; Kuskowski, M.A.; Owens, K.; Gajewski, A.; Winokur, P.L. (2003). Phylogenetic origin and virulence genotype in relation to resistance to fluoroquinolones and/or extended-spectrum cephalosporins and cephamycins among *Escherichia coli* isolates from animals and humans. *Journal of Infectious Diseases*, Vol. 188, No. 5, pp. 759–768, ISSN 0022-1899.

Johnson, J.R.; Kuskowski, M.A.; Gajewski, A.; Soto, S.; Horcajada, J.P.; Jimenez de Anta, M.T.; Vila, J. (2005). Extended virulence genotypes and phylogenetic background of *Escherichia coli* isolates from patients with cystitis, pyelonephritis, or prostatitis. *Journal of Infectious Diseases*, Vol. 191, No. 1, pp. 46-50, ISSN 0022-1899.

Justice, S. S.; Hung,C.; Theriot, J.A.; Fletcher, D.A.; Anderson, G.G.; Footer, M.J.; et al. (2004). Differentiation and developmental pathways of uropathogenic *Escherichia coli* in urinary tract pathogenesis. *Procedings of the National Academy of Sciences of the United States of America*, Vol. 101, No. 5, pp. 1333-1338, ISSN 0027-8424.

Kahlmeter G. (2003). An international survey of the antimicrobial susceptibility of pathogens from uncomplicated urinary tract infections: the ECO-SENS Project. International Journal of Antimicrobial Agents, Vol. 22, No. 1, pp. S49-S52, ISSN 0924-8579.

Kravchick, S.; Cytron, S.; Agulansky, L.; Ben-Dor, D. (2004). Acute prostatitis in middle-aged men: a prospective study. British Journal of Urology International, Vol. 93, No. 1, pp. 93-96, ISSN 1464-410X.

Lai, X.H.; Arencibia, I.; Johansson, A.; Wai, S.N.; Oscarsson, J. (2000). Cytocidal and apoptotic effects of the ClyA protein from *Escherichia coli* on primary and cultured monocytes and macrophages. Infection and Immunity, Vol. 68, No. 7, pp. 4363-4367, ISSN 0019-9567.

Mitsumori, K.; Terai, A.; Yamamoto, S.; Ishitoya, S.; Yoshida, O. (1999). Virulence characteristics of *Escherichia coli* in acute bacterial prostatitis. *Journal of Infectious Diseases*, Vol. 180, No. 4, pp. 1378-1381, ISSN 0022-1899.

Molin, S.; Tolker-Nielsen, T. (2003). Gene transfer occurs with enhanced efficiency in biofilms and induces enhanced stabilisation of the biofilm structure. *Current Opinion on Biotechnology,* Vol. 14, No. 3, pp. 255-261, ISSN 0958-1669.

Mulvey, M.A.; Schilling, J.D.; Martinez, J.J.; Hultgren, S.J. (2000). Bad bugs and beleaguered bladders: interplay between uropathogenic *Escherichia coli* and innate host defenses. *Procedings of the National Academy of Sciences of the United States of America,* Vol. 97, No. 16, pp. 8829-35, ISSN 0027-8424.

Phillips, I.; Culebras, E.; Moreno, F.; Baquero, F. (1987). Induction of the SOS response by new 4-quinolones. *Journal of Antimicrobial Chemotherapy,* Vol. 20, No. 5, pp. 631-638, ISSN 0305-7453.

Pratt, L. A.; Kolter, R. (1998). Genetic analysis of *Escherichia coli* biofilm formation: roles of flagella, motility, chemotaxis and type I pili. *Molecular Microbiology,* Vol. 30, No. 2, pp. 285-293, ISSN 0950-382X.

Prüss, B.M.; Besemann, C.; Denton, A.; Wolfe, A.J. (2006). A complex transcription network controls the early stages of biofilm development by *Escherichia coli. Journal of Bacteriology,* Vol. 188, No. 11, pp. 3731-3739, ISSN 0021-9193.

Redfield, R. J. (2002). Is quorum sensing a side effect of diffusion sensing? *Trends in Microbiology,* Vol. 10, No. 8, pp. 365-370, ISSN 0966-842X.

Reisner, A.; Haagensen J.A.; Schembri, M.A.; Zechner, E.L.; Molin, S. (2003). Development and maturation of *Escherichia coli* K-12 biofilms. *Molecular Microbiology,* Vol. 48, No. 4, pp. 933-946, ISSN 0950-382X.

Ruiz, J.; Simon, K.; Horcajada, J.P.; Velasco, M.; Barranco, M.; Roig, G.; Moreno-Martinez, A.; Martinez, J.A.; Jimenez de Anta, M.T.; Mensa, J.; Vila, J. (2002). Differences in virulence factors among clinical isolates of *Escherichia coli* causing cystitis and pyelonephritis in women and prostatitis in men. *Journal of Clinical Microbiology,* Vol. 40, No. 12, pp. 4445–4449, ISSN 0095-1137.

Schembri, M. A.; Christiansen, G.; Klemm, P. (2001). FimH-mediated autoaggregation of *Escherichia coli. Molecular Microbiology,* Vol. 41, No. 6, pp. 1419-1430, ISSN 0950-382X.

Schembri, M.A.; Hjerrild, L.; Gjermansen, M.; Klemm, P. (2003). Differential expression of the *Escherichia coli* autoaggregation factor antigen 43. *Journal of Bacteriology,* Vol. 185, No. 7, pp. 2236-2242, ISSN 0021-9193.

Smith, H. W. (1963). The haemolysins of *Escherichia coli. Journal of Pathology and Bacteriology,* Vol. 85, pp. 197-211, ISSN 0368-3494.

Soto, S.M.; Smithson, A.; Horcajada, J.P.; Martinez, J.A.; Mensa, J.; Vila, J. (2006). Implication of biofilm formation in the persistence of urinary tract infection caused by uropathogenic *Escherichia coli. Clinical Microbiology and Infection,* Vol. 12, No. 10, p.p. 1034-1036, ISSN 1198-743X.

Soto, S.M.; Jimenez de Anta, M.T.; Vila, J. (2006). Quinolones induce partial or total loss of pathogenicity islands in uropathogenic *Escherichia coli* by SOS-dependent or -independent pathways, respectively. *Antimicrobial Agents and Chemotherapy,* Vol. 50, No. 2, pp. 649-653, ISSN 0066-4804.

Soto, S.M.; Smithson, A.; Martinez, J.A.; Horcajada, J.P.; Mensa, J.; Vila, J. (2007). Biofilm formation in uropathogenic *Escherichia coli* strains: relationship with prostatitis, urovirulence factors and antimicrobial resistance. *Journal of Urology*, Vol. 177, No. 1, pp. 365-368, ISSN 0022-5347.

Terai, A.; Yamamoto, S.; Mitsumori, K.; Okada, Y.; Kurazono, H.; Takeda, Y.; et al. (1997). *Escherichia coli* virulence factors and serotypes in acute bacterial prostatitis. *International Journal of Urology*, Vol. 4, No. 3, pp. 289-294, ISSN 0919-8172.

Toth, I.; Oswald, E.; Mitsumori, K.; Szabo, B.; Barcs, I.; Emody, L. (2000). Virulence markers of human uropathogenic *Escherichia coli* strains isolated in Hungary. *Advances in Experimental and Medical Biology*, Vol. 485, pp. 335-338, ISSN 0065-2598.

Uhlich, G. A.; Cooke, P.H.; Solomon, E.B. (2006). Analyses of the red-dry-rough phenotype of an *Escherichia coli* O157:H7 strain and its role in biofilm formation and resistance to antibacterial agents. *Applied Environmental Microbiology*, Vol. 72, No. 4, pp. 2564-2572, ISSN 0099-2240.

Ulett, G. C.; Mabbett,A.N.; Fung, K.C.; Webb, R.I.; Schembri, M.A. (2007a). The role of F9 fimbriae of uropathogenic *Escherichia coli* in biofilm formation. *Microbiology*, Vol. 153, Pt. 7, pp. 2321-2331, ISSN 1350-0872.

Ulett, G. C.; Valle, J.; Beloin, C.; Sherlock, O.; Ghigo, J.M.; Schembri, M.A. (2007b). Functional analysis of antigen 43 in uropathogenic *Escherichia coli* reveals a role in long-term persistence in the urinary tract. *Infection and Immunity*, Vol. 75, No. 7, pp. 3233-3244, ISSN 0099-9567.

Velasco, M.; Horcajada, J.P.; Mensa, J.; Moreno-Martinez, A.; Vila, J.; Martinez, J.A.; Ruiz, J.; Barranco, M.; Roig, G.; Soriano, E. (2001). Decreased invasive capacity of quinolone-resistant *Escherichia coli* in patients with urinary tract infections. *Clinical of Infectious Diseases*, Vol. 33, No. 10, pp. :1682–1686, ISSN 1058-4838.

Vidal, O.; Longin, R.; Prigent-Combaret, C.; Dorel, C.; Hooreman, M.; Lejeune, P. (1998). Isolation of an *Escherichia coli* K-12 mutant strain able to form biofilms on inert surfaces: involvement of a new *omp*R allele that increases curli expression. *Journal of Bacteriology*, Vol. 180, No. 9, pp. 2442-2449, ISSN 0021-9193.

Vila, J.; Simon, K.; Ruiz, J.; Horcajada, J.P.; Velasco, M.; Barranco, M.; et al. (2002). Are quinolone-resistant uropathogenic *Escherichia coli* less virulent? *Journal of Infectious Diseases*, Vol. 186, No. 7, pp. 1039-1042, ISSN 0022-1899.

Warren, J. W.; Abrutyn, E.; Hebel, J. R.; Johnson, J. R.; Schaeffer, A. J.; Stamm, W. E. (1999). Guidelines for antimicrobial treatment of uncomplicated acute bacterial cystitis and acute pyelonephritis in women. Infectious Diseases Society of America (IDSA). *Clinical Infectious Diseases*, Vol. 29, No. 4, pp. 745–758, ISSN 1058-4838.

Welch, R. A.; Burland, V.; Plunkett, G.; Redford, P.; Roesch, P.; Rasko, D.; et al. (2002). Extensive mosaic structure revealed by the complete genome sequence of uropathogenic *Escherichia coli*. *Procedings of the National Academy of Sciences of the United States of America*, Vol. 99, No. 26, pp. 17020-17024, ISNN 0027-8424.

White, A.P.; Gibson, D.L.; Collinson, S.K.; Banser, P.A.; Kay, W.W. (2003). Extracellular polysaccharides associated with thin aggregative fimbriae of *Salmonella enterica* serovar *enteritidis*. *Journal of Bacteriology*, Vol. 185, No. 18, pp. 5398-407, ISSN 0021-9193.

Wu, X.R.; Sun, T.T.; Medina, J.J. (1996). In vitro binding of type 1-fimbriated *Escherichia coli* to uroplakins Ia and Ib: Relation to urinary tract infections. *Procedings of the National*

Academy of Sciences of the United States of America, Vol. 93, No. 18, pp. 9630-9635, ISSN 0027-8424.

Zhanel, G. G.; Hisanaga, T. L.; Laing, N. M.; DeCorby, M. R.; Nichol, K. A.; et al. (2006). Antibiotic resistence in *Escherichia coli* outpatient urinary isolates: final results from the North American Urinary Tract Infection Collaborative Alliance (NAUTICA). International Journal of Antimicrobial Agents, Vol. 27, No. 6, pp. 468-75, ISSN 0924-8579.

11

Rheumatoid Arthritis is Caused by Asymptomatic Proteus Urinary Tract Infections

Taha Rashid and Alan Ebringer
King's College, Analytical Sciences Group, London
U.K

1. Introduction

Urinary tract infections (UTI) are considered as one of the most common groups of infections in humans and affecting either the upper (kidneys--pyelonephritis) or the lower (bladder--cystitis) part of the urinary tract (Thomson and Armitage, 2010).

The gastrointestinal tract is a reservoir from which uropathogens emerge. Reflecting this, *Enterobacteriaceae* are the most important cause of UTI in all population groups, accounting for more than 95% of all UTIs. Among these microbes, *E. coli* is by far the most common invader, causing some 90% of UTIs in outpatients and approximately 50% in hospitalized patients. Whilst, the frequency of *P. mirabilis* causing outpatient and inpatients UTIs were 3.2% and 12.7% respectively, these value were reversed to 26.6% and 9.3% when all strains of *Proteus* species were examined (Talkoff-Robin et al, 2008). In a most recent multicentre study involving nine Spanish hospitals, 784 women with uncomplicated cystitis were evaluated for the frequencies of isolated uropathogens and their susceptibility to antibiotics. Among the 650 pathogens isolated, the first group of the most frequent bacterial agents was *Escherichia coli* (79.2%) followed by *Staphylococcus saprophyticus* (4.4%), *Proteus mirabilis* (4.3%), *Enterococcus faecalis* (3.3%), and *Klebsiella pneumoniae* (2.3%) (Palou et al, 2011).

In contrast to *E. coli* strains, it appears that all strains of *P. mirabilis*, regardless of isolate origin, are capable of infecting the urinary tract (Sosa et al, 2006). *Proteus* is particularly significant as a renal pathogen especially in causing upper UTI because of its propensity to promote struvite renal calculi (Ronald and Nicolle, 2007).

2. Asymptomatic bacteriuria and subclinical urinary infections

Bacteriuria might be either symptomatic or asymptomatic. An estimated 40% of women and 12% of men will experience at least one attack of symptomatic or overt UTI during their lifetime, and approximately a quarter of affected women will suffer recurrent UTIs within 6-12 months (Nielubowicz and Mobley, 2010).

Asymptomatic bacteriuria (ABU) is considered as one of the most common findings in women all over the world. It is defined as the presence of $\geq 10^5$ cfu/ml of the same bacterial species in two consecutive midstream urine samples (Schmiemann et al, 2010). Although in the majority of patients with ABU the site of infection is in the lower urinary tract, some individuals with ABU, however, do have upper tract involvement (Ronald and Nicolle, 2007). In a cross-sectional longitudinal study, Kunin and associates have found that among 16,000 schoolgirls with ages ranging between 6 to 18 years the prevalence of UTI was 1.2%, and two-third of 5% girls who had one or more episodes of bacteriuria were asymptomatic (Kunin, 1970). It also appears that the prevalence of asymptomatic bacteriuria increases with age and this has been reported by Gaymans et al (1976), where in a study of 1,758 Dutch women, the prevalence of bacteriuria was found to be increased from 2.7% of women aged 15 to 24 years to 9.3% of women aged 65 years or older.

Although it is usually true to say that bacteriuria is a valid indicator of either bacterial localization or infection of the urinary tract, studies in animals (Mulvey et al, 1998) and humans (Elliott et al, 1985) have indicated that bacteria may reside in the urothelium in the absence of bacteriuria. The majority of patients with kidney or upper tract infection show the clinical signs and symptoms of pyelonephritis, but in others this might not be the case. In a study by Stamey et al (1965), using ureteral catheterization it was shown that 50 percent of women with asymptomatic bacteriuria had infection in their upper tracts, and that a small but significant proportion of women with preliminary associated cystitis also had upper UTI. It is possible that bacteria within the kidney or upper urinary tract may remain latent in a nidus of infection for any length of time (Cattell, 2005). For example *Proteus* spp. can form urinary calculi and remain dormant inside these infected stones undetected and resistant to the effects of antibiotics used. It should also be stressed that *P. mirabilis* is probably the second most common microbe among the family of *Enterobacteriaceae* after *E. coli* in causing UTI, especially of the upper tract in middle-aged and elderly women (Senior, 1979).

3. Rheumatoid arthritis and urinary tract infections

Rheumatoid arthritis (RA) is a potentially disabling chronic systemic polyarthropathy with a world-wide distribution and an increased likelihood to have a considerable amount of negative impacts on the economical status of the patient and society (Zhang and Anis 2011). The cause of this disease is generally agreed to be due to a combined action of genetic and environmental (mainly microbial) factors (Firestein, 2009).

Among the urologists and rheumatologists, the evidence of the link between UTIs and RA is not apparently recognized because of the consistent lack of data supporting this association and more probably because of the possibility for an existing hidden infection expressed in the form of asymptomatic bacteriuria in patients with RA.

In a preliminary study carried out by a group from Tel Aviv, it has been found that 35 percent of patients with RA and secondary Sjogren's syndrome had recurrent attacks of UTIs (Tishler et al, 1992). Furthermore, another group from Edinburgh, using a necroscopic examination of kidneys from dead patients with RA, found that approximately 17.6 percent of males and 22.7 percent of female patients showed signs of chronic pyelonephritis (Lawson and Maclean, 1966). A similar result was found in a previous study carried out by a group from Copenhagen, where a considerably high degree of associated non-obstructive pyelonephritis and renal papillary necrosis was detected among the renal autopsy materials from patients with RA (Clausen and Pedersen, 1961). However, this kind of association between RA and UTIs was not always observed (Vandenbroucke et al, 1987). This discrepancy in the results with an apparent lack of the epidemiological link between urinary infections and RA could be due to the occurrence of sub-clinical or occult infections, which are merely characterized by bacteriuria.

4. *Proteus* in the urine of patients with RA

RA is most probably caused or initiated by an upper urinary tract infection with *Proteus* bacteria. Regarding this particular subject, more than 100 articles have been published by our and various other collaborative as well as independent groups throughout the world (Ebringer et al, 2010).

The first evidence of a link between *Proteus* microbe and RA was reported nearly three decades ago where in a study by Chandler and co-workers, it was shown that among a panel of 30 microbial agents tested, the mean geometric titres of antibodies were raised only against *Proteus* OXK and herpes virus hominis microbes in 22 newly diagnosed RA patients when compared to 22 control subjects (Chandler et al, 1971). Meanwhile, this disease-microbe association was established fourteen years later in a study by our group, where a significant elevation of *Proteus* antibodies ($p<0.001$) was shown in 30 patients with RA compared to 41 healthy controls (Ebringer et al, 1985). To search for the source of this microbe in urinary tract of RA patients various studies were carried out by our and other independent groups:

1. In a controlled study of 89 patients with RA from London, *P. mirabilis* was isolated from the urine of 63% of female and 50% of male patients and these results were found to be significant in comparison to female (32%) ($p<0.001$) or male (11%) ($p<0.001$) healthy subjects. However, the frequency of the isolation of *Proteus* from urine of men and women patients without RA (osteoarthritis, fibromyalgia, psoriasis, gout, and systemic lupus erythematosus) was 7% and 35% respectively, which were similar to those obtained from healthy men (11%) and women (32%) individuals (Figure 1). Furthermore, a positive correlation was found between high anti-*Proteus* antibody levels in sera of RA patients and the number of colony-forming units obtained from urine specimens of these patients (Wilson et al, 1997).
2. In another study carried out by a group of scientists from Dundee in the UK, a significantly increased isolation rate of *Proteus* microbes from the urine of 76 patients (33%) were detected when compared to those of 48 gender-matched healthy individuals (4%) (Senior et al 1999) and this isolation rate was found to be occurring twice more frequently as *E. coli*. In the same study significant elevations ($p<0.001$) of antibodies against *P. mirabilis* were detected in the urine and serum samples of patients with RA when compared to the corresponding healthy subjects.

Another group, however, was unable to find a significant increase in the isolation of *Proteus* microbes from the urine or faeces of RA patients (McDonagh et al, 1994).

5. *Proteus* virulence factors and cross-reactive antigens

The main virulence factors which have been involved in the uropathogenetic mechanisms and utilized by the major group of uropathogens, namely *E. coli* and *P. mirabilis* include motility, adherence, biofilm formations, β-lactamase productions, toxin productions, hydrolytic enzyme productions, metal acquisitions and evasion of the host immune defenses (Dobrindt, 2010).

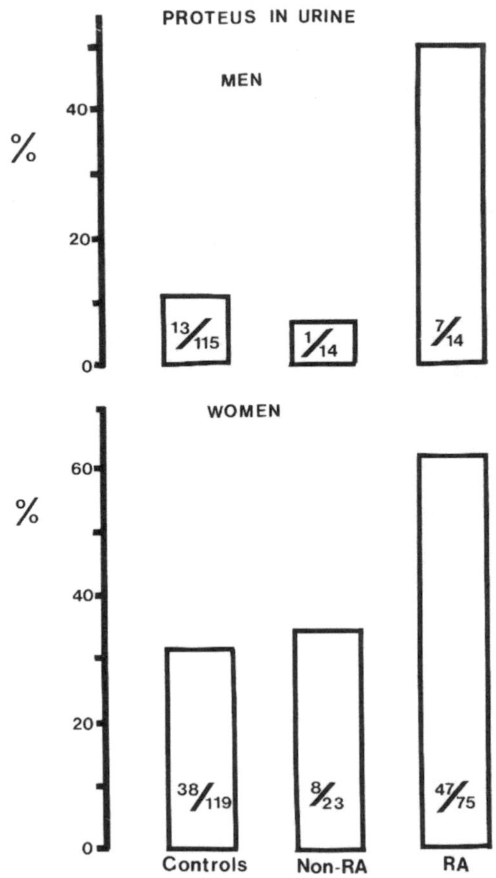

Fig. 1. Percentage isolation of *Proteus* bacteria from the urine of rheumatoid arthritis (RA) and non-RA patients and healthy controls. (Urine cultures were measured down to the level of 1 cfu/ml of urine, to determine presence or absence of bacterial signal).

In contrast to *E. coli*, *P. mirabilis* is the main producer of the urease enzyme (Rozaliski et al, 1997), which hydrolyzes urea into ammonia and carbonate. One of the hallmarks of UTI caused by *P. mirabilis* is the production of urinary stones through action of urease. These stones which are a composite of magnesium ammonium phosphate crystals (struvite), might act as infective reservoirs of *Proteus* microbes, and basically protected from host defenses and antibiotic treatment (Li et al, 2002).

Proteus microbes possess various different antigens. Two of these were found to resemble self tissue antigens. The *Proteus* haemolysin protein possesses six amino acid molecules "ESRRAL" which resembles a similar amino acid motif "EQRRAA" present in the HLA-DR1/4 genetic molecules (Wilson et al, 1995) frequently found in association with RA (Stastny, 1976). Whilst another group of antigens comprising five amino acid molecules "IRRET" which is present in *Proteus* urease resembles the "LRREI" motif present in type XI collagens (Wilson et al, 1995), which is found in hyaline cartilage of the joint tissues.

6. *Proteus* antibodies and their role in the pathogenetic mechanism of RA

Elevated levels of antibodies to *P. mirabilis* have been detected in patients with RA among many populations from 14 different countries including UK, USA, France, and Netherlands (Ebringer et al, 2010). These results have been detected by using various immunological methods carried out by collaborative (Table 1) and other independent (Tables 2) groups. The specificity of *Proteus* antibodies in patients with RA was shown in many studies. Deighton et al, found that antibodies to *P. mirabilis* but not to four different viruses (Deighton[1] et al, 1992) were elevated significantly in RA patients. Moreover, in a review analysis it was shown that in patients with RA there were significant elevations of antibodies to *Proteus* but not against more than 20 other enterobacterial or uropathogenic microbes, including *E. coli* (Rashid et al, 2007).

As the result of molecular mimicry or similarity between *Proteus* and self antigens, patients infected with *Proteus* microbes will produce not only antibodies against this microbe but also against the self tissue molecules carrying the cross-reactive antigens. These antibodies will bind to and be cytopathic to the joint tissues which carry *Proteus* cross-reactive antigens (Wilson et al, 2003) and this immune reaction will lead to the release of more self tissue antigens with a consequent production of further autoantibodies, propagation of the pathological process and the development of classical RA, in the same way that *Streptococcus* causes rheumatic fever and valvular lesions in the heart (Guilherme et al, 2011).

7. A proposal for a new treatment in RA—eradication of *Proteus* microbes

Currently the pharmacologic treatment of RA mainly involves the use of disease modifying anti-rheumatic drugs and biological agents (Haraoui and Pope, 2011). In concurrent use with these medical treatments other therapeutic measures can be employed in order to eradicate *Proteus* bacteria from the urinary tract which could help to prevent further tissue and joint damages in patients with RA. These measures could involve the use of cranberry juice products, antibiotics or even vaccination.

Cranberry products have been used widely for several decades for the prevention and treatment of UTIs. A meta-analysis has established that recurrence rates of UTIs over 1 year are reduced approximately by 35% in young to middle-aged women (Guay, 2009). Other studies, however, either supported (Ferrara et al, 2009) or disputed (Barbosa-Cesnik et al, 2011) the effect of cranberry preparations in the prevention of UTIs.

Although the use of anti-microbial agents has not been recognized in the management of RA, some antibiotics have already been tried with encouraging results. Among these are sulphasalazine, metronidazole, rifampicin and minocycline (Ebringer et al, 2003). Some problems, however, exist in regard to the use of antibiotics against *Proteus* microbes. Firstly, *Proteus* infection affects mainly the kidneys and upper urinary tract (Fairley, et al, 1971) where the use of ordinary sterilizing substances and antibiotics can be less effective. Secondly, *P. mirabilis* possesses various virulence factors which enhance its urinary epithelial invasiveness rendering this microbe resistant to antibiotics (Mathoera et al, 2002). Thirdly, when an infected struvite stone is present in the kidney, none of the antibiotic agents seems to be effective unless the stone is removed by surgery or shock-wave therapy.

In order to test the effects of antibiotics in patients with RA through prospective longitudinal studies, the search for an effective anti-*Proteus* chemotherapeutic agent is mandatory. In a most recent study from Japan it was shown that all of the *P. mirabilis* strains including extended system β-lactamase (ESBL)-producing strains were susceptible to penicillin derivatives combined with β-lactamase inhibitors (Ishikawa et al, 2011). In another study, it was shown that among the three carbapenems tested, meropenem was the most potent antibiotic being effective against the majority of the *Proteus* species isolates (Lee et al, 2011). If patients with RA respond to anti-microbial measures, prophylaxis of susceptible individuals could be instigated by the mean of immunization with attenuated antigens from causative microbe or other cross-reactive microbes among the *Enterobacteriaceae* group (Scavone et al, 2011).

It is logical to start treating patients with RA from early stages of the disease in order to prevent further irreversible joint damages from occurring. If such early therapy is undertaken the possibility arises that RA may be eradicated in the same way that rheumatic fever has been eliminated in the Western World by the means of early treatment of *Streptoccocal* tonsillitis with penicillin and other related antibiotics.

8. General discussion

It generally appears that there is an apparent relationship between *Proteus* asymptomatic UTIs and RA. The main hallmark of this association is based on showing the linkage between RA and *Proteus* but not other microbes in the majority of studies carried out by various groups throughout the world. The combination of isolation of *Proteus* microbes in the urine and elevation of antibodies in sera of RA patients as well as the evidence for the cytopathic effects of these antibodies against the joint tissue cross-reactive antigens, forms the major evidence for the role of this microbe in the development of RA. Elimination of *Proteus* microbes by using cranberry juice, antibiotics could have a remarkable effect in the management of RA patients alongside currently used anti-rheumatic drugs. It would appear that the management of RA may be relevant to urologists as well as to rheumatologists.

YEAR	RA	HC	METHOD	P VALUE	REFERENCE
1985	30	41	AM	P<0.001	Ebringer et al
1988	32	18	ELISA	P<0.05	Khalafpour et al
1995	50	49	ELISA	P<0.001	Fielder et al
1995	40	30	ELISA	P<0.001	Wilson et al
1995	34	33	ELISA+IIF	P<0.001	Subair et al
1996	66	60	ELISA	P<0.001	Tiwana et al
1997	50	50	ELISA	P<0.001	Tani et al
1997	89	234	ELISA	P<0.001	Wilson et al
1997	60	60	ELISA	P<0.001	Tiwana et al
1998	25	34	IIF	P<0.001	Blankenberg-Sprenkels et al
1999	114	69	IIF	P<0.001	Rashid et al
2003	51	38	ELISA	P<0.001	Wilson et al
2004	159	53	IIF	P<0.001	Rashid et al
2006	50	38	ELISA	P<0.0001	Rashid et al
2007	70	20	ELISA	P<0.001	Rashid et al

RA = rheumatoid arthritis; HC = healthy controls; AM = agglutination method ; ELISA = enzyme-linked immunosorbent assay; IIF = indirect immunofluorescence.

Table 1. Studies carried out by various collaborative groups showing increased anti-*Proteus* antibodies in patients with RA compared to HC individuals (number of subjects indicated in each study).

YEAR	RA	CONTROLS*	METHOD	P VALUE	REFERENCE
1988	29	30	ELISA	P<0.01	Rogers et al
1991	9	10+10 (AS+HC)	ELISA	p<0.01; NS	Murphy et al
1992	142	121	IIF	P<0.0001	Deighton[2] et al
1994	87	29 (non-RA)	IIF	P<0.003	McDonagh et al
1995	27	27 (non-RA)	ELISA; IB	P<0.0001	Senior et al
1996	40	40	ELISA	P<0.001	Dybwad et al
1997	70	82	AM	P<0.001	Wanchu et al
1999	39	51	ELISA	p<0.001	Chou et al
2003	50	25	AM	P<0.001	Gautam et al
2005	59	63	IB	P<0.01	Weisbart et al
2005	246	43+90 (SpA+UA)	ELISA	P<0.0003; p<0.015	Newkirk et al

*Controls are always healthy individuals unless otherwise stated; RA = rheumatoid arthritis; AS = ankylosing spondylitis; HC = healthy control; SpA = spondyloarthropathy; UA = undifferentiated arthritis; ELISA = enzyme-linked immunosorbent assay; IIF = indirect immunofluorescence; AM = agglutination method; IB = immunoblot; NS = not significant.

Table 2. Studies carried out by independent groups showing increased anti-*Proteus* antibodies in patients with RA compared to controls.

9. Acknowledgements

This work was supported by the "American Friends of King's College".

10. References

Barbosa-Cesnik C, Brown MB, Buxton M, Zhang L, DeBusscher J, Foxman B. Cranberry juice fails to prevent recurrent urinary tract infection: results from a randomized placebo-controlled trial. Clin Infect Dis 2011;52:23-30.

Blankenberg-Sprenkels SH, Fielder M, Feltkamp TE, Tiwana H, Wilson C, Ebringer A. Antibodies to *Klebsiella pneumoniae* in Dutch patients with ankylosing spondylitis and acute anterior uveitis and to *Proteus mirabilis* in rheumatoid arthritis. J Rheumatol 1998;25:743–747.

Cattell WR. Lower and upper urinary tract infections. In: Davison AM, Cameron JS, Grunfeld J, Ponticelli C, Ritz E, Winearls CG, van Ypersele C (editors). Oxford Textbook of Clinical Nephrology. Oxford University Press, Oxford, 2005;1111-1129.

Chandler RW, Robinson H, Masi AT. Serological investigations for evidence of an infectious aetiology of rheumatoid arthritis. Ann Rheum Dis 1971;30:274-278.

Chou CT, Uksila J, Toivanen P. Enterobacterial antibodies in Chinese patients with rheumatoid arthritis and ankylosing spondylitis. Clin Exp Rheumatol 1998;16:161-164.

Clausen E, Pedersen J. Necrosis of the renal papillae in rheumatoid arthritis. Acta Med Scand 1961;170:631-633.

Deighton[1] CM, Gray JW, Bint AJ, Walker DJ. Specificity of the *Proteus* antibody response in rheumatoid arthritis. Ann Rheum Dis 1992;51:1206–1207.

Deighton[2] CM, Gray JW, Bint AJ, Walker DJ. Anti-*Proteus* antibodies in rheumatoid arthritis same-sexed sibships. Br J Rheumatol 1992;31:241-245.

Dobrindt U. Virulence factors of uropathogens. Urologe A 2010;49:598-605.

Dybwad A, Forre O, Sioud M. Increased serum and synovial fluid antibodies to immunoselected peptides in patients with rheumatoid arthritis. Ann Rheum Dis 1996;55:437-441.

Ebringer A, Ptaszynska T, Corbett M, Wilson C, Macafee Y, Avakian H, Baron P, James DC. Antibodies to *Proteus* in rheumatoid arthritis. Lancet 1985;ii:305–307.

Ebringer A, Rashid T, Wilson C. Rheumatoid arthritis: proposal for the use of anti-microbial therapy in early cases. Scand J Rheumatol 2003;32:2–11.

Ebringer A, Rashid T, Wilson C. Rheumatoid arthritis, *Proteus*, anti-CCP antibodies and Karl Popper. Autoimm Rev 2010;9:216-223.

Elliott TS, Reed L, Slack RC, Bishop MC. Bacteriology and ultrastructure of the bladder in patients with urinary tract infections. J Infect 1985;11:191-199.

Fairley KF, Carson NE, Gutch RC, Leighton P, Grounds AD, Laird EC, et al. Site of infection in acute urinary tract infection in general practice. Lancet 1971;ii:615-618.

Ferrara P, Romaniello L, Vitelli O, Gatto A, Serva M, Cataldi L. Cranberry juice for the prevention of recurrent urinary tract infections: a randomized controlled trial in children. Scand J Urol Nephrol 2009;43:369-372.

Fielder M, Tiwana H, Youinou P, Le Goff P, Deonarian R, Wilson C et al. The specificity of the anti-*Proteus* antibody response in tissue-typed rheumatoid arthritis (RA) patients from Brest. Rheumatol Int 1995;15:79–82.

Firestein GS. Etiology and pathogenesis of rheumatoid arthritis. In: Firestein GS, Budd RC, Harris Jr ED, McInnes IB, Ruddy S, Sergent JS (editors). Kelly's Textbook of Rheumatology. Saunders—Elsevier, Philadelphia, 2009;1035-1380.

Gautam V, Sehgal R, Paramjeet SG, Arora DR. Detection of anti-*Proteus* antibodies in sera of patients with rheumatoid arthritis. Indian J Pathol Microbiol 2003;46:137-141.

Gaymans R, Haverkorn MJ, Valkenburg HA, Goslings WR. A prospective study of urinary tract infections in a Dutch general practice. Lancet 1976;ii:674-677.

Guay DR. Cranberry and urinary tract infections. Drugs 2009;69;775-807.

Guilherme L, Kohler KF, Kalil J. Rheumatic heart disease: mediation by complex immune events. Adv Clin Chem 2011;53:31-50.

Haraoui B, Pope J. Treatment of early rheumatoid arthritis: concepts in management. Semin Arthritis Rheum 2011;40:371-388.

Ishikawa K, Matsumoto T, Yasuda M, Uehara S, Muratani T, Yagisawa M, et al. The nationwide study of bacterial pathogens associated with urinary tract infections conducted by the Japanese Society of Chemotherapy. J Infect Chemother 2011;17:126-138.

Khalafpour S, Ebringer A, Abuljadayel I, Corbett M. Antibodies to *Klebsiella* and *Proteus* microorganisms in ankylosing spondylitis and rheumatoid arthritis patients measured by ELISA. Br J Rheumatol 1988;27 (Suppl. II):86–89.

Kunin CM. The natural history of recurrent bacteriuria in schoolgirls. N Engl J Med 1970:282:1443-1448.

Lawson AA, Maclean N. Renal disease and drug therapy in rheumatoid arthritis. Ann Rheum Dis 1966 ;25:441–449.

Lee H, Ko KS, Song JH, Peck KR. Antimicrobial activity of doripenem and other carbapenems against gram-negative pathogens from Korea. Microb Drug Resist 2011;17:37-45.

Li X, Zhao H, Lockatell CV, Drachengberg CB, Johnson DE, Mobley HL. Visualization of *Proteus mirabilis* within the matrix of urease-induced bladder stones during experimental urinary tract infection. Infect Immun 2002;70:389-394.

Mathoera RB, Kok DJ, Verduin CM, Nijman RJ. Pathological and therapeutic significance of cellular invasion by *Proteus mirabilis* in an enterocystoplasty infection stone model. Infect Immun 2002;70:7022-7032.

McDonagh J, Gray J, Sykes H, Walker DJ, Bint AJ, Deighton CM. Anti-*Proteus* antibodies and *Proteus* organisms in rheumatoid arthritis: a clinical study. Br J Rheumatol 1994;33:32-35.

Mulvey MA, Lopez-Boado YS, Wilson CL, Roth R, Parks WC, Heuser J, Hulgren SJ. Induction and evasion of host defenses by type 1-pillated uropathogenic *Escherichia coli*. Science 1998;282:1494-1497.

Murphy EA, Mowat L, Sturrock RD. Antibodies to *Proteus* in rheumatoid arthritis. Br J Rheumatol 1991;30:390.

Newkirk MM, Goldbach-Mansky R, Senior BW, Klippel J, Schumacher HR Jr, El-Gabalawy HS. Elevated levels of IgM and IgA antibodies to *Proteus mirabilis* and IgM antibodies to *Escherichia coli* are associated with early rheumatoid factor (RF)-positive rheumatoid arthritis. Rheumatology 2005;44:1433–1441.

Nielubowicz GR, Mobley HR. Host-pathogen interactions in urinary tract infection. Nat Rev Urol 2010;7:430-441.

Palou J, Pigrau C, Molina I, Ledesma JM, Angulo J. Etiology and sensitivity of uropathogens identified in uncomplicated lower urinary tract infections in women (ARESC Study): implications on empiric therapy. Med Clin (Barc) 2011;136:1-7.

Rashid T, Darlington G, Kjeldsen-Kragh J, Forre O, Collado A, Ebringer A. *Proteus* IgG antibodies and C-reactive protein in English, Norwegian and Spanish patients with rheumatoid arthritis. Clin Rheumatol 1999;18:190–195.

Rashid T, Leirisalo-Repo M, Tani Y, Hukuda S, Kobayashi S, Wilson C, Bansal S, Ebringer A. Antibacterial and antipeptide antibodies in Japanese and Finnish patients with rheumatoid arthritis. Clin Rheumatol 2004;23:134–141.

Rashid T, Ebringer A, Wilson C, Bansal S, Paimela L, Binder A. The potential use of antibacterial peptide antibody indices in the diagnosis of rheumatoid arthritis and ankylosing spondylitis. J Clin Rheumatol 2006;12:11–16.

Rashid T, Ebringer A. Rheumatoid arthritis is linked to *Proteus*—the evidence. Clin Rheumatol 2007;26:1036-1043.

Rogers P, Hassan J, Bresnihan B, Feighery C, Whelan A. Antibodies to *Proteus* in rheumatoid arthritis. Br J Rheumatol 1988;27 (Suppl.2):90–94.

Ronald AR, Nicolle LE. Infections of the upper urinary tract. In: Schrier RW (editor). Diseases of the Kidney and Urinary Tract. Wolters Kluwer | Lippincott Williams & Wilkins, Philadelphia 2007: pp 847-869.

Rozalski A, Sidorczyk Z, Kotelko K. Potential virulence factors of *Proteus* bacilli. Microbiol Mol Biol Rev 1997;61:65-89.

Scavone P, Umpierrez A, Maskell DJ, Zunino P. Nasal immunization with attenuated *Salmonella typhimurium* expressing an MrpA-TetC fusion protein significantly reduced *Proteus mirabilis* colonization in the mouse urinary tract. J Med Microbiol 2011; Mar 17: [Epub ahead of print].

Schmiemann G, Kniehl E, Gebhardt K, Matejczyk MM, Hummers-Pradier E. The diagnosis of urinary tract infection: a systematic review. Dtsch Arztebl Int 2010;107:361-367.

Senior BW. The special affinity of particular types of *Proteus mirabilis* for the urinary tract. J Med Microbiol 1979;12:1–8.

Senior BW, McBride PDP, Morley KD, Kerr MA. The detection of raised levels of IgM to *Proteus mirabilis* in sera from patients with rheumatoid arthritis. J Med Microbiol 1995;43:176–84.

Senior BW, Anderson GA, Morley KD, Kerr MA. Evidence that patients with rheumatoid arthritis have asymptomatic 'non-significant' *Proteus mirabilis* bacteriuria more frequently than healthy controls. J Infect 1999;38:99–106.

Stamey TA, Govan DE, Palmer JM. The localization and treatment of urinary tract infection: the role of bactericidal urine levels as opposed to serum levels. Medicine (Baltimore) 1965;44:1-36.

Stastny P. Mixed lymphocyte cultures in rheumatoid arthritis. J Clin Invest 1976;57:1148–1157.

Subair H, Tiwana H, Fielder M, Binder A, Cunningham K, Ebringer A et al. Elevation in anti-*Proteus* antibodies in patients with rheumatoid arthritis from Bermuda and England. J Rheumatol 1995;22:1825–1828.

Talkoff-Rubin NE, Cotran RS, Rubin RH. Urinary tract infection, pyelonephritis, and reflux nephropathy. In: Brenner BM (editor). Brenner and Rector's The Kidney. Saunders Elsevier, Philadelphia, 2008;1203-1238.

Tani Y, Tiwana H, Hukuda S, Nishioka J, Fielder M, Wilson C et al. Antibodies to *Klebsiella*, *Proteus* and HLA-B27 peptides in Japanese patients with ankylosing spondylitis and rheumatoid arthritis. J Rheumatol 1997;24:109–114.

Thomson C, Armitage A. Urinary tract infection. In: Warrell DA, Cox TM, Firth JD (editors). Oxford Textbook of Medicine. Oxford University Press, Oxford, 2010;4103-4122.

Tishler M, Caspi D, Aimog Y, Segal R, Yaron M. Increased incidence of urinary tract infection in patients with rheumatoid arthritis and secondary Sjogren's syndrome. Ann Rheum Dis 1992;51:604–606.

Tiwana H, Wilson C, Cunningham P, Binder A, Ebringer A. Antibodies to four gram-negative bacteria in rheumatoid arthritis which share sequences with the rheumatoid arthritis susceptibility motif. Br J Rheumatol 1996;35:592–594.

Tiwana H, Wilson C, Walmsley RS, Wakefield AJ, Smith MS, Cox NL et al. Antibody response to gut bacteria in ankylosing spondylitis, rheumatoid arthritis, Crohn's disease and ulcerative colitis. Rheumatol Int 1997;17:11–16.

Vandenbroucke JP, Kaaks R, Valkenburg HA, Boersma JW, Cats A, Festen JJ, et al. Frequency of infections among rheumatoid arthritis patients, before and after disease onset. Arthritis Rheum 1987;30:810-813.

Wanchu A, Deodhar SD, Sharma M, Gupta V, Bambery P, Sud A. Elevated levels of anti-*Proteus* antibodies in patients with active rheumatoid arthritis. Ind J Med Res 1997;105:39–42.

Weisbart RH, Min Y, Wong AL, Kang J, Kwunyeun S, Lin A, et al. Selective IgA immune unresponsiveness to *Proteus mirabilis* fumarate reductase A-chain in rheumatoid arthritis. J Rheumatol 2005;32:1208-1212.

Wilson C, Ebringer A, Ahmadi K, Wrigglesworth J, Tiwana H, Fielder M et al. Shared amino acid sequences between major histocompatibility complex class II glycoproteins, type XI collagen and *Proteus mirabilis* in rheumatoid arthritis. Ann Rheum Dis 1995;54:216–220.

Wilson C, Thakore D, Isenberg D, Ebringer A. Correlation between anti-*Proteus* antibodies and isolation rates of *P. mirabilis* in rheumatoid arthritis. Rheumatol Int 1997;16:187–189.

Wilson C, Rashid T, Tiwana H, Beyan H, Hughes L, Bansal S et al. Cytotoxicity responses to peptide antigens in rheumatoid arthritis and ankylosing spondylitis. J Rheumatol 2003;30:972–978.

Zhang W, Anis AH. The economic burden of rheumatoid arthritis: beyond health care costs. Clin Rheumatol 2011;30 (Supp 1):S25-32.

Part 4

Infection and Urinary Stones

12

Infected Urinary Stones, Endotoxins and Urosepsis

Joel Gustavo Gómez-Núñez[1], Ulises M. Alvarez[2], Francisco Fernández[3], Jorge Gutiérrez-Aceves[1], Luz María López-Marín[3] and Achim M. Loske[3]
[1]*Nuevo Hospital Civil de Guadalajara, Universidad de Guadalajara, Guadalajara Jal. and Instituto de Endourología, Hospital Puerta de Hierro, Zapopan Jal.,*
[2]*Posgrado en Ciencias Químicas, Facultad de Química, Universidad Nacional Autónoma de México*
[3]*Centro de Física Aplicada y Tecnología Avanzada, Universidad Nacional Autónoma de México, México*
México

1. Introduction

Urinary tract infections (UTIs) and their complications represent one of the most common causes of medical consultation with high cost to medical services and high morbidity and mortality. Urinary stones are another medical challenge that represents an acute or chronic clinical setting for patients requiring most of the time active treatment, either as an invasive or as a non-invasive management, thus increasing costs and risks. The combination of both clinical scenarios —urinary tract infection and urinary stone— is common and can trigger a systemic inflammatory response syndrome (SIRS) before, during or after medical treatment (i.e. antibiotics) and/or surgical manipulation of infected urinary stones. It is believed that SIRS is due to the release of endotoxins from infected urinary stones, developing endotoxemia, bacteremia and urosepsis. If not controlled, multiple organ failure syndrome (MOF) and death of the patient may occur. Urologists are familiar with these scenarios where not only prevention and diagnosis but also an early and appropriated treatment is crucial. Unfortunately, the use of prophylactic antibiotics does not guarantee prevention of these fatalities. The aim of this chapter is to review the evidence of possible endotoxin release during invasive and non-invasive treatment of infected urinary stones as a trigger of SIRS and sepsis.

2. Urinary tract infections

Urinary tract infections are the second most frequent infections in developed countries and uropathogenic *Escherichia coli* (*E. coli*) a non-urea-splitting bacterium represents 80 % of uncomplicated UTIs (Oelschlaeger et al., 2002). There is a geographic variation about *E. coli* and several other Gram-negative, as well as Gram-positive bacteria and fungi causing complicated and uncomplicated UTIs among specific populations. Virulence of bacteria causing UTIs is determinant for progression of the disease. Some virulence factors in uropathogenic *E. Coli*, as adhesins (Type 1 pili, Dr-family pili, P fimbriae, F1C fimbriae, S fimbriae) and toxins (CNF1, Hemolysin and Sat) (Oelschlaeger et al., 2002), could explain the systemic forms of invasion of the bloodstream by some *Enterobacteriaceae* in possible synergism with the release of endotoxins that may result in SIRS and urosepsis. These virulence factors are reviewed elsewhere in this book.

2.1 Urinary bacterial epidemiology

Urinary tract infections in Western countries are mainly caused by *E. coli* (90 %), *Proteus* spp, *Klebsiella* spp, and *Pseudomonas* spp (McRae & Shortliffe, 2000; Bochud & Calandra, 2003). Variation in proportions and specific populations have been reported and described (Foxman, 2003; Savas et al., 2006). Bacterial resistance is another important issue that increases morbidity and mortality. For further details and specific information about bacterial epidemiology in UTIs we invite the reader to consult other sections of this book.

2.1.1 Endotoxins

To invade hosts, bacteria use a variety of substances, some of them are essential for their survival. In Gram-negative bacteria, specific molecular patterns composed of lipid and sugar moieties represent some of the most toxic virulence factors of bacterial origin. Structurally classified as lipopolysaccharides (LPS), these substances have no chemical homologs among human cells, and are known as endotoxins, to denote their ability for causing fever, shock and organ injury when released in mammalian endothelial vessels (Beutler, 2000). The presence of endotoxins in the blood-stream is named endotoxemia and can trigger SIRS. LPS have specific structural motifs which are typical of different bacterial species. However, all of them are known to induce endotoxemia and sepsis (Bochud & Calandra, 2003). Endotoxins are known to be recognized by cell-surface proteins, the LPS receptors, which are widely distributed in animals as part of their immune systems (from insects to vertebrates). However, a strong inflammatory reaction after LPS recognition is restricted to a handful of species, including humans (Beutler, 2000). According to numerous studies in cellular and animal models, recognition of LPS by their receptors initiate a cascade of intracellular signals guiding the secretion of pro-inflammatory mediators (Beutler, 2000; Triantafilou & Triantafilou, 2005). An emerging concern is the toxicity of LPS after microbial death, especially in the context of hospital-acquired infections. In fact, released LPS keep their full toxic potential, unless inactivation processes take place in the host to degrade endotoxins (Munford et al., 2009).

3. Urinary stones

Urinary stones have been reported in human history since antiquity. Traditionally, stones have been classified according to their main mineral content. The etiology of urinary stones is wide, including chronic dehydration, urinary tract malformations, obstructed uropathy, metabolic diseases (i.e. hyperparathyroidism, gout, and obesity), foreign body inside urinary tract, infections, etc. The risk for stone disease in patients of developed countries is close to 10 % life-long. An increase in the incidence of stone disease related with changes in the life style, modifications on the diet, morbid obesity surgery syndrome and new drugs has been reported in Western countries in recent years. For example, in the United States, an increase of 37 % in stone disease was observed over the last 20 years (Straub & Hautmann,

2005). A variation in the frequency and in the composition of the minerals forming the urinary stones was also observed.
There is a large variety of urinary stone compositions. If the main component is more than 80 % of the total mass, the stone is named "pure". If the main component is at least 50 % of the stone, it is named mixed. In Western countries, struvite stones used to represent 15-30 % of cases. Nowadays only 2 % of stones are struvite (McALeer et al., 2003; Kramer et al., 2000). The explanation of that decrease is unknown. In developing countries and Eastern countries there is a large variation among incidence, prevalence and stone composition. For example, in India a report including 1050 urinary calculi from surgically treated patients (900 renal and 150 ureteral) revealed 93.04 % oxalate calcium stones (80 % calcium oxalate monohydrate [COM] and 20 % calcium oxalate dihydrate [COD]), 1.92 % struvite stones, 1.48 % apatite stones, 0.95 % uric acid stones and 2.96 % mixed stones. Surprisingly, 89.98 % of the staghorn stones consisted of oxalates and only 4.2 % were struvite (Ansari et al., 2005). A study in Japan showed that the most common stone composition was struvite (32.1 %) and mixed calcium oxalate phosphate (22.2 %) (Akagashi et al., 2004). These differences could be explained by variations in ethnics, epigenetics, geographical area, diet, life-style, and different metabolism.

3.1 Infected stones

It has been suggested that urinary stones can be infected mainly in two ways. Stones develop due to several mechanisms which may or may not be associated to obstructive uropathy (i.e. hyperparathyroidism). The first way in which a stone can be infected is by ascending bacteria. Once the stone is formed, ascending bacteria may reach its surface, invade the interstice and become part of it (Takeuchi et al., 1984; Abrahams & Stoller, 2003). Adherence of new minerals could cover and paste bacteria layers. In this case, the stone acts as a reservoir for bacteria. Due to the poor penetration of drugs into the stone matrix the action of antibiotics is limited (Prabakharan et al., 1999). This phenomenon can be the reason of bacterial resistance, repeated, chronic or complicated UTIs in several patients, therefore increasing the risk of urosepsis. The most possible scenario according to the most frequent stone component and urinary bacteria in our Western world is a calcium stone infected with *E. coli*. In this case, the urinary stone forms first and gets infected by bacteria afterwards.
The second scenario is that bacteria living inside the urinary tract and causing chronic UTIs produce the stones. These bacteria are named urea-splitting bacteria. Members of this group are *Proteus, Klebsiella, Pseudomonas, Providencia, Serratia* spp, *Staphylococcus aureus* and *Ureaplasma urealyticum*, among others. *P. mirabilis* accounts for more than half of all urease-positive urinary infections (Kramer et al., 2000). Urea-splitting bacteria change the urine pH (> 7.2) and allow easier precipitation of phosphate with several compounds, mainly ammonium and magnesium (Abrahams & Stoller, 2003). The result is a compound phosphate named struvite (magnesium-ammonium-phosphate [MAP] stones and/or triple phosphate stones). Another type of phosphate stones are apatite stones (calcium phosphate). The terms "infectious stones" or "infection stones" are used as synonymous of struvite stones and represent up to 15 % of all stones sent for analysis in the Western world (Kramer et al., 2000). Infected stones that contain struvite may originate *de novo*, but often pre-existing stones are infected with urea-splitting bacteria (Kramer et al., 2000). There is evidence that urinary tract infections caused by urease-producing microorganisms are not exclusively related to the formation of struvite stones. Considering this scenario, *Proteus*

mirabilis and struvite stones are the most likely combination. In this case, the risk for urosepsis is also patent.

It has been suggested that some agents named nanobacteria could have a role in the development of calcium-based urinary stones (Kajander & Çiftçioglu, 1998); however, this is not yet well established (Kramer et al., 2000). A prevalence of nanobacteria in 0.5 % of 1000 stones was reported; but nanobacteria are still difficult to identify (Abrahams & Stoller, 2003).

3.1.1 Bacterial epidemiology of infected urinary stones

Urinary stone cultures from fragments retrieved during stone surgery were not a common practice until recently. Negative urine culture before urinary surgery was considered safe. In general urology it has been a routine to have a negative midstream urine culture before doing any endoscopic procedure. Recent studies suggest that voiding urine culture is not representative of upper urinary tract pelvis infection or pelvis infected stone bacteria (Mariappan & Loong, 2004; Mariappan et al., 2005a). A group of 73 patients with unilateral stone-obstructed ureter were treated with ureterorenoscopy and lithotripsy. Midstream urine (MSU) sample culture and sensitivity were performed the morning of the endoscopic surgery. During the procedure a pelvis urine sample and stone fragments were collected for culture and sensitivity with an aseptic technique in a retrograde approach. The authors reported that 25 (34.3 %) patients had positive stone culture, 43 (58.9 %) had positive pelvic urine and 21 (28.8 %) had positive MSU culture. The most common isolated bacterium was *E coli*. The MSU culture and sensitivity test had 30.2 % sensitivity and 73 % specificity to detect pelvic urine culture and sensitivity. The same test had a low positive predictive value and negative predictive value in relation to infected pelvic urine (positive predictive value = 0.62, negative predictive value = 0.42) (Mariappan & Loong, 2004). According to these authors, in case of a ureteral obstructive uropathy secondary to a stone, MSU culture and sensitivity do not represent infected urine proximal to the obstruction or infected stone. Stone components were not analyzed. In conclusion, pelvic urine and stone cultures were considered as a more appropriate indicator of upper urinary tract infection. Collection of the obstructed urine for culture and sensitivity are recommended.

Mariappan and colleagues (2005a) studied a group of 54 patients with renal stones who were candidates for percutaneous nephrolithotomy (PCNL). Various specimens were collected for culture and sensitivity, i.e., MSU sample, bladder urine sample, renal pelvic urine sample and crushed stone sample. The objective of the study was to identify the most predictive analysis of urosepsis. MSU culture was positive in 11.1 % of cases, stone culture was positive in 35.2 % and pelvic urine was positive in 20.4 % of cases. A wide variety of bacteria were isolated. In 37 % of the patients SIRS was developed and 5.5 % experienced septic shock. Pelvic urine culture predicted infected stones better than bladder urine culture. Patients with infected stones or pelvic urine were found to be at a relative risk for urosepsis that was at least four times greater ($P = 0.0009$). The authors concluded that positive stone and pelvic urine are better predictors of potential urosepsis than bladder urine and recommend routine collections of these specimens. Stone components were not analyzed.

The bacterial epidemiology of infected urinary stones also depend on differences in geographic area, strains, bacterial resistance, bacterial virulence, exposure to some kind of antibiotics and environment.

4. Sepsis and urosepsis

Sepsis is an extreme health condition that threatens life of patients with a high cost for the healthcare systems. Reports from US and European surveys have estimated that severe sepsis accounts for 2–11 % of all admissions to hospitals or intensive care units. The most common microbes isolated from patients with severe sepsis and septic shock are Gram negative bacilli (mainly *E. coli, Klebsiella* species and *Pseudomonas aeruginosa*) and Gram positive cocci (mainly *Staphylococci* and *Streptpcocci* spp). Most cases of Gram negative sepsis are caused by *E coli* and *Klebsiella* species followed by *P. aeruginosa*. Infections usually occur in the lung, abdomen, bloodstream, or urinary tract (Bochud & Calandra, 2003). In a trial performed in an intensive care unit with 142 septic patients having a urinary catheter, urosepsis occurred in 15.8 % of them (Rosser et al., 1999). Urosepsis in adults comprises approximately 25 % of all sepsis cases and in most cases is due to complicated urinary tract infections (Wagenlehner et al., 2007). An incidence of sepsis associated with obstructed uropathy and urinary stones treated surgically has also been reported in 1.28 % of cases (O'Keeffe et al., 1993). Rao et al. (1991) found an incidence of septic shock after endoscopic manipulation for urinary stone in about 1% of treated patients. Sepsis is an advanced stage of uncontrolled systemic inflammatory response syndrome that may turn toward irreversible multiple organ failure and death.

5. Endotoxins and sepsis

Activation of local and systemic metabolic response to trauma and SIRS is mainly caused by activation of IL-1 and tumor necrosis factor-α (TNF-α). It is well established that after recognition by cognate receptors, LPS trigger the synthesis and release of pro-inflammatory cytokines (Triantafilou & Triantafilou, 2005). Once IL-1 and TNF are secreted, they activate several other reactions like complement factors, exacerbating the host inflammatory response. As a consequence, MOF or death may result. *In vitro* human blood monocytes produce IL-1 and TNF-α when they are exposed to 25 to 50 pg/mL of endotoxin concentration. These endotoxin levels have been reported in the bloodstream of patients during septic shock (Dinarello & Cannon, 1993). In a clinical report of 97 consecutive patients, 56 % developed sepsis syndrome with about 26 pg/mL of TNF-α.; 37 % had 20 pg/mL of IL-1 and in 80 %, 415 pg/mL of IL-6 was detected, including a LPS mean concentration of 2.6 endotoxin units (EU)/mL (1 EU/mL = 0.6 ng/mL) (Casey et al., 1993). The level of procalcitonin has also been used as a sepsis marker. Another assay with healthy volunteers demonstrated elevation of procalcitonin (peak up to about 4 ng/mL at 6 hours) after I.V. administration of 4 ng/kg of body weight of endotoxin derived from *E coli* 0113:H10:k (Dandona et al., 1994). In a new human model of low grade inflammation, 10 healthy male subjects were exposed to 3 ng/kg body weight of endotoxin (LPS) derived from *E. coli* in I.V. bolus injection versus I.V. infusion during 4 hours. Results revealed that TNF-α, IL-6 and neutrophil response were earlier and more pronounced in the bolus trial, suggesting that sudden release of endotoxins triggers faster and higher release of cytokines and inflammatory mediators similar to sepsis. Changes in cytokines measured in the infusion trial would be a more representative model of human systemic low-grade inflammation in chronic disease (Taudorf et al., 2007).

6. Infected urinary stones and urosepsis

In a study on 700 patients, the prevalence of sepsis related with obstructed uropathy and urinary stones treated surgically was 1.28 %. These nine patients developed SIRS and sepsis during 6 hours postoperative. Although males and females were treated in roughly equal proportions, all of the patients who developed severe sepsis were females. There were six deaths accounting for 66 % mortality (O'Keeffe et al., 1993). Septic shock following urinary stone manipulation was reported with an incidence of 1 % and mortality up to 80 % (Rao et al., 1991).

In an effort to predict septicemia following endourological manipulation for stones in the upper urinary tract, 117 patients were studied and classified according to the procedure performed (Rao et al., 1991): Percutaneous nephrolithotomy, push-back/push-bang procedure, double-J and extracorporeal shock wave lithotripsy (SWL), ureteroscopy, SWL alone and only cystoscopy. Blood samples for bacterial culture, endotoxin and tumor necrosis factor assay were collected before, at onset, at the end and one hour after completing the procedure. Preoperative bacteriuria was present in 35 % of the patients. The mean endotoxin level of the entire group —except the cystoscopy group— was 16.2 pg/mL (range 11 to 58.3 pg/mL). In the cystoscopy group the mean endotoxin level was 11.7 pg/mL (range 11 to 12.2 pg/mL). All patients (16) with preoperative endotoxemia had increased levels of endotoxin detected in subsequent samples (mean increase 15 pg/mL, range 0.5 to 64 pg/mL). The tumor necrosis factor was greater than 15 pg/mL in four cases preoperatively. Postoperatively there was elevation of the tumor necrosis factor only in 12 patients. The authors reported that in case of upper urinary tract manipulation, the risk of bacteremia was higher. The risk was greatest after performing the push-back method and least after cystoscopy. Combination of preoperative endotoxemia, bacteriuria and the type of procedure had 85 % of sensitivity, 84 % of specificity and a positive predictive value of 52 % for the development of postoperative bacteremia. A total of 41 patients had pyrexia and 17 patients had rigors and fever 2 to 3 hours after the end of the procedure. No patient suffered septic shock; however, this complication developed in a female patient one week after percutaneous nephrolithotomy. Serum endotoxin and tumor necrosis factor levels after admission of this patient to the intensive care unit were 67.7 pg/mL and 3,827.5 pg/mL, respectively (Rao et al., 1991).

Measurements of LPS were done in 34 renal stones, stored for several months and classified as infection stones (16), i.e., struvite and calcium apatite, and non-infection stones (18) composed of 50 % calcium oxalate monohydrate (McALeer et al., 2003). All stones were weighed, aseptically crushed and aliquots were tested for endotoxins. Four stones of each group were aseptically washed and crushed separately. Washed materials and crushed stones were processed in MacConkey agar culture to recover bacteria colonizing the stones. Mean endotoxin concentration in the infection group was 12,223 ng per gram of stone and 340.3 ng per gram of stone in the non-infection group. The difference was statistically significant (P = 0.001). These results reveal an almost 36 times higher concentration of endotoxins in the infection stones. No living bacteria were recovered on the MacConkey plates from crushed stones from neither group. The authors concluded that large amounts of endotoxins can be found in infected renal stones even months after they were removed from the body, and long after viable bacteria could be detected. Furthermore, endotoxin may remain after bacteria are no longer viable or have been killed with antibiotic therapy (Munford et al., 2009). Non-infectious stones can also contain endotoxin but in a lower amount (McALeer et al., 2003). McALeer et al. (2002) published a case report of an 8 year old boy with a left staghorn calculus treated with holmium laser percutaneous nephrolithotripsy (PCNL). Culture specific antibiotic were administered to the patient, both orally and intravenously, before, during and after surgery. Intraoperative fluid and pleural fluid cultures (urologists lost percutaneous access from lower pole calyx with intraperitoneal extravasation and pleural effusions) were obtained. A urine culture was performed before and after stone manipulation. All samples grew a few colonies of *Proteus mirabilis*. Blood cultures were requested but could not be obtained; serum endotoxin results could not be obtained either. Two hours after procedure the patient developed disseminated intravascular coagulopathy. Twelve hours after stone manipulations the patient died despite aggressive support care. Stone composition was apatite (80%) and struvite (10%). Post-mortem culture of the stone grew several colonies of *Proteus mirabilis*. The assay of the stone fragments for endotoxin showed concentrations of 285,600 pg per gram, suggesting that endotoxemia can induce sepsis syndrome without concomitant bacteremia. The authors concluded that the outstanding endotoxin concentration of the renal stone was the source of the fatal outcome.

There is not a general consensus on how to best prevent sepsis in patients undergoing surgical treatment of urinary stones. Pre-surgical, trans-surgical and post-surgical strategies have been proposed. The combination of multiple factors can prevent, trigger or worsen sepsis. For example, control of metabolic or cardiopulmonary diseases is important. Although antibiotic prophylaxis does not completely avoid the risk of developing sepsis, it is a recommendation for stone surgery according to the American Urological Association (AUA) and the European Association of Urology (EAU) guidelines on urinary tract infection (Grabe et al., 2011; Wolf et al., 2010). It is suggested to define an antibiotic prophylaxis according to local bacterial populations, resistance and antibiotic sensitivity patterns. In a prospective controlled trial, Mariappan et al. (2006) and Bag et al. (2011) reported the beneficial use of one week ciprofloxacin and nitrofurantoin regimen respectively, before percutaneous nephrolithotomy. Furthermore it has been found that renal stones larger than 20 mm are more likely to be culture positive (Mariappan et al., 2005a; 2005b). Mariappan and colleagues (2005a) suggested to obtain pelvic urine and stone samples for culture and sensitivity as a routine during surgical stone procedures, with the aim of administering proper antibiotic regimen if later urosepsis develops. If an unusual urine sample (i.e. turbidity, foully) is obtained, culture and sensitivity is a must. In this case, a nephrostomy tube should be left in place and the initial procedure rescheduled until sterile urine is confirmed.

An increase of pressure inside the urinary tract system generated by the irrigation fluid results in a potential bacterial and endotoxin translocation into the bloodstream. Auge et al. (2004) reported significant reduction in urinary tract pressures using ureteral access sheath if working both in distal ureter and inside the renal pelvis. Bacteria and likely endotoxins may emerge from several kinds of urinary stones and not exclusively from struvite stones (Hugosson et al., 1990; McALeer et al., 2003). In post-surgical stage, the most critical evidences of SIRS are during the first 6 hours post-procedure and seem to correlate with cytokines release into the bloodstream after endotoxin stimulus (Dandona et al., 1994; O'Keeffe et al., 1993; Rao et al., 1991; Taudorf et al., 2007). It has been suggested that if other causes of SIRS different than infection (i.e. cardiogenic or pulmonary events, atelectasis, hypovolemia and pain) have been ruled out and if SIRS persists, then sepsis could be the explanation (Monga, 2005). Close vital signs and symptoms monitoring and high suspicious index for sepsis is crucial at this stage. Once urosepsis is diagnosed, an early tissue oxygenation, appropriate initial antibiotic therapy, inotropic and nutritional support with invasive monitoring at intensive therapy unit is required. Empirical broad-spectrum antibiotics regimen is prescribed according to local bacteria, sensitivity and resistance patterns. If cultures were performed from bladder urine, pelvis urine or stone sample, direct therapy must be installed as soon as results are obtained (Mariappan et al., 2005b). Wagenlehner and his group (2007) reported that the treatment of urosepsis comprises four major aspects: Early goal-directed therapy, optimal pharmacodynamics exposure to antimicrobials both in blood and in the urinary tract, control of complicating factors in the urinary tract and specific sepsis therapy. They considered that interdisciplinary approach is necessary to achieve an optimal goal of treatment. At any of these stages, it is very important to act as soon as possible if any evidence of initial SIRS and urosepsis is addressed. It is necessary to instruct the patient and relatives once discharged from the hospital, that if SIRS develops, urgent evaluation in an emergency unit is crucial (Rao et al., 1991). There is no doubt that further research is required and that several other issues have to be considered; however, these do not fall within the scope of this chapter.

7. Research on bacterial suspensions and extracorporeal shock wave lithotripsy

Several articles report the bactericidal effect of shock waves *in vitro*; however, results remain controversial. Elbers et al. (1988) observed no effect of shock waves on calculi inoculated with urease-positive calculogenic bacteria. Bacteria from different genera and species have different resistances to physical, chemical and environmental factors; such variations in bacteria may determine the degree of susceptibility to shock waves. For instance, we have previously found that shock wave-induced cavitation contributes to *L. monocytogenes*, *S. typhimurium* and *E. coli* O157:H7 inactivation; however, *L. monocytogenes* was more sensitive to shock waves than *E. coli* O157:H7 (Alvarez et al., 2004). Kerfoot and colleagues (1992) found no effect of shock wave application on *S. aureus*; however von Eiff et al. (2000) reported inactivation of a different strain of the same bacteria. Similarly, whereas Ohshima et al. (1991) observed no effect of shock waves on the viability of *E. coli* strains DSM 1077 and JM 109/pKPDH2, Loske et al. (1999) reported inactivation of *E. coli* strain ATCC 10536. Patel et al. (2005) reported no effect of shock waves on a five-stain cocktail of *E. coli* O157:H7, whereas Podolak et al. (2005) reported shock wave inactivation of a slightly different cocktail of the same *E. coli*. Various shock wave generators were used by these authors, which may explain their different results. When performing *in vitro* exposure of bacteria in suspension by shock waves generated with electrohydraulic shock wave generators, the electromagnetic radiation produced at the spark gap contributes to microorganism inactivation. During SWL this radiation (visible and UV) does not penetrate into the calculus. Besides, electromagnetic radiation, compression, tensile stress, and cavitation may also damage bacteria. Cavitation is produced by the trailing tensile pulse of the shock wave. A cloud of bubbles forms at the focus of every lithotripter after the passage of each shock wave. During collapse, they create secondary shock waves, powerful jet blasts of fluid (microjets), high temperature gradients, and free radicals (Crum, 1988). If a second shock wave is sent during, or shortly after, the stable phase of the bubbles, their collapse can be intensified. This technique, referred to as "tandem SWL" has proven to reduce *in vivo* SWL treatment time by 50 % (Fernández et al., 2009). To test the efficiency of tandem shock waves to inactivate bacteria, Alvarez and colleagues (2008) used an experimental piezoelectric tandem shock wave generator that generates two shock waves shifted in time. The effects of single and tandem shock waves on the viability of *L. monocytogenes* and *E. coli* O157:H7 suspensions were studied. Tandem shock waves were generated at delays of 450 and 900 microseconds. No effect on bacteria viability was reported after exposure to 8,000 single shock waves, but significant bacteria inactivation was reported after 3,400 tandem shock waves. The delay yielding the highest inactivation was 900 microseconds.

8. Research with stone models

Efforts to develop an ideal stone model have been done worldwide to perform *in vitro* and *in vivo* fragmentation tests exposing artificial stone models to different lithotripter energy settings. To study the inactivation of bacteria by shock waves and the bactericidal effect of different intracorporeal lithotripters, we developed an artificial calcium sulphate stone model infected homogenously with *E. coli*, a mixed struvite-calcium sulphate stone infected with *P. mirabilis* and a calcium sulphate stone infected with *P. mirabilis*.

8.1 The bactericidal effect of intracorporeal lithotripters

Only a few authors report results on the interaction of infected urinary stones with intracorporeal lithotripters. Artificial kidney stones, infected with *E. coli*, were manufactured by our research group to evaluate the bactericidal effect of shock waves, and the differences on intra-bacterial protein release produced by four different intracorporeal lithotripters. The stone models were exposed to a holmium laser, an electrohydraulic, a pneumatic and an ultrasonic intracorporeal lithotripter using two energy settings. Non-infected control stones were manufactured by casting a mixture of gypsum cement, Velmix-stone (Kerr Division of Syborn Corp., Romulus, MI, USA) and distilled water in cylindrical molds (diameter = 10 mm, height = 10 mm). A saline solution containing *E. coli* was used instead of distilled water to manufacture the infected stones. Cells were obtained in the stationary phase of growth. Stones were placed on a copper mesh with 1.8 mm by 1.8 mm openings at the bottom of a specially designed lucite test tube. The lucite tube was placed inside a standard laboratory test tube, containing 10 mL of saline solution. The tip of the lithotripter was introduced inside the lucite tube (see Figure 1). Five infected stones were fragmented with each lithotripter at each energy level (low and high) during a fixed time. After treatment all remaining stone fragments were crushed with a hand press. The suspension containing stone powder and bacteria was centrifuged, serially diluted and incubated on agar plates. Viable counts were made by plating on trypticase soy agar supplemented with 0.6 % (w/v) yeast extract (TSAY). Bactericidal action was defined as the logarithmic difference of colony forming units (CFU) per milliliter between untreated and treated stones. To study the effect of the lithotripters on bacteria living outside the stone, an *E. coli* suspension was exposed to the action of each lithotripter, using the same energy settings and exposure times as for infected stones. The process was repeated five times for each lithotripter at each energy setting. Stone fragmentation of infected stones was repeated as described before, in order to measure the release of protein (LPS) as a result of *in vitro* lithotripsy. After treatment, certain amount of the suspension was centrifuged and placed inside a spectrophotometer to measure absorbance at 280 nm. Results revealed that the variation in the amount of bacteria inside the stones was not significant. Complete inactivation resulted with the electrohydraulic lithotripter at both energy levels. No difference was observed between inactivation obtained with the other lithotripters at their low energy settings. Increasing the energy resulted in higher bacteria inactivation for the laser, pneumatic and ultrasonic lithotripter. The laser lithotripter produced the lowest bacteria inactivation. Inactivation increased as the energy setting of the laser, pneumatic and ultrasonic lithotripter was changed from low to high. No bacteria inactivation was observed using the pneumatic lithotripter in an *E. coli* suspension alone. No viable bacteria could be observed after using the laser, the electrohydraulic and the ultrasonic lithotripter in the infected suspension (without stone). Maximum protein release occurred at low energy with the electrohydraulic lithotripter and protein was denaturized by this lithotripter at the high energy setting. No difference was observed between the amount of protein released with the laser, the pneumatic, and the ultrasonic lithotripters at both energy levels. The four lithotripters inactivated more than 99 % of the initial amount of bacteria; however, this antibacterial effect does not necessarily indicate that lithotripters sterilize stone fragments. The presence of free endotoxins liberated from bacteria after lithotripsy may increase the risk of sepsis. These findings could explain local and systemic inflammation response by the immune system of some patients developing in SIRS and sepsis (Gutiérrez et al., 2008).

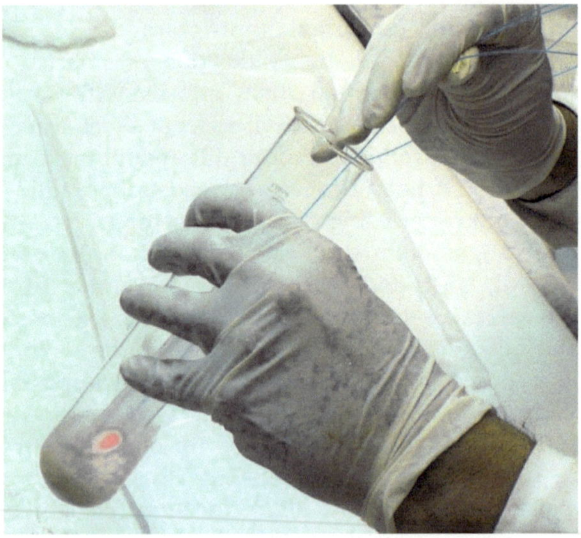

Fig. 1. Photograph of the special lucite test tube with copper mesh bottom (not seen) placed inside a standard glass laboratory test tube during *in vitro* fragmentation of an artificial infected kidney stone with a laser lithotripter.

Our group also studied the effect of the four above-mentioned intracorporeal lithotripters on the bacterial inactivation of artificial struvite stones inoculated with *Proteus mirabilis*. Again two energy settings were tested with each lithotripter, with exception of the pneumatic lithotripter, which was used only at one intensity. Calcium sulphate stones and struvite-gypsum stones were manufactured and homogeneously infected with *P. mirabilis*. Details on the methodology of producing infected stones can be found in the literature (Gutiérrez et al., 2008; Gómez-Núñez et al., 2009). Infected calcium sulphate and infected struvite-gypsum stones were exposed to each device at each intensity level until complete fragmentation. The treatment time was dependant on the lithotripter and the intensity level. After *in vitro* lithotripsy, the suspension containing stone debris and *P. mirabilis* was diluted and incubated on agar plates. A sham group of non-treated infected stones was crushed with a hand press to determine the amount of bacteria surviving inside the artificial stones. The whole experiment was repeated three times. The initial viable count in the sham group was about 6.02 log_{10} CFU/mL. Results revealed that all lithotripters inactivated a high percentage of *P. mirabilis*. No statistically significant difference was observed between calcium sulphate and infected struvite-gypsum stones (Gómez-Núñez et al., 2009). Prabakharan and colleagues (1999) reported an *in vitro* assay using 46 "natural" struvite stone models (fragments), sterilized in an autoclave and reinfected with *P. mirabilis*, coming from patients treated for urinary stones. The stones were exposed to shock waves generated with an extracorporeal lithotripter, as well as to the action of an ultrasonic, an electrohydraulic, a pneumatic, and a Holium:YAG laser intracorporeal lithotripter. No bacterial inactivation was observed, except for the laser intracorporeal lithotripter. A possible lack of this trial could be the variability of stone shape, composition, and non-homogeneous bacteria colonization of the stone.

In conclusion, it seems that the stone material plays a minor role regarding bacterial inactivation due to intracorporeal lithotripsy. Furthermore, according to our results, intracorporeal lithotripters are very harmful to bacteria; however, whether bacterial destruction is desirable or not is still unknown.

8.2 The bactericidal effect of extracorporeal lithotripters

A reduction in bacteriuria and resolution of urinary tract infection after SWL has been reported by several authors (Beck & Riehle, 1991; Gerdesmeyer et al., 2005; Michaels et al., 1988; Pode et al., 1988); however, it is not known if the stone protects bacteria or if other mechanisms, such as shear, contribute to the bactericidal effect of shock waves. To answer these questions, infected stones were exposed *in vitro* to shock waves from both an electrohydraulic and a piezoelectric lithotripter. Energy comparable to that used in SWL was used, so that the stress on the bacteria was similar to that experienced by bacteria living inside calculi during shock wave treatment. Two types of artificial kidney stones (soft and hard) were manufactured by mixing different amounts of gypsum cement and Velmix-stone, as explained in the previous section. In this case the length and diameter of the models were about 7 mm and 8 mm, respectively. *Salmonella enterica* serovar *typhimurium* in the stationary phase of growth was used to inoculate the stones. Stones to be treated were placed inside a translucent polypropylene bag, filled with deionized water, heat sealed, and centered at the lithotripter focus. All fragments from shock wave treated stones, as well as a set of intact control stones, were completely crushed using a hand press until stone powder was obtained. All bags were opened and dilutions of the suspension containing stone powder and bacteria were inoculated on TSAY plates and incubated at 35 °C. About 29 % of all bacteria were inactivated with the piezoelectric lithotripter and 14 % with the electrohydraulic lithotripter. This study demonstrated that the bactericidal action of shock waves is weaker inside the stones than in the fluid outside them (Quintero et al., 2008). Whether it is desirable for a lithotripter to inactivate instead of destroying bacteria is still to be answered.

9. Conclusions

Sepsis is a serious health condition with high mortality and cost. Advances in the manufacture of standardized infected stone models and *in vitro* assays could help to better understand the pathophysiology of sepsis associated to urinary tract infection alone and UTIs with infected stones. *In vitro* fragmentation of artificial stones could also help to understand and prevent the pathophysiology and phases of Gram negative sepsis. According to our initial results, living bacteria infecting urinary stones release endotoxins as part of their metabolic activity or as a consequence of bacteria lysis during intracorporeal and extracorporeal lithotripsy. Bacteria fragments could be a source of endotoxin even in the case of urine voiding and urine pelvis negative cultures. Further research related with release of LPS during lithotripsy and its relation with triggering sepsis is urgently needed. Absorption of LPS into the bloodstream by reflux due to open pyelolymphatic and pyelovenous channels during obstructive uropathy, bacterial translocation, interaction with lithotripters, increased irrigation pressure during endoscopic surgery, and rupture of the hemato-urinary barrier (microtrauma) should be studied. On the other hand, recent investigations (Soriano et al., 2005; Opal, 2003) have been revealing valuable information about sepsis mediators, such as cytokines, including tumor necrosis factor (TNF), interferons, complement factors or nitric oxide, anti-LPS host hydrolases, and bacterial factors. Translational studies focusing clinical strategies based on benchmark discoveries regarding LPS-triggered toxemia therefore represent a major task for the urologist. The main highlights of this chapter are summarized in Table 1.

Highlights
• During sepsis, a 25 - 50 pg/mL LPS concentration has been reported in the bloodstream. • LPS concentrations of up to 285,600 pg per gram stone have been reported in a fatal case of urosepsis. • Release of LPS has been observed after *in vitro* lithotripsy to infected artificial kidney stones. • *In vitro* application of conventional single-pulse shock waves revealed a limited bactericidal effect against bacteria in suspension and bacteria inoculated inside artificial stones. • *In vitro* application of tandem shock waves to bacterial suspensions inactivates bacteria efficiently. • *In vitro* intracorporeal lithotripsy revealed an outstanding effect against bacteria in artificial infected urinary stones. • The bactericidal effect of both extra- and intracorporeal lithotripsy should be studied carefully due the possible release of large amounts of LPS. • Under certain circumstances, this initial evidence could explain triggering of SIRS, urosepsis and MOF.

Table 1. Infected Urinary Stones, Endotoxins and Urosepsis. LPS. Lipopolysaccharide; SWL. Extracorporeal shock wave lithotripsy; SIRS. Systemic inflammatory response syndrome; MOF. Multiple organ failure.

10. Acknowledgments

The authors would like to thank Carmen Clapp, Carmen Wacher-Rodarte, Eduardo Fernández-Escartín, Concepción Arredondo, Olivia Vázquez, Marisol Moreno, Daniel Marín, Mauricio Díaz-Muñóz, Rodolfo Galeana, Arturo Méndez, and René Preza for important assistance. This research was supported by the PAPIIT-UNAM grant IN108410.

11. References

Abrahams H.M. & Stoller M.L. (2003) Infection and urinary stones. *Current Opinion in Urology* 13:63-67.

Akagashi K., Tanda K., Kato S., Ohnishi S., Nakajima H., Nambu A., Nitta T., Koroku M., Sato Y. & Hanzawa T. (2004) Characteristics of patients with staghorn calculi in our experience. *International Journal of Urology* 11(5):276-281.

Alvarez U.M., Loske A.M., Castaño-Tostado E. & Prieto F.E. (2004) Inactivation of *Escherichia coli* O157:H7, *Salmonella typhimurium* and *Listeria monocytogenes* by underwater shockwaves. *Innovative Food Science and Emerging Technologies* 5:459-463.

Alvarez U.M., Ramírez A., Fernández F., Méndez A. & Loske A.M. (2008) The influence of single-pulse and tandem shock waves on bacteria. *Shock Waves* 17:441-447.

Ansari M.S., Gupta N.P., Hemal A.K., Dogra P.N, Seth A., Aron M. & Singh T.P. (2005) Spectrum of stone composition: structural analysis of 1050 upper urinary tract calculi from northern India. *International Journal of Urology* 12(1):12-16.

Auge B.K., Pietrow P.K., Lallas C.D., Raj G.V., Santa-Cruz R.W., & Preminger G.M. (2004) Ureteral access sheath provides protection against elevated renal pressures during routine flexible ureteroscopic stone manipulation. *Journal of Endourology* 18:33-36.

Bag S., Kumar S., Taneja N., Sharma V., Mandal A.K. & Singh S.K. (2011) One week of nitrofurantoin before percutaneous nephrolithotomy significantly reduces upper tract infection and urosepsis: a prospective controlled study. *Urology* 77(1):45-49.

Beck E.M. & Riehle R.A. Jr (1991) The fate of residual fragments after extracorporeal shock wave lithotripsy monotherapy of infection stones. *Journal of Urology* 145:6-10.

Beutler B. (2000) Endotoxin, Toll-like receptor 4, and the afferent limb of innate immunity. *Current Opinion in Microbiology* 3:23-28.

Bochud P.-Y. & Calandra T. (2003) Pathogenesis of sepsis: new concepts and implications for future treatment. *British Medical Journal* 326:262-266.

Casey L.C., Balk R.A. & Bone R.C. (1993) Plasma cytokine and endotoxin levels correlate with survival in patients with the Sepsis Syndrome. *Annals of Internal Medicine* 119(8):771-778.

Crum L.A. (1988) Cavitation microjets as a contributory mechanism for renal calculi disintegration in ESWL. *Journal of Urology* 140:1587–1590.

Dandona P., Nix D., Wilson M.F., Aljada A., Love J., Assicot M. & Bohuon C. (1994) Procalcitonin increase after endotoxin injection in normal subjects. *Journal of Clinical Endocrinology & Metabolism* 79:1605-1608.

Dinarello C.A. & Cannon J.G. (1993) Cytokine Measurements in Septic Shock. *Annals of Internal Medicine* 119(8):853-854.

Elbers J., Seline P. & Clayman R.V. (1988) Effect of shock wave lithotripsy on urease-positive calculogenic bacteria. *Journal of Endourology* 2:83-88.

Fernández F., Fernández G. & Loske A.M. (2009) Treatment time reduction using tandem shockwaves for lithotripsy: an *in vivo* study. *Journal of Endourology* 23(8):1247-1253.

Foxman B. (2003) Epidemiology of urinary tract infections: incidence, morbidity, and economic costs. *Disease-a-Month* 49(2):53-70.

Gerdesmeyer L., von Eiff C., Horn C., Henne M., Roessner M., Diehl P. & Gollwitzer H. (2005) Antibacterial effects of extracorporeal shock waves. *Ultrasound in Medicine & Biology* 31:115-119.

Gómez-Núñez J.G., Alvarez U.M., Fernández F., Gutiérrez-Aceves J. & Loske A.M. (2009) Interaction of intracorporeal lithotripters with *Proteus mirabilis* inoculated inside artificial calcium and struvite stones. *Journal of Endourology* 23(3):519-522.

Grabe M. (Chairman) (2011) Guidelines on Urological Infections. In: European Association of Urology (EAU) Date of access: May 18th, 2011, Available from: http://www.uroweb.org/gls/pdf/15_Urological_Infections.pdf

Gutiérrez-Aceves J., Alvarez U.M., Mues E., Fernández F., Gómez G. & Loske A.M. (2008) Inactivation of bacteria inoculated inside urinary stone-phantoms using intracorporeal lithotripters. *Urological Research* 36:67-72.

Hugosson J., Grenabo L., Hedelin H., Pettersson S., & Seeberg S. (1990) Bacteriology of upper urinary tract stones. *Journal of Urology* 143:965-968.

Kajander E. O. & Çiftçioglu N. (1998) Nanobacteria: An alternative mechanism for pathogenic intra- and extracellular calcification and stone formation. *Proceedings of the National Academy of Sciences of the United States of America* 95(14): 8274–8279.

Kerfoot W.W., Beshai A.Z. & Carson C.C. (1992) The effect of isolated high-energy shock wave treatments on subsequent bacterial growth. *Urological Research* 20:183-186.

Kramer G., Klingler H. C. & Steiner G.E. (2000) Role of bacteria in the development of kidney stones. *Current Opinion in Urology* 10:35-38.

Loske A.M., Prieto F.E, Zavala M.L., Santana A.D. & Armenta E. (1999) Repeated application of shock waves as a possible method for food preservation. *Shock Waves* 9:49-55.

Loske A.M., Alvarez U.M. Hernández-Galicia C., Castaño-Tostado E. & Prieto F.E. (2002) Bactericidal effect of underwater shockwaves on *Escherichia coli* ATCC 10536 suspensions. *Innovative Food Science and Emerging Technologies* 3:321-327.

Mariappan P. & Loong Ch.W. (2004) Midstream urine culture and sensitivity test is a poor predictor of infected urine proximal to the obstructing ureteral stone or infected stones: A prospective clinical study. *Journal of Urology* 171:2142-2145.

Mariappan P., Smith G., Bariol S.V., Moussa S.A. & Tolley M.A. (2005a). Stone and pelvis urine culture and sensitivity are better than bladder urine as predictors of urosepsis following percutaneous nephrolithotomy: a prospective clinical study. *Journal of Urology* 173(5):1610-1614.

Mariappan P. & Tolley D.A (2005b) Endoscopic stone surgery: minimizing the risk of post-operative sepsis. *Current Opinion in Urology* 15:101-105.

Mariappan P., Smith G., Moussa S.A. & Tolley D.A. (2006) One week of ciprofloxacin before percutaneous nephrolithotomy significantly reduces upper tract infection and urosepsis: a prospective controlled trial. *British Journal of Urology International* 98(5):1075-1079.

McALeer I.M., Kaplan G.W., Bradley J.S. & Carroll S.F. (2002) Staghorn calculus endotoxin expression in sepsis. *Urology* 59(4):601iv-601v.

McALeer I.M., Kaplan G.W., Bradley J.S., Carroll S.F. & Griffith D.P. (2003) Endotoxin content in renal calculi. *Journal of Urology* 169:1813-1814.

McRae S.N. & Shortliffe L.M.D. (2000). Bacterial infections of the genitourinary tract, In: *Smith´s General Urology*, Emil A. Tanagho & Jack W. McAninch, pp 237-264, McGraw-Hill, ISBN 0-8385-8607-4, USA.

Michaels E.K., Fowler J.E. Jr & Mariano M. (1988) Bacteriuria following extracorporeal shock wave lithotripsy of infection stones. *Journal of Urology* 140:254-256.

Monga M., (2005) Re: Stone and pelvis urine culture and sensitivity are better than bladder urine as predictors of urosepsis following percutaneous nephrolithotomy: a prospective clinical study. *Journal of Urology* 174:2069.

Munford R., Lu M. & Varley A. (2009) Kill the bacteria…and also their messengers? *Advances in Immunology* 103:29-48.

Oelschlaeger T.A., Dobrindt U. & Hacker J. (2002) Virulence factors of uropathogens. *Current Opinion in Urology* 12:33-38.

Ohshima T., Tanaka S. & Teshima K. (1992). Effects of shockwaves on microorganisms: an evaluation method of the effects. In: *Shock Waves*, Takayama K. pp. 1215-1219, Springer Verlag, Berlin, Heidelberg.

O'Keeffe N.K., Mortimer A.J., Sambrook P.A. & Rao PN (1993) Severe sepsis following percutaneous or endoscopic procedures for urinary tract stones. *British Journal of Urology* 72(3):277-283.

Opal S.M. (2003) Clinical Trial design and outcomes in patients with severe sepsis. *Shock* 20 (4):295-302.

Patel J.R., Williams-Campbell A.C., Liu M.N. & Solomon M.B. (2005) Effect of hydrodynamic pressure treatment and cooking on inactivation of *Escherichia coli* O157:H7 in blade-tenderized beef steaks. *Journal of Muscle Foods* 16(4):342-353.

Pode D., Lenkovsky Z., Shapiro A. & Pfau A. (1988) Can extracorporeal shock wave lithotripsy eradicate persistent urinary infections associated with infected stones? *Journal of Urology* 140:257-59.

Podolak R., Solomon M.B., Patel J.R. & Liu M.N. (2005) Effect of hydrodynamic pressure processing on the survival of *Escherichia coli* O157:H7 in ground beef. *Innovative Food Science & Emerging Technologies* 7:28-31.

Prabakharan S., Teichman J.M.H., Spore S.S., Sabanegh E., Glickman R.D. & McLean R.J.C. (1999) *Proteus mirabilis* viability after lithotripsy of struvite calculi. *Journal of Urology* 162:1666-1669.

Quintero M.D.S., Alvarez U.M., Wacher C., Gutiérrez-Aceves J., Castaño-Tostado E., Fernández F. & Loske A.M. (2008) Interaction of shockwaves with infected kidney stones: is there a bactericidal effect? *Journal of Endourology* 22(8):1629-1637.

Rao P.N., Dube D.A., Weightman N.C., Oppeinheim B.A. & Morris J. (1991) Prediction of septicemia following endourological manipulation for stones in the upper urinary tract. *Journal of Urology* 146:955-960.

Rosser C.J., Bare R.L. & Meredith J.W. (1999) Urinary tract infections in the critically ill patient with urinary catheter. *American Journal of Surgery* 177(4):287-290.

Savas L., Guvel S., Onlen Y., Savas N. & Duran N. (2006) Nosocomial urinary tract infections: micro-organisms, antibiotic sensitivities and risk factors. *West Indian Medical Journal* 55(3):188-193.

Soriano A.O., Jy W., Chirinos J.A., Valdivia M.A., Velasquez H.S., Jimenez J.J., Horstman L.L., Kett D.H., Schein R.M.H. & Ahn Y.S. (2005) Levels of endothelial and platelet microparticles and their interactions with leukocytes negatively correlate with organ dysfunction and predict mortality in severe sepsis. *Critical Care Medicine.* 33(11):2540-2546.

Straub M. & Hautmann R.E. (2005) Developments in stone prevention. *Current Opinion in Urology* 15:119-126.

Takeuchi H., Konishi T., Takayama H., Tomoyoshi T., Okada Y., Kiriyama T., Yoshida O.(1984) Bacteriological and architectural studies of infected stones. *Hinyokika Kiyo* 30(4):479-487. (Abstract in English, article in Japanese).

Taudorf S., Krabbe K.S., Berg R.M.G., Pedersen B.K. & Møller K. (2007) Human models of low-grade inflammation: bolus versus continuous infusion of endotoxin. *Clinical and Vaccine Immunology* 14(3):250-255.

Triantafilou M. & Triantafilou K. (2005) The dynamics of LPS recognition: complex orchestration of multiple receptors. *Journal of Endotoxin Research* 11(1):5-11.

von Eiff C., Overbeck J., Haupts G., Herrmann M., Winckler S., Richter K.D., Peters G., Spiegel H.U. (2000) Bactericidal effect of extracorporeal shock waves on *Staphylococcus aureus*. *Journal of Medical Microbiology* 49:709-712.

Wagenlehner F.M., Weidner W. & Naber K.G. (2007) Optimal management of urosepsis from the urological perspective. *International Journal of Antimicrobial Agents* 30(5):390-397.

Wolf J.S. (Chairman) (2010) Best Practice Policy Statement on Urologic Surgery antimicrobial prophylaxis. In: American Urological Association (AUA) Date of access: May 18th, 2011, available from:
http://www.auanet.org/content/media/antimicroprop08.pdf

Part 5

Urological Problem and Urinary Tract Infection

13

Chronic Prostatitis / Chronic Pelvic Pain Syndrome

Nikhil Vasdev and Andrew C Thorpe
Department of Urology, Freeman Hospital, Newcastle upon Tyne
UK

1. Introduction

Chronic prostatitis (CP) refers to "inflammation" of the prostate and is thought to be related to either an acute or chronic infection of the prostate gland. It is important to distinguish chronic prostatitis / chronic pelvic pain syndrome (CPPS) from other forms of infections of the prostate gland which include chronic bacterial prostatitis and acute bacterial prostatitis [1]. The aetiology, pathogenesis, and optimal treatment of CP/CPPS continue to be evaluated. In addition to an infective and inflammatory pathogenesis hypothesized for patients with CP/CPPS, it is important to highlight a variable degree of neuropathic pain. We present the current definition, pathogenesis and new treatment methodologies being developed to treat CP/CPPS, which continue to be a challenging clinical entity to treat worldwide by Urologist.

2. Definition and classification

The European Urology Association [EAU] 2010 guidelines use the term "Painful Prostate Syndrome (PPS)" instead of the initial terminology by the National Institute of Diabetes and Digestive and Kidney Diseases (NIDDK) of CP/CPPS. PPS or CP/CPSS is defined as PPS is persistent discomfort or pain in the pelvic region with sterile specimen cultures and either significant or insignificant white blood cell counts in prostate-specific specimens (i.e., semen, expressed prostatic secretions, and urine collected after prostate massage) [2]. As there are no clinically relevant diagnostic or therapeutic consequences arising from differentiating between inflammatory and noninflammatory subtypes, CP/CPPS can be regarded as one entity.
The National Institute of Health (NIH) International Collaborative Prostatitis Network developed a prostatitis classification system in 1995, which termed CP/CPPS as 'Category III prostatitis' defined by its abacterial nature and occurrence with or without prostatic inflammation [3, 4]. A summary of this classification is presented in Table 1.
As per the NIH classification in actual clinical practice, both Type I (Acute Bacterial Prostatitis) and Type II (Chronic Bacterial Prostatitis) only account for approximately 5-10% of patients [5]. Acute prostatitis is characterized by a sudden onset of fever and dysuria. Chronic prostatitis is clinically characterized by recurrent episodes associated with recurrent same organism. Patients tend to be asymptomatic in-between episodes of infections.

NIH Consensus	Clinical descriptor	Clinical details
Type I	Acute bacterial prostatitis	Severe symptoms of prostatitis, symptoms of systemic infection and acute bacterial urinary tract infection with bacteriuria and pyuria
Type II	Chronic bacterial prostatitis	Chronic bacterial infection of the prostate gland with or without symptoms of prostatitis, usually with recurrent UTI's cause by the same bacteria
Type III A	Inflammatory subtype [a] (CP/CPPS)	Characterized by chronic pelvic pain and possibly voiding symptoms with no bacterial infection; leucocytes present in expressed prostatic secretions or semen
Type III B	Non-Inflammatory subtype	Characterized by chronic pelvic pain and possibly voiding symptoms with no bacterial infection; leukocytes present in expressed prostatic secretion or semen
Type IV	Asymptomatic Inflammatory prostatitis	Evidence of inflammation without symptoms of prostatitis or UTI
[a]WBC semen > 10^6/ml, WBC EPS > 5 p hpf, WBC VB3 > 10 p hpf		

Table 1. NIH classification of prostatitis syndromes.

Type III is classified as CP/CPPS and PPS as per the latest EAU guidelines. Patients within this category constitute about 90% of cases and it is hence very important to understand the definition of Type IIIA and Type IIIB categories. Type IIIA refers to the presence of white blood cells (WBC) in semen, after a prostate massage urine specimen (VB3) or expressed prostatic secretion (EPS). Type IIIB refers to patients with pelvic pain with no evidence of inflammation on semen, VB3 or EPS.

Type IV patients are asymptomatic and are commonly diagnosed during work up for infertility and lower urinary tract symptoms (LUTS) where they have an elevated PSA. In the MTOPS study, there is a strong link between prostatic inflammation to increased LUTS or the risk of acute urinary retention in a cohort of BPH subjects [6]. This may suggest that Type IV prostatitis may not be "asymptomatic" after all.

3. Epidemiology

Prostatitis is a significant health problem with prevalence rates of 11-16%.[7,8] More than 2 million consultations for prostatitis are required every year in the United States[9]. Prostatitis has a significant impact on the quality of life (QoL) comparable to active Crohn's disease or a recent myocardial infarction.[10] with up to 50% of men affected by it at some stage of their lives.[11,12].

In a large recent review by Krieger et al [13], the prevalence of prostatitis symptoms in 10,617 men was 8.2% (873). Amongst these patients the prevalence of prostatitis symptoms ranged from 2.2% to 9.7%, with a median rate of 8.7%.

Prostatitis-like symptoms result in a substantial number of physician visits. Sixty percent of participants with prostatitis-like symptoms seek medical help [13, 14]. The odds of a prostatitis diagnosis is 13-fold greater during visits to urologists than during visits to primary care physicians [15]. Additionally, patients with prostatitis tend to receive antimicrobials therapy in 45% of cases compared to 27% of the time for patients with no genitourinary symptoms [15]. Men with prostatitis symptoms appear to be at increased risk for persistent symptoms and for recurrent episodes. Although the pathogenesis of prostates is still being evaluated, it is common in clinical practice to see patients recurrently with acute episodes of prostatitis with a background of chronic prostatitis. These patients hence have a substantially higher cumulative probability of subsequent episodes of prostatitis [16].

4. Pathogenesis

The aetiology and pathophysiology of CP/CPPS remains a mystery, although central neurological mechanisms probably play a role. Patients with PPS show no evidence of infection; they do not have urethritis, urogenital cancer, urethral stricture, or neurologic disease involving the bladder, and they do not exhibit any overt renal tract disease [17]. Hence, the exact aetiology of CP/ CPPS is unknown. The main factor that continues to be evaluated in patients with CP / CPPS is whether infection and inflammation are responsible for the clinical symptomology of these patients. The difficulty in pinpointing etiologic mechanisms and obtaining efficacious therapies is probably due to the heterogeneity of factors that contribute to CP/CPPS. Despite this complexity, most experts agree that pain is the defining feature of the condition.

The initial concept of infection and inflammation arose when True et al [18], analyzed the outcome of Prostate histopathology in 368 biopsies from 97 patients with the CP/CPPS. In these patients prostatic inflammation was detected in only 33% of patients, including 29% with mild (less than 10 leukocytes per 1 mm. field) and 4% with moderate (between 10 and 200) or severe (more than 200) infiltrate. Of the 3 patients with moderate inflammation 1 had glandular, 1 periglandular and 3 multifocal or diffuse distribution of leukocytes in the interstitium. Although 33% of patients had inflammation on prostate biopsies, only 5% of 97 patients had moderate to severe inflammation. This study questioned the assocaition and role of inflammation in the pathogenesis of CP/CPPS. Despite this CP/CPPS continues to be diagnosed on the basis of symptoms. It is diagnosed from a history of persistent genitourinary pain and an absence of other lower urinary tract pathologies. The severity of disease, its progression and treatment response can be assessed only by means of a validated symptom-scoring instrument [19, 20].

Patients with CP/CPPS are diagnosed traditionally using the gold-standard four-glass test for bacterial localisation [21]. However, as this test is cumbersome to perform and hence the diagnostic efficiency may be enhanced cost effectively by a simple screening procedure, that is, the two-glass test, or by pre- and post-massage test (PPMT) [22], with PPMT able to indicate the correct diagnosis in >96% of patients [23]. These tests use the concept of White blood cells (WBC) as a marker on inflammation. White blood cells can be found in seminal plasma and prostatic fluid of asymptomatic patients and in patients with pelvic pain [24].

Schaeffer et al [24], examined whether leukocytes and bacteria correlate with symptom severity in men with chronic prostatitis/chronic pelvic pain syndrome. In this landmark publication, 488 men were classified into the CP/CPPS criteria NIH criteria. Participants were classified as category IIIa based on WBC counts of 5 or more, or 10 or more (5+, 10+) in the expressed prostatic secretion, or 1+ or 5+ either in the post-expressed prostatic secretion urine (voided urine 3) or semen. Uropathogens were classified as localizing if the designated bacterial species were absent in voided urine 1 and voided urine 2 but present in expressed prostatic secretion, voided urine 3 or semen, or present in expressed prostatic secretion, voided urine 3 or semen at 2 log concentrations higher than at voided urine 1 or 2. Associations between symptoms and inflammation and infection were investigated using generalized Mantel-Haenszel methods. Of all participants 50% had urethral leukocytes and of 397 with expressed prostatic secretion samples 194 (49%) and 122 (31%) had 5+ or 10+ WBCs in expressed prostatic secretion, respectively. The prevalence of category IIIa ranged from 90% to 54%, depending on the composite set of cut points. None of the index measures were statistically different (p >0.10) for selected leukocytosis subgroups. Based on prostate and semen cultures, 37 of 488 men (8%) had at least 1 localizing uropathogen. None of the index measures were statistically different (p >0.10) for selected bacterial culture subgroups. The authors thus concluded that men with chronic prostatitis routinely receive anti-inflammatory and antimicrobial therapy despite leukocytes and bacterial counts which do not correlate with severity of symptoms. These findings suggest that factors other than leukocytes and bacteria also contribute to symptoms associated with chronic pelvic pain syndrome.

Based on current studies the initiator of the inflammatory process in CP / CPPS within the prostate is thought to be a local infection, chemical irritation, dysfunctional voiding, intraductal reflux, neuromuscular disturbances or an immunological process. Regardless of the triggering factor, the resultant inflammatory process causes tissue oedema and increased intra-prostatic pressure leading to local hypoxia and varied mediator-induced tissue damage. This leads to altered neurotransmission in sensory nerve fibres thereby resulting in the pain and other symptoms associated with the condition [25]. We now present each aetiology associated with CP / CPPS.

The common etiologies associated with CP / CPPS include

- 4A. Infection
- 4B. Inflammation and Autoimmunity
- 4C. Neurological
- 4E. Psychological
- 4F. Additional Conditions

4A. Infection

An acute episode of prostatitis and recurrent episodes of chronic prostatitis can be caused by organisms that are commonly responsible for Urinary Tract Infections (UTI). The majority of organisms isolated within both patients groups include Escherichia coli in the community. Additionally bacteria responsible for both acute and chronic prostatitis include *Pseudomonas* and *Streptococcus faecalis*. The symptoms of CP / CPPS are identical to those of prostatic infection. Pontari et al [26], conducted a questionnaire to evaluate the demographic, behavioural, clinical and medical history characteristics of men with chronic prostatitis/chronic pelvic pain syndrome (CP/CPPS) and asymptomatic controls. In their study they analyzed the outcome of 463 men with CP/CPPS and 121 asymptomatic age-matched controls. Interestingly, compared to controls, men with CP/CPPS reported a significantly greater lifetime prevalence of nonspecific urethritis (12% vs 4%, P = 0.008), cardiovascular disease (11% vs 2%, P = 0.004), neurological disease (41% vs 14%, P < 0.001), psychiatric conditions (29% vs 11%, P < 0.001), and haematopoietic, lymphatic or infectious disease (41% vs 20%, $P < 0.001$). Hence, the outcome of this publication suggested that a range of self-reported medical conditions are associated with CP/CPPS with a higher proportion reporting a history of nonspecific uretheritis caused due to gonorrhoeal, trichomonal and henital herpetic infections. It was also suggested that rare episodes of recurrent cystitis in young males is caused due to secondary infections of the prostatic ducts. An important factor associated with recurrent infections in CP is ascending urethral infection and reflux of urine into ejaculatory and prostatic ducts [27]. Bacteria can be isolated preferentially from an expressed prostatic secretion (EPS) or a post-prostatic massage urine specimen rather than from the mid-stream urine (MSU) sample or can be demonstrated on the prostatic biopsy specimen [28,29]. The concept of intraprostatic reflux was demonstrated by Kirby et al [30]. In this publication the authors injected carbon particles into the bladders of men about to undergo a transurethral resection of prostate (TURP). On histological analysis of the resected TURP specimen, carbon particles could be demonstrated which suggested a intraprostatic reflux.

Blacklock et al [31], noted that some patients with CP / CPPS had some pathogens identified in vaginal cultures of their sexual partners. Magri et al [32], evaluated 55 symptomatic patients with CP / CPPS they were subjected to segmented tests to localise Chlamydia trachomatis in first voided urine (VB1), prostatic secretions (EPS), post-massage voided (VB3) or semen specimens. Patients were divided in three treatment groups: the 'urethral involvement' group (VB1 positive, EPS/VB3/Semen negative) was treated with 500 mg day(-1) azithromycin for 3 days. The 'prostatitis' group (VB1 negative, EPS/VB3/semen positive) with 4-week levofloxacin-azithromycin combination. A third group, 'Urethral and Prostate group' (VB1, EPS/VB3/semen positive) received both treatments in sequence. In patients prosatitis, eradication of Chlamydia trachomatis was paralleled by marked, sustained symptom improvement and by significant decrease of serum prostate-specific antigen (PSA) levels. Compared with Urethral patients, undergoing rapid regression of symptoms related to painful micturition after short-term azithromycin, U+P patients showed symptom and pathogen persistence in VB3/EPS/semen and required additional treatment with 4-week levofloxacin-azithromycin to achieve pathogen eradication, symptom regression, and decrease of PSA. The results from this publication support a causative role of Chlamydia trachomatis in CP / CPPS.

Mardh et al [33], evaluated the role of Chlamydia trachomatis in non-acute prostatitis was investigated by cultural and serological techniques in a study of 53 adult males. C. trachomatis was isolated from the urethra of only one of the 53 patients and from none of the 28 specimens of prostatic fluid from the same patients. By means of a modified microimmunofluorescent test, serum chlamydial IgG antibodies at a titre of 1/64 or greater, or IgM antibodies at a titre of 1/8 or greater, or both were detected in six of the patients, suggesting a recent or current chlamydial infection, while IgG or IgA antibodies at a titre of 1/8 or greater were detected in the specimens of prostatic fluid from two of the 28 men studied. In the seven patients with evidence of chlamydial infection, as well as in a further 13 of the 53 patients studied, the presenting symptoms suggested non-gonococcal urethritis (NGU) rather than prostatitis. Thus in this study, C. trachomatis would appear to play a minor aetiological role, if any, in CP / CPPS.

Based on current literature and evidence, there continues to be inconsistencies in the response to antibacterial treatment and the inability to consistently isolate any pathogenic organisms in the appropriate specimens in patients with CP / CPPS.

4B. Inflammation and autoimmunity

Both acute and chronic inflammation is now thought to be associated with CP / CPPS. The core of Inflammation lies with the presence of both pro and anti-inflammatory cytokines present with the prostate in comparison to normal asymptomatic patients. The main cytokines linked with CP / CPPS are Interleukin - 8 [34], Interleukin - 10 [35] and Tumour Necrosis Factor - alpha (TNF-α) [36].

The concentration of citric acid is a significant parameter of prostate gland function [37]. Substantial amounts of citric acid are produced and stored in the gland. A decrease in its concentration is observed in cases of inflammation or cancer of the prostate gland [38]. In addition to citric acid there is now a new interest in the evaluation of polymorphonuclear (PMN) leukocytes and PMN elastase levels in patients with PC / CPPS. Zdrodowska-Stefanow et al [39], evaluated PMN leukocytes , PMN elastase and citric acid concentrations in chronic prostatitis patients regardless of aetiology and in a parallel group with C trachomatis infection. In this paper the analysis of expressed prostatic secretions (EPC) of 46 patients with chronic prostatitis was evaluated for leukocyte count, PMN elastase (ELISA) and citric acid concentrations. All patients have an additional analysis for C. trachomatis infection (ligase chain reaction). Analysis confirmed increased PMN cell counts (≥10 per high-power field) in 73.9% of patients and increased PMN elastase concentration (<250 ng/ml) in 78.3%. In 44.4% of the patients the elastase concentration indicated moderate (250–1000 ng/ml) and in 55.6% acute infection (≥1000 ng/ml). Decreased citric acid concentration (<18.12 mg/ml) in the EPS was found in 65.2% of the men. C. trachomatis prostate infection was detected in 17.4% of the patients and all of these men had higher inflammation parameters and lower citric acid concentrations. The authors concluded that CP /CPSS associated with C. trachomatis infection were accompanied by an increase in inflammation markers and a decrease in citric acid concentration.

Autoimmunity is characterized by recognition of self by the immune system with the resulting immune response destroying or damaging normal cells and tissues. T lymphocytes are principally responsible for the recognition of antigens by the immune system. CD4 T cells recognize processed peptide antigens in association with the MHC class II molecule and play a significant role in the effector function of CD8 T-cells and B-cell activation. In previous work we have shown that soluble components in normal semen can be recognized by CD4 T lymphocytes in men with CP/CPPS [40, 41]. The current concept of autoimmunity is best recognized in patients with non-specific granulomatous prostatitis (NSGP). Within this group of patients it is the HLA class II allele DRB1*1501 in Caucasian men is associated with CP/CPPS [42].

In a landmark paper evaluating the link between autoimmunity and CP / CPPS, Kouiavskaia et al [40], aimed to assess whether T cells from a group of men with CP/CPPS would recognize peptides derived from the normal self prostatic proteins prostate specific antigen (PSA) and prostatic acid phosphatase (PAP). The authors used purified CD4 T cells from the peripheral blood of 31 patients with CP/CPPS and from the buffy coat preparation of 27 normal male blood donors that were stimulated *in vitro* with a panel of immunogenic peptides from PSA and PAP and assayed for reactivity with the peptides by IFN-γ ELISPOT assay. The data from this study suggested that the peptides such as $PAP_{133\text{-}152}$, $PAP_{173\text{-}192}$, $PSA_{171\text{-}190}$, $PSA_{221\text{-}240}$ represent promiscuous epitopes able to be presented by different HLA-DR alleles. High level of the peptides promiscuity was supported by the results of both analysis of MHC class II allele expression by the individuals responding to the peptides in the IFN-γ ELISPOT assay and analysis of the direct binding of the peptides to MHC class II molecules. *In vitro* functional assays showed that autoreactive T cells specific for the peptides are present and can be activated in the patients with CP/CPPS and normal male blood donors, identified PAP as a possible target protein for autoimmune reactivity in the patients with CP/CPPS and demonstrated that autoimmune reactions to the immunodominant peptide $PAP_{173\text{-}192}$ might be involved in the disease development. The data supported autoimmunity as a potential aetiology for CP/CPPS in some patients and suggest that immunosuppressive therapies might logically be tested in the treatment of this complex and frustrating disorder. The authors found that Peptide $PAP_{173\text{-}192}$ was more frequently recognized by CD4 T cells from the patients with CP/CPPS compared to the healthy donors. Peptide reactivity was more commonly observed in cases compared to normal male blood donors for any PSA peptide or any tested peptides. This study demonstrated a strong link between autoimmunity and CP / CPPS in that CD4 T cells from patients with CP/CPPS had a higher frequency of recognition of the self prostatic proteins PAP and PSA compared to normal male blood donors.

4C. Neurological

CP/CPPS is associated with the patient developing pain and this suggests a possible neurological link with the diagnosis. The pain perceived by these patients can be a combination of either local pain within the pelvis or more central pain. Hence, one further hypothesis in the development of CP/CPPS includes dysfunction of the nervous system that attributes to the patients symptoms. Despite attributing a strong neurological link few of the agents that have been studied in clinical trials target pain pathways directly, particularly those in the central nervous system (CNS). Recent animal model studies on retrograde labelling of the prostate and pelvic floor indicates that there are double labelled cells in the dorsal root ganglion in the lumbar and sacral cord [42]. Patients with CPPS are thought to have an altered sensation of the perineum in comparison to control patients without CP/CPPS. The mechanism of this 'altered' innervations is poorly understood and is thought to be related to reflex sympathetic dystrophy of the perineum and pelvic floor [43-45].

4E. Psychological

Psychological stress is also commonly associated with the exacerbation of symptoms related to CP/CPPS. The initial evidence of a strong psychological link was after Wallner et al [46], collected data from 703 men enrolled in the Flint Men's Health Study, a population-based health study of African American men. Participants were interviewed about their health history and lifestyle factors, such as physical activity. They also answered questions about stress and emotional health. In this study poor emotional health, high levels of stress (as perceived by study participants), and a lack of social support were associated with a history of CP. The findings were consistent with a previous study by Collins et al [47], which also reconfirmed that patients with severe stress at work or home were 1.2 and 1.5 times more likely to report CP, respectively, than those whose lives were relatively stress-free.

Ullrich et al [48], associated stress to be an important factor responsible for the development of CP/CPPS. In this study , 200 men were interviewed about the level of stress and degree of pain intensity by telephone a month after the men were diagnosed with CP and then again three, six, and 12 months later. This publication concluded that the men with more perceived stress during the six months following diagnosis were in more pain after a year than those who experienced less stress. Despite the limitations of the study, such as the lack of health data on participants prior to diagnosis, the paper concluded that treatment in patients with CP / CPPS should include stress management techniques.

4F. Additional health conditions

Additional health conditions associated with CP / CPPS include - Irritable bowel syndrome, Fibromyalgia and chronic fatigue syndrome .

5. Diagnosis

There is no gold standard for diagnostic testing for the CPPS [49]. The 4-glass or 2-glass test may provide information on prostatic inflammation (e.g., the number of white cells per high-power field), but this finding is not helpful in the diagnosis or management of the condition. Among men with presumed chronic pelvic pain syndrome and no history of urinary tract infection, up to 8% have been found to have positive prostatic localization cultures, but these findings have also been reported in a similar percentage of asymptomatic men [50].

The current EAU 2008 guidelines highlight that CP/CPPS is more of a symptomatic diagnosis. To facilitate in the diagnosis the following an initial sterile pre-massage urine (voided bladder urine-2 [VB2]) is collected, patient with CP/CPPS shows less than 10,000 colony-forming units of uropathogenic bacteria in expressed prostatic secretions (EPS) and insignificant numbers of leucocytes or bacterial growth in ejaculate. Diagnostic efficiency may be enhanced cost-effectively by a simple screening procedure, i.e. the two-glass test or pre-post-massage test (PPMT) [49]. In an extensive analysis of both tests, PPMT was able to indicate the correct diagnosis in more than 96% of patients [50].

Additional tests performed to facilitate diagnosis include a flowrate studies, urodynamic assessments and a transrectal ultrasound to exclude an obstructed seminal vesicle. A transrectal ultrasound is indicated in patients with CP/CPPS and painful ejaculation. In these patients a transrectal ultrasonography may reveal enlargement of the seminal vesicle caused by obstruction of the ejaculatory duct; such an obstruction may be associated with or exacerbate the chronic pelvic pain syndrome. Isolated case reports suggest that the correction of the obstruction may relieve pain, although this cannot be proved because of a lack of data [51]. A urodynamic assessment can be performed when patients have concomitant lower urinary tract symptoms that are refractory to treatment.

To assess the accurate symptomology at the time of diagnosis it is essential for patients tom complete the The NIH Chronic Prostatitis Symptom Index. This 9 item, self-administered tool leads to the development of a score between is 0 to 43 points [52]. A summary of the current investigations from our department based on current European Association of Urology guidelines summarized in Figure 1.

6. Treatment

The treatment of CP/CPPS continues to be challenging. We divide the Urological treatment into Medical and Surgical categories.

6A. Urological medical treatment

Effective treatment for the CP/CPPS remains uncertain. Factors complicating the management of this condition include its probably multifactorial pathogenesis, lack of a gold standard for diagnostic testing, and the methodological limitations of many treatment

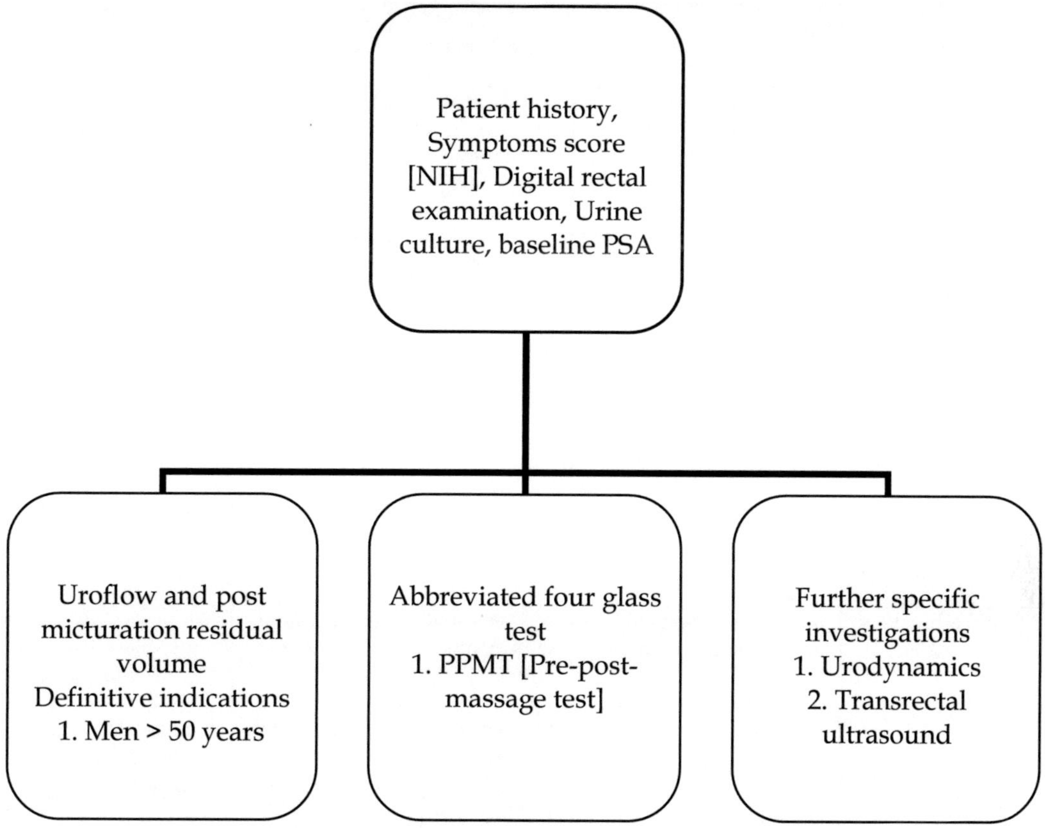

Fig. 1. Our departments guidelines for the initial investigating patients with CP/CPPS.

studies. Most current treatment strategies focus on symptomatic relief. Despite of numerous advocated strategies and new drugs being developed, the US Preventive Services Task Force system best summarizes current treatments for CP/CPSS as grade 1 which is defined as "drug therapy where current evidence is insufficient to assess the balance of benefits and harms of the service. Evidence is lacking, of poor quality, or conflicting, and the balance of benefits and harms cannot be determined."

The predominant medical treatment of drugs include:-

1. Antibiotics
2. Alpha blockers
3. Anti-inflammatories
4. 5 α reductase inhibitors
5. Pentosulphan Polyphosphate
6. Additional therapies [Physical therapy, Myofascial and trigger point therapy]

The current mechanism of action and evidence to support the above mentioned treatment is summarized in Table 2.

The Urological Surgery Treatment in patients with CP/CPPS include

1. Prostatic Massage
2. Transurethral Microwave therapy
3. Transurethral resection of prostate

Drug	Mechanism of action	Evidence for treatment/Recommended agents	Side effects
1. Antibiotics	Reduces and cures infections. This further reduces inflammation and hence improves symptoms of CP/CPPS.	A. Levofloxacin in 80 patients for 6 weeks. Outcome - 6 point decrease in NIH symptoms [53] B. Ciprofloxacin in 196 patients for 4-6 weeks. Outcome - Significant symptomatic improvement [54]	A. Side effects of fluroquinolones including central nervous system (CNS) toxicity, phototoxicity, cardiotoxicity, arthropathy, and tendon toxicity. B. RCTs have failed to show significant beneficial effects of antibiotics compared to placebo in patients who have already failed antibiotic treatment
2. Alpha blockers	Inhibit neurological activation induced by sympathetic overactivation	A. Meta-analysis of treatment with Alpha blockers in men with CP/CPPS showed significant reduction in symptoms over a duration of 3 months [55].	Adverse effects of alpha-blockers include dizziness, fatigue, hypotension and decreased ejaculate volume
3. Anti-inflammatories	Reduce systemic or prostatic inflammation, autoimmunity, CNS transmission of pain signals, and central sensitization	A. Main symptom of CP/CPPS is pain. Hence, it is very important to control this symptom. B. Tricyclic Antidepressants are widely used for pain and act by inhibiting central neuronal reuptake of Norepinephrine and Serotonin. Both substances linked to pain. C. Current medication recommenced includes - Gabapentin, Pregabalin and Amitriptyline D. COX 2 inhibitors are now being investigated as these drugs regulate prostaglandin production. In an RCT of the COX2 inhibitor rofecoxib, the NIH-CPSI total and pain scores showed improvement in the rofecoxib group, but the difference between rofecoxib and placebo was not statistically significant [56].	Adverse effects of Tricyclic include dry mouth, dry nose, and increased body temperature. Other side effects may include drowsiness, anxiety, akathisia, , tachycardia. Twitching, hallucinations, delirium and coma are also some of the toxic effects caused by overdose. Rhabdomyolysis or muscle breakdown has been rarely reported.

Drug	Mechanism of action	Evidence for treatment/Recommended agents	Side effects
4. 5 α reductase inhibitors	Reduction in prostatic volume	A. One randomized, placebo-controlled trial of Finasteride showed that scores on the Prostatitis Symptom Severity Index and the International Prostatitis Symptom Survey decreased significantly after 1 year of treatment, but pain scores did not change significantly [57]. B. Response rates at 6 months (defined as an improvement of more than 25% in scores on the NIH Chronic Prostatitis Symptom Index) were not significantly better for Finasteride than for placebo (33% vs. 16%) [58].	Adverse effects of 5 α reductase inhibitors include impotence, decreased libido, and decreased ejaculate volume. Rare side effects include breast tenderness and enlargement.
5. Pentosulphan Polyphosphate	Replenish the glycosaminoglycan layer of the bladder, stabilize prostatic stromal mast cells	CP/CPPS is thought to be related conditions, and Pentosan Polysulfate has been tested in an RCT for CP/CPPS . The results showed some clinical benefit in the treatment arm, but the change in total NIH-CPSI score was not statistically significant [59].	Pentosan Polysulfate has minimal side effects and is well tolerated.
6. Additional therapies [Physical therapy, Myofascial and trigger point therapy	Reduce pelvic floor muscle dysfunction	A. Physical therapy, Myofascial therapy and trigger point therapy reduce symptoms related to CP/CPPS. B. A recent study has demonstrated a statistically significant improvement in symptoms in the patients receiving myofascial therapy for CP/CPPS in comparison to the pharmacological medication mention in category 1-3.	None reported

Table 2. Urological Medical Treatment of CP/CPPS.

6B. Urological Surgery Treatment

The latter two treatments have side effects including reterograde ejaculation and erectile dysfunction. These must be highlighted to patients being offered Urological Surgery for medically refractory CP/CPPS which continues to be a clinically challenging category of patients to manage.

1. Prostate Massage

The rationale of this procedure is to try to expel dense prostatic secretion and/or to force an obstructed outlet duct. In order to avoid damage to the integrity of a prostatic acinus which could lead to worsening of the inflammation, it should be done with care, and in my opinion, not before the patient has had hot baths and drugs for a couple of days. It seems very helpful in those patients in whom TRUS has shown a sectorial oedema in the prostate. In my experience, patients with massive calcifications in the veru-region are rarely helped by this manoeuvre; this seems understandable, as those calcifications cannot be removed by massage, but, on the contrary, manipulation can traumatize this area and worsen the situation. I see my patients 2-3 times a week for a total of about 6-8 sessions.

2. Transurethral Microwave therapy

Transurethral microwave thermotherapy, which is widely available, can achieve temperatures of more than 45°C within prostatic tissue. One small randomized trial (20 patients) suggested that transurethral microwave thermotherapy significantly improved the quality of life at 3 months, as compared with sham treatment [61]; four patients reported transient adverse effects, including hematuria, urinary tract infection, impotence, urinary retention, urinary incontinence, and premature ejaculation, but whether these patients received active or sham treatment was not stated.

3. Transurethral Resection of Prostate

Transurethral resection of the prostate (TURP) is advocated for CP/CPPS based on a few anecdotal experiences, but there are absolutely no reliable data or experiences to substantiate a treatment effect [62]. Patient with significant lower urinary tract symptoms with a background of CP/CPPS may benefit from this therapy.

7. Conclusion

Chronic Prostatitis / Chronic Pelvic pain syndrome continues to be a challenging clinical entity for urologists. A thorough clinical evaluation and organizing appropriate clinical investigations are essential to establish a potentially treatable cause, although this is not found in all patients. With new avenues of autoimmunity and inflammation being explored as a strong link in the pathogenesis of CP/CPPS, we envisage that this may well direct future treatment strategies. However, based on current clinical practice a combination of treatment trial including newer biomarkers, genomic, immunological, imaging studies, epidemiologic and symptom-based assessments, will maximize the ability to identify an effective treatment strategy in the future.

8. References

[1] Schaeffer, AJ; Datta, NS; Fowler Jr, JE; Krieger, JN; Litwin, MS; Nadler, RB; Nickel, JC; Pontari, MA et al. (2002). "Overview summary statement. Diagnosis and

management of chronic prostatitis/chronic pelvic pain syndrome (CP/CPPS)". Urology 60 (6 Suppl): 1–4.
[2] Nickel JC, Weidner W. Chronic prostatitis: current concepts and antimicrobial therapy. Infect Urol 2000;13:S22–8.
[3] Krieger JN, Nyberg L, Jr, Nickel JC. NIH consensus definition and classification of prostatitis.JAMA.1999;282:236–237
[4] Schaeffer AJ. Clinical practice. Chronic prostatitis and the chronic pelvic pain syndrome. N Engl J Med. 2006;355:1690–1698
[5] De la Rosette JJ, Hubregtse MR, Meuleman EJ, Stolk-Engelaar MV, Debruyne FM. Diagnosis and treatment of 409 patients with prostatitis syndromes. Urology. 1993 Apr;41(4):301-7
[6] Kaplan SA, Lee JY, Meehan AG, Kusek JW; MTOPS Research Group. Long-Term Treatment With Finasteride Improves Clinical Progression of Benign Prostatic Hyperplasia in Men With an Enlarged Versus a Smaller Prostate: Data From the MTOPS Trial. J Urol. 2011 Apr;185(4):1369-73
[7] Roberts RO, Lieber MM, Rhodes T, Girman CJ, Bostwick DJ, Jacobsen SJ. Prevalence of a physician-assigned diagnosis of prostatitis: The Olmstead County study of urinary symptoms and health status among men. Urology. 1998;51:578–84.
[8] Collins MM, Meigs JB, Barry MJ, Walker Corkery E, Giovannucci E, Kawachi I. Prevalence and correlates of prostatitis in the health professionals follow-up study cohort. J Urol. 2002;167:1363–6.
[9] Collins MM, Stafford RS, O'Leary MP, Barry MJ. How common is prostatitis? A national survey of physician visits. J Urol. 1998;159:1224–8
[10] Wenninger K, Heiman J, Rothman I, Berguis JP, Berger BE. Sickness impact on chronic nonbacterial prostatitis and its correlates. J Urol. 1996;155:965–8.
[11] Lobel B, Rodriguez A. Chronic prostatitis: What we know, what we don't know and what we should do! World J Urol. 2003;21:57–63.
[12] Stamey TA. Periurethral or perineal bacteria in urinary tract infections? JAMA. 1981;245:127–8
[13] Krieger JN, Lee SW, Jeon J, Cheah PY, Liong ML, Riley DE. Epidemiology of prostatitis. Int J Antimicrob Agents. 2008 Feb;31 Suppl 1:S85-90
[14] Nickel JC, Downey J, Hunter D, Clark J. Prevalence of prostatitis-like symptoms in a population based study using the National Institutes of Health chronic prostatitis symptom index. J Urol. 2001;165:842–5
[15] Collins MM, Stafford RS, O'Leary MP, Barry MJ. How common is prostatitis? A national survey of physician visits. J Urol. 1998;159:1224–8.
[16] Turner JA, Ciol MA, Von Korff M, Berger R. Prognosis of patients with new prostatitis/pelvic pain syndrome episodes. J Urol. 2004;172:538–41
[17] Nickel JC, Weidner W. Chronic prostatitis: current concepts and antimicrobial therapy. Infect Urol 2000;13:S22–8.
[18] True LD, Berger RE, Rothman I, Ross SO, Krieger JN. Prostate histopathology and the chronic prostatitis/chronic pelvic pain syndrome: a prospective biopsy study. J Urol. 1999 Dec;162(6):2014-8
[19] Barry MJ, Fowler Jr FJ, O'Leary MP, et al. The American Urological Association symptom index for benign prostatic hyperplasia. The Measurement Committee of the American Urological Association. J Urol 1992;148:1549–57, discussion 1564.

[20] Nickel JC. Effective office management of chronic prostatitis. Urol Clin North Am 1998;25:677–84.

[21] Meares EM, Stamey TA. Bacteriologic localization patterns in bacterial prostatitis and urethritis. Invest Urol 1968;5:492–518.

[22] Nickel JC. The pre and post massage test (PPMT): a simple screen for prostatitis. Tech Urol 1997;3:38–43.

[23] Nickel JC, Shoskes D, Wang Y, et al. How does the pre-massage and postmassage 2-glass test compare to the Meares-Stamey 4-glass test in men with chronic prostatitis/chronic pelvic pain syndrome?J Urol 2006;176:119–24.

[24] Schaeffer AJ, Knauss JS, Landis JR, Propert KJ, Alexander RB, Litwin MS, Nickel JC, O'Leary MP, Nadler RB, Pontari MA, Shoskes DA, Zeitlin SI, Fowler JE Jr, Mazurick CA, Kusek JW, Nyberg LM; Chronic Prostatitis Collaborative Research Network Study Group. Leukocyte and bacterial counts do not correlate with severity of symptoms in men with chronic prostatitis: the National Institutes of Health Chronic Prostatitis Cohort Study. J Urol. 2002 Sep;168(3):1048-53.

[25] Vaidyanathan R, Mishra VC. Chronic prostatitis: Current concepts. Indian J Urol. 2008 Jan;24(1):22-7.

[26] Bartoletti R, Mondaini N, Pavone C, Dinelli N, Prezioso D. Introduction to chronic prostatitis and chronic pelvic pain syndrome (CP/CPPS). Arch Ital Urol Androl. 2007 Jun;79(2):55-7

[27] Nickel JC, Bruce AW, Reid G. Pathogenesis, diagnosis and treatment of the prostatitis syndromes. In: Krane RJ, Siroky MB, editors. Clinical urology. Philadelphia: Lippincott; 1994. p. 925.

[28] Berger RE, Krieger JN, Rothman I, Muller CH, Hillier SL. Bacteria in the prostate tissue of men withidiopathic prostatic inflammation. J Urol. 1997;157:863–5.

[29] Nickel JC, Costerton JW. Bacterial localization in antibiotic-refractory chronic bacterial prostatitis. Prostate. 1993;23:107–14.

[30] Kirby RS, Lowe D, Bultitude MI, Shuttleworth KE. Intra-prostatic urinary reflux: an aetiological factor in abacterial prostatitis. Br J Urol. 1982 Dec;54(6):729-31

[31] Blacklock NJ. Anatomical factors in prostatitis. Br J Urol.1974 Feb;46(1):47-54

[32] Magri V, Marras E, Skerk V, Markotić A, Restelli A, Garlaschi MC, Perletti G. Eradication of Chlamydia trachomatis parallels symptom regression in chronibacterial prostatitis patients treated with a fluoroquinolone-macrolide combination.Andrologia. 2010 Dec;42(6):366-75

[33] Mårdh PA, Ripa KT, Colleen S, Treharne JD, Darougar S. Role of Chlamydia trachomatis in non-acute prostatitis. Br J Vener Dis. 1978 Oct;54(5):330-4.

[34] Hochreiter WW, Nadler RB, Koch AE, Campbell PL, Ludwig M, Weidner W, Schaeffer AJ. Evaluation of the cytokines interleukin 8 and epithelial neutrophil activating peptide 78 as indicators of inflammation in prostatic secretions. Urology. 2000 Dec 20;56(6):1025-9.

[35] Miller LJ, Fischer KA, Goralnick SJ, Litt M, Burleson JA, Albertsen P, Kreutzer DL. Interleukin-10 levels in seminal plasma: implications for chronic prostatitis-chronic pelvic pain syndrome. J Urol. 2002 Feb;167(2 Pt 1):753-6.

[36] Nadler RB, Koch AE, Calhoun EA, Campbell PL, Pruden DL, Bennett CL, Yarnold PR, Schaeffer AJ. IL-1beta and TNF-alpha in prostatic secretions are indicators in the evaluation of men with chronic prostatitis. J Urol. 2000 Jul;164(1):214-8.

[37] Kavanagh J. P., Darby C. and Costello C. B. (1982): The response of seven prostatic fluid components to prostatic disease. Int. J. Androl., 5, 487–496

[38] Kammer H., Scheit K. H., Weidner W. and Cooper T. G. (1991): The evaluation of markers of prostatic function. Urol. Res., 19, 343–347

[39] Zdrodowska-Stefanow B, Ostaszewska-Puchalska I, Badyda J, Galewska Z. The evaluation of markers of prostatic inflammation and function of the prostate gland in patients with chronic prostatitis. Arch Immunol Ther Exp (Warsz). 2008 Jul-Aug;56(4):277-82. Epub 2008 Jul 29.

[40] Kouiavskaia DV, Southwood S, Berard CA, Klyushnenkova EN, Alexander RB. T-cell recognition of prostatic peptides in men with chronic prostatitis/chronic pelvic pain syndrome. J Urol. 2009 Nov;182(5):2483-9

[41] Alexander RB, Brady F, Ponniah S. Autoimmune prostatitis: Evidence of T cell reactivity with normal prostatic proteins. Urology. 1997;50:893.

[42] Yang CC, Lee JC, Kromm BG, Ciol MA, Berger RE. Pain sensitization in male chronic pelvic pain syndrome: why are symptoms so difficult to treat? J Urol. 2003 Sep;170(3):823-6; discussion 826-7.

[43] Andersen JT. Treatment of prostatodynia. In: Nickel JC (ed). Textbook of Prostatitis. London: ISIS Medical Media Ltd. 1999; pp. 357-364.

[44] Egan KJ, Krieger JL. Chronic abacterial prostatitis–a urological chronic pain syndrome? Pain 1997Feb;69(3):213-8.

[45] Osborn DE, George NJ, Rao PN, Barnard RJ, Reading C, Marklow C, Blacklock NJ. Prostatodynia– physiological characteristics and rational management with muscle relaxants. Br J Urol 1981 Dec;53(6):621-3.

[46] Wallner LP, Clemens JQ, Sarma AV. Prevalence of and Risk Factors for Prostatitis in African American Men: The Flint Men's Health Study. Prostate 2009;69:24–32

[47] Collins MM, Meigs JB, Barry MJ, et al. Prevalence and Correlates of Prostatitis in the Health Professionals Follow-Up Study Cohort. Journal of Urology 2002;167:1363–66.

[48] Ullrich PM, Turner JA, Ciol M, Berger R. Stress Is Associated with Subsequent Pain and Disability Among Men with Nonbacterial Prostatitis/Pelvic Pain. Annals of Behavioral Medicine 2005;30:112–18.

[49] McNaughton Collins M, MacDonald R, Wilt TJ. Diagnosis and treatment of chronic abacterial prostatitis: a systematic review. Ann Intern Med 2000;133:367-81.

[50] Nickel JC, Alexander RB, Schaeffer AJ, Landis JR, Knauss JS, Propert KJ. Leukocytes and bacteria in men with chronic prostatitis/chronic pelvic pain syndrome compared to asymptomatic controls. J Urol 2003;170:818-22.

[51] Nadler RB, Rubenstein JN. Laparoscopic excision of a seminal vesicle for the chronic pelvic pain syndrome. J Urol 2001;166:2293-4.

[52] Litwin MS, McNaughton-Collins M, Fowler FJ Jr, et al. The National Institutes of Health chronic prostatitis symptom index: development and validation of a new outcome measure. J Urol 1999;162:369-75.

[53.Nickel JC, Downey J, Clark J, et al. Levofloxacin for chronic prostatitis/chronic pelvic pain syndrome in men: a randomized placebo-controlled multicenter trial. Urology 2003;62:614-7.

[54] Alexander RB, Propert KJ, Schaeffer AJ, et al. Ciprofloxacin or tamsulosin in men with chronic prostatitis/chronic pelvic pain syndrome: a randomized, double-blind trial. Ann Intern Med 2004;141:581-9.

[55] Yang G, Wei Q, Li H, Yang Y, Zhang S, Dong Q. The effect of alpha-adrenergic antagonists in chronic prostatitis/chronic pelvic pain syndrome: a meta-analysis of randomized controlled trials. J Androl. 2006 Nov-Dec;27(6):847-52. Epub 2006 Jul 26.

[56] Zeng X, et al. Clinical evaluation of celecoxib in treating type IIIA chronic prostatitis [Chinese] Zhonghua Nan Ke Xue. 2004;10:278–281

[57] McNaughton Collins M, MacDonald R, Wilt TJ. Diagnosis and treatment of chronic abacterial prostatitis: a systematic review. Ann Intern Med 2000;133:367-81.

[58] Nickel JC, Downey J, Pontari MA, Shoskes DA, Zeitlin SI. A randomized placebo-controlled multicentre study to evaluate the safety and efficacy of finasteride for male chronic pelvic pain syndrome (category IIIA chronic nonbacterial prostatitis). BJU Int 2004;93:991-5.

[59] Nickel JC, et al. Pentosan polysulfate sodium therapy for men with chronic pelvic pain syndrome: a multicenter, randomized, placebo controlled study. J Urol. 2005;173:1252–1255.

[60] FitzGerald MPS. Randomized multicenter feasibility trial of myofascial physical therapy for the treatment of urological chronic pelvic pain syndromes. J Urol. 2009;182:570–580

[61] McNaughton Collins M, MacDonald R, Wilt TJ. Diagnosis and treatment of chronic abacterial prostatitis: a systematic review. Ann Intern Med 2000;133:367-81.

[62] Kaplan SA, Te AE, Jacobs BZ. Urodynamic evidence of vesical neck obstruction in men with misdiagnosed chronic nonbacterial prostatitis and the therapeutic role of endoscopic incision of the bladder neck. J Urol. 1994;152:2063–5

14

Transposition of Distal Urethra in Female Patients with Recurrent Lower UTI Associated with Sexual Intercourse

Natalia Sumerova, Dmitry Pushkar and Mikhail Gvozdev
Moscow Medical Stomatological University, Russia

1. Introduction

The treatment of recurrent lower urinary tract infections in young female patients remains controversial (Naber, 2000; Stamatiou, 2005; Wagenlehner, 2009). Recurrent lower UTI is often associated with sexual intercourse. The association of UTI with sexual intercourse poses both medical and psychological problems for these patients (Stamatiou, 2005). Usually these patients are young females. Repeated courses of antibiotic therapy and postcoital antibiotics prophylactic help some, but not all patients. Conventional antimicrobial therapy has limited success and often has to be repeated (Naber, 2000). A remarkable increase of antibiotic resistance is also noted in uncomplicated UTI (Wagenlehner, 2009).

"Intravaginal urethral displacement" during sexual intercourse appears to play a role in both the development of these symptoms and the recurrence of UTI symptoms by contamination of microbial agents in the distal urethra (Stamatiou, 2005), which may often lead to cystitis. The repositioning of the distal part of the urethra may potentially minimize microbial contamination in this area. The operation makes it possible to withdraw the meatus from the area concerned. Careful mobilization of the distal part of the urethra with modern technology and fine absorbable suture materials provides minimal invasion and may be considered an option for patients with recurrent UTI associated with sexual intercourse.

In this chapter we shall present detailed surgical techniques and long-term results of distal urethral transposition in female patients with recurrent UTI associated with sexual intercourse.

2. Methods

2.1 Patients

From 1995 to 2010 two hundred and seventy one female patients underwent surgical treatment in the Urology Department of MSMSU for recurrent UTI associated mainly with sexual intercourse. The patients' age ranged from 16 to 48 years (mean 25.9 years) - Group I. All of them exhibited failure of standard drug therapy, including UTI prophylaxis (three-day antimicrobial treatment is recommended for simple cystitis (Valiquette, 2001). All patients had practiced additional prophylactic methods, such as perineal hygiene, post-coital micturition, with sufficient fluid intake, but with little benefit. The patients themselves also believed that the conservative treatments being used were of little benefit. The mean duration of symptoms before urethral transposition was scheduled 2,7 years (13 months - 4,5 years). After the failure of traditional medical and conservative therapies (hygiene, antibiotic therapy) all patients underwent surgery.

Table 1 shows the age distribution of patients scheduled for surgery.

All patients had long suffered from recurrent infections of the lower urinary tract, mainly from symptoms of acute cystitis. Usually these were cases of classic "honeymoon" cystitis. In all cases, the manifestation of the disease coincided with the beginning of regular sexual life. The UTI symptoms were related directly to sexual intercourse, with the duration of recurrences increasing with time and the efficiency of conservative treatment progressively decreasing. It should be noted that sexual sensation became dull in all women, with decreased sexual activity due to the fear of a recurrence of UTI and discomfort in the perineal area.

57 patients (mean age 26, 9) with the same histories, anatomical findings, symptoms and signs of lower UTI, receiving conventional antibiotic treatment, served as controls - Group II. Repeated short and long-term courses of antibiotics were used according to urinary culture. It should be noted that this group served as a control for the first year. These patients were advised to have surgery as they showed the same anatomical features, but they initially refused to undergo surgical treatment.

The mean follow up time of the 271 patients from Group I was 52.5 months (48 - 57 months). 183 patients were available for additional examinations after three and five years, (mean 52,5 months).

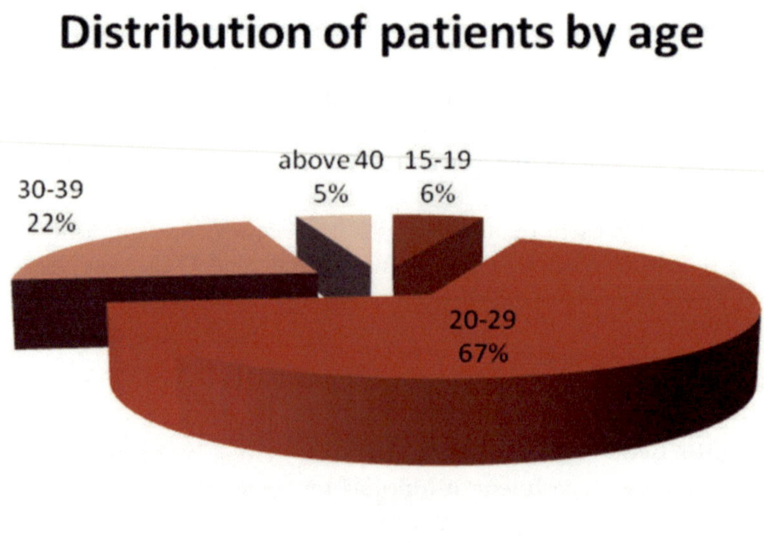

Table 1. Age distribution of patients scheduled for surgery.

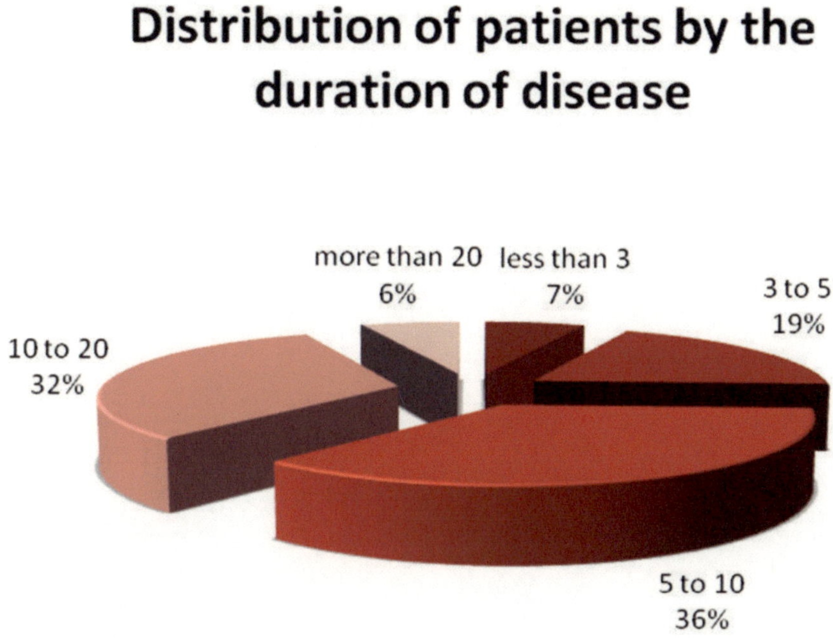

Table 2.

2.2 Preoperative evaluation

Full medical histories were obtained. During vaginal examinations, special emphasis was given to the position of the distal urethra. A plastic penile imitator was introduced vaginally to evaluate urethral movements simulating intercourse. Detailed pelvic examination was described by Hrischhorn in 1966. We believe that a finger exam and stretching the fingers widely apart does not provide adequate understanding or a complete assessment of the meatal movements. For this reason we decided to use a plastic penile imitator. Urinalysis (including nitrite dipstick and leukocyte esterase test), urinary culture and urinary tract ultrasonography to exclude anatomical abnormalities were performed in all patients. Cystoscopy, carried out in all cases, was always normal apart from the occasional finding of urethrotrigonitis. All patients were counseled extensively regarding anatomy and the technique of this procedure.

2.3 Surgical techniques

This technically simple operation allows the elimination of peculiar «lateral tractions» that permanently displace the meatus into the vaginal lumen during intercourse and subsequent frictions by causing retrograde infection of the urinary tract by vaginal microflora. The operation makes it possible to withdraw the meatus from the area concerned and hence create conditions for further adequate anti-microbal therapy.

The patient is placed in the standard lithotomy position and a conventional cleansing preparation with a sterile covering is used. The procedure starts by analyzing existing urethral-hymenal fusions. In cases where these fusions are well-developed, and limit the mobilization of the distal part of the urethra, they should be dissected widely in the transverse fashion.

In order to mobilize the distal part of the urethra and create a submucosal bed for subsequent urethral transposition, an inverse tennis racket incision is performed with a fine 11 blade scalpel. The distal portion of the urethra should be exposed widely in order to be fixed as close as possible to the clitoral area in the submucosal bed already created. (Fig.1).

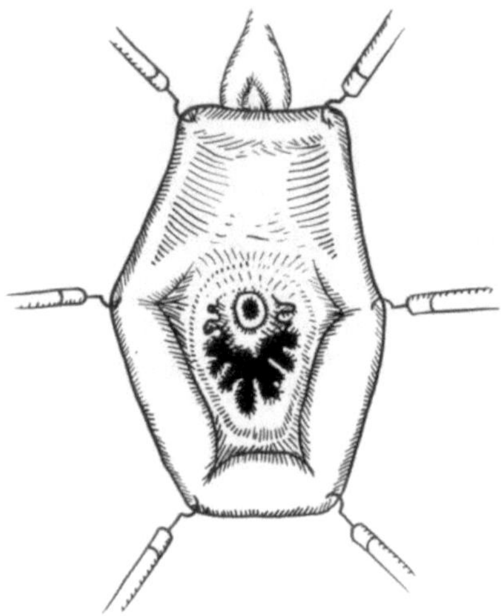

(1)

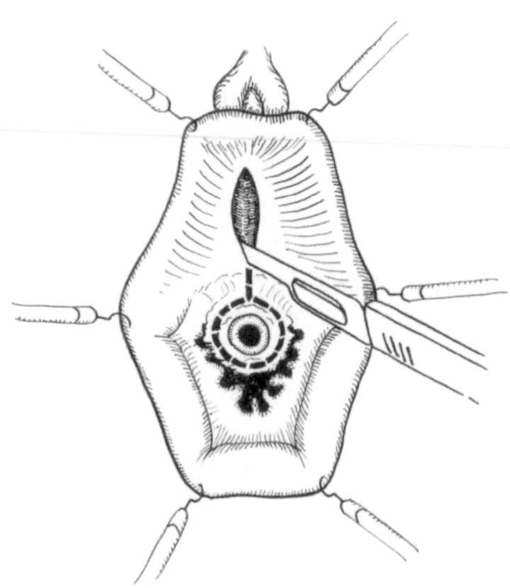

(2)

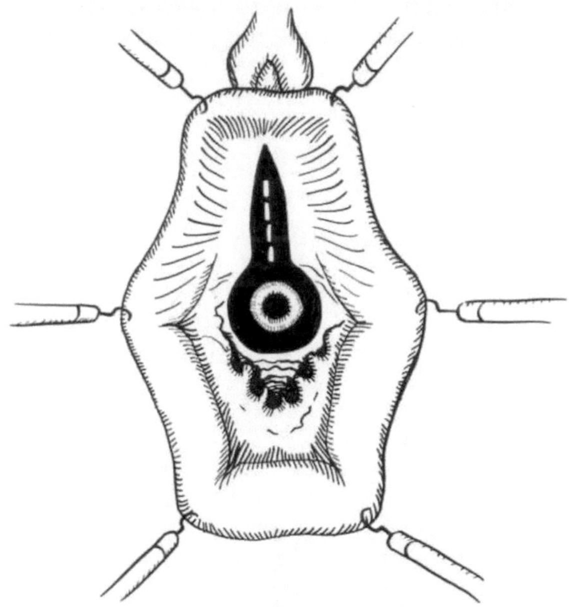

(3)

Fig. 1. Incision used for mobilization of the distal urethra.

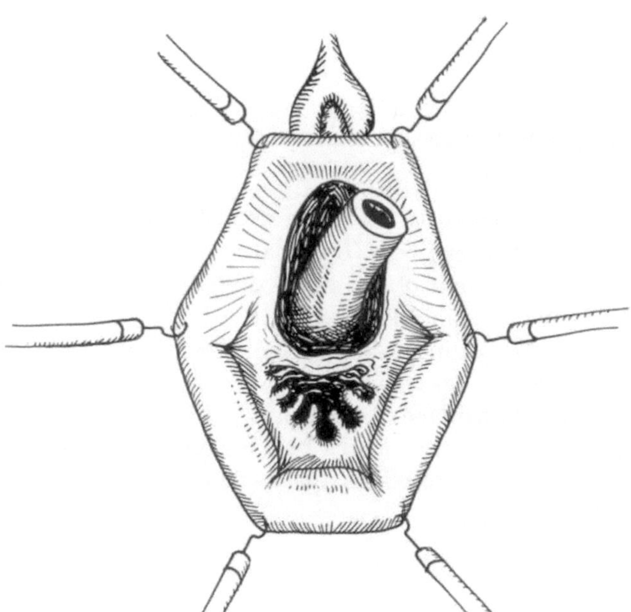

Fig. 2. Exposed distal urethral portion.

The edges of the distal urethra are fixed by interrupted sutures from synthetic absorbable material (Vicryl, Monocryl 4/0) to the tissue of the vaginal vestibule in the formed bed (Fig. 2).

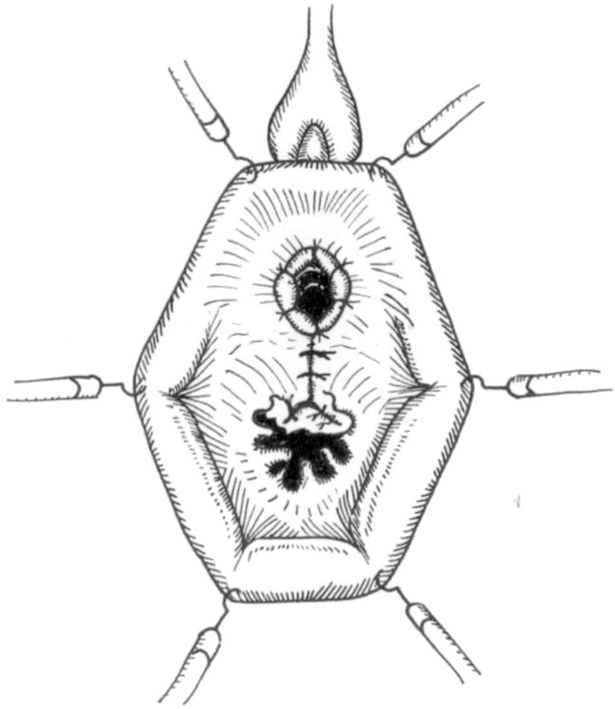

Fig. 3. The initial step of fixing the urethra: the exposed part of the urethral tube is fixed to the apex of the incision.

Sufficient mobilization of the distal part of the urethra should provide tension-free fixation in the apical part of the submucosal bed. (Fig.3). Tension-free fixation can be achieved by both careful and wide mobilization of the distal urethra and the suturing of previously transversely dissected hymenal fusions longitudinally.
Care must be taken to provide secure fixation of the external meatus in a new area with the final step of the operation being vaginal mucosa closure.
In cases of vaginal anatomical narrowness, encountered in nulliparas, or marked hymenal ring, the described operation is supplemented by a hymenectomy that enlarges the vaginal orifice and creates the optimal conditions for further sexual life, minimizing bacterial contamination.

2.4 Follow up

A 16 Fr. Foley catheter was placed for three days. All patients were treated postoperatively with standard antibiotic therapy course for a mean time of three weeks. Patients were required to avoid sexual intercourse postoperatively for one month. The mean hospital stay was 2,6 days.

3. Results

Patients from Group I were evaluated after three months, showing no postoperative complications. Those who wished to begin sexual activity were able to do so after one month. Coital activity was resumed with no further recurrence of pre op. dyspareunia. Examinations of 204 (75,3%) patients from Group I one year later showed no symptoms and signs of UTI. 67 (24,7%) patients required further antimicrobial prophylaxis after the procedure because of the longer preoperative duration of their symptoms. 19 patients (7,1%) showed poor results. 183 patients were available for additional examinations after three and five years, (mean 52,5 months) revealing stable results with no lower UTI for these patients. It should be noted that the flow rate remained unchanged postoperatively, with no signs of obstruction or dysfunctional voiding. Patients did not complain about sexual dysfunction postoperatively, although it should be noted that we did not conduct in-depth evaluations.
Group II patients were followed up for one year. 46 (80,7%) of them were found to have recurrent symptoms with poor response to the therapy, and had to undergo repeated treatment.

4. Discussion & conclusion

Recurrent UTI and dysuria associated with sexual intercourse represent a common urological problem. The relationship of lower urinary tract symptoms with sexual activity is well recognized in terms of onset and recurrence. This condition automatically leads to dyspareunia (Valiquette, 2001).
It seems that distal urethral vaginal ectopy with intravaginal movements of the external meatus during sexual intercourse plays an important role in the development of acute UTI with symptoms of acute cystitis (Reed, 1970). The antimicrobal defense mechanism of the urethra is altered by frequent recurrences, and conventional antimicrobal therapy may not help. Careful physical examination may provide a detailed evaluation of distal urethral position and assess urethral-hymenal fusions. Initial work done by Hirshhorn in early 1966 concluded that bilateral hymenotomies may provide a stable effect with no further recurrence of urethritis or cystitis (Hirshhorn, 1966). This type of procedure has been used in our department for many years with limited success. We feel that simple finger evaluation of the distal urethra movements will not provide adequate information in order to select candidates for surgery. We have developed a simple method of assessment of the urethral position by simulating sexual intercourse with a plastic penile imitator. We now believe that all younger sexually active females who develop dysuria after sexual intercourse should be evaluated by this method in order to exclude intravaginal movements of the distal urethra.
In 1972 Alan R. Alexander et al. published a limited study on bilateral hymenectomy alone or with urethral transposition, achieving good results (Alexander et al, 1970). They considered urethral transposition a radical operation which should be reserved for only those cases in which the patients failed to respond to simple bilateral hymenectomy. We may understand that at that time there was not such a wide variety of antibiotics. Therefore some cases could have benefited from simple bilateral hymenectomy. We now try to prescribe longer courses of antibiotic treatment with stronger agents. We may therefore assume that our patients would not benefit from a simple bilateral hymenectomy.
Careful mobilization of the distal part of the urethra with modern technology and fine absorbable suture materials provides minimal invasion and may be considered an option for

patients with recurrent UTI associated with sexual intercourse. It should be emphasized that we do not advocate this procedure as a primary choice. This means that all patients showing this type of UTI should be initially treated conservatively, and scheduled for surgery only if this treatment is unsuccessful.

5. References

Alan R. Alexander, Paul M. Morrisseau - Urethral-hymenal adhesions and recurrent post-coital cystitis: treatment by hymenoplasty. The Journal of Urology, Vol. 107, April 1970 Hirschhorn R. C. Urethral - hymeneal fusion: a surgically correctable cause of recurrent cystitis. Obstetrics and Gynecology. Vol. 26, №6, 1965. pp. 903 - 908.

Naber KG. Treatment options for acute uncomplicated cystitis in adults. Urological Clinic, Hospital St Elisabeth, Straubing, Germany. J Antimicrob Chemother. 2000 Sep;46 Suppl 1:23-7; discussion 63-5

Reed J. F. Urethral - hymenal fusion: a cause of chronic adult female cystitis. The Journal of Urology. 1970, vol. 103, №4 pp. 374 - 378.

Reziciner S. Prevention of recurrent post-coital cystitis using hymenoplasty. Ann Urol (Paris). 1988;22(6):446-51

Santucci RA, Payne CK, Saigal CS - Office dilatation of the female urethra: a quality of care problem in the field of urology. J Urol. 2008 Nov;180(5):2068-75.

Scotti R. J. Ostergard D. R. The urethral syndrome. Obstetrics and Gynecology Vol. 27, №2, pp. 515 - 529.

Smith PJ, Roberts JB, Ball AJ - "Honeymoon cystitis" : a simple surgical cure. BJU, 1982, 54, 708-710

Stamatiou C, Bovis C, Panagopoulos P - Sex-induced cystitis - patient burden and other epidemiological features. Clin Exp Obstet Gynecol. 2005;32(3):180-2.

O' Donnell R. P. Relative hypospadias potentiated by inadequate rupture of the hymen. Int. Coll. V 32, p 374 - 388. 1959.

Valiquette L. - Urinary tract infections in women. Can J Urol. 2001 Jun; 8 Suppl 1:6-12

15

Nosocomial Urinary Tract Infections

Sonia Isabel Cuervo Maldonado and Jorge Alberto Cortés Luna
Universidad Nacional de Colombia, Bogotá
Colombia

1. Introduction

Healthcare-associated urinary infection is one of the most frequent infections and it is responsible for more than 40% of nosocomial or healthcare-associated infections (HAIs) and nursing homes for the elderly. The complexity and diversification of health services currently offered has motivated an enlargement in literature about infectious complications that may happen in each one of these scenarios; and according to the recommendations from literature since 2007 (1), in this chapter, urinary tract infection will be approached as a result of the care provided at hospitals or nosocomial care (NUTI).

Due to the fact that most of NUTIs are associated to urinary tract instrumentation, i.e. secondary to either indwelling or intermittent vesical catheterization, cystoscopies or any invasive urologic procedures, or to nephrostomy tube placement, this chapter will emphasize in the most recurrent complication derived from the use of these medical devices: urinary catheter-associated bacteriuria (UCAB).

2. Epidemiology

The risk to acquire a NUTI depends on: location of Urinary Catheter (UC), catheterization's period of time, catheter care measures and host's susceptibility. 13.2 % of inpatients, 4.9% in nursing homes for the elderly and 3.9% of home care patients have urinary catheters (14). After just one catheterization of the urinary tract, infection rates vary from 1% to 5% to 100% in patients who have indwelling urinary catheter with open drainage system. Likewise, and regardless of the use of closed drainage system, more than 20% of patients with urinary catheters might become infected when mishandling of closed drainage system (3, 4). Among risk factors that increase acquiring a catheter-associated urinary tract infection (CAUTI) are: advanced age, debilitating disease and postpartum.

In the National Nosocomial Infections Surveillance in United States, between 1992 and 1997, data from 112 medical intensive care units was includes with 181.993 patients and 715.930 patient-days of follow up. They found 14.177 HAIs, where NUTI was the most frequent diagnosis, with 31% of the cases, followed by nosocomial pneumonia and primary bloodstream infection (5).

Information about the epidemiology of nosocomial infections is provided in developing countries by the International Nosocomial Infection Control Consortium (INICC). This multicenter, international surveillance system proceeded data in 2008 about 98 intensive care units around the world. Those units belonged public and private hospitals in 18 countries in Latin-America, Africa, Asia and Europe. Between 2002 and 2007 a total of 1212

NUTI were reported in 202.311 patient-days, with a median rate of 6.49 per 1.000 catheter-days. Those ICU that had medical and neurosurgical patients had the highest rates, with 9.63 and 8.29 infection per 1.000 catheter-days, respectively (6). Previous studies have shown that different kinds of patients had different rates of infections because of different risk factors that need to be addressed with different control strategies.

Urinary Catheter-associated NUTIs are caused by a variety of pathogens: *E. coli, Klebsiella, Proteus, Enterococcus, Pseudomonas, Enterobacter, Serratia and Candida.* Many of these microorganisms constitute intestinal flora, but they can also be acquired through cross contamination from other patients or hospital personnel, or through exposure to contaminated solutions or non-sterile equipment. NUTIs produced by *Serratia marcescens y Pseudomonas cepacia* have great epidemiologic meaning since its isolation from catheterized patients clearly suggest that they are obtained from exogenous flora, as normally these organisms are not part of the intestinal flora.

Secondary becteremia for NUTI can be present even in a 4% of the patients and it occupies the second place among bacteremias of secondary cause; it has even been related to mortality rates ranging from 13 to 30%, nonetheless, in a study performed in a ICU to determine the impact on UC use in death outcomes, it showed that once all confounding variables were controlled, mortality was not higher in patients with UC --mortality in ICU patients OR 0,846 (IC 95% 0,695-1,086) versus mortality in hospitals OR 0,949 (IC 95% 0,763-1,181) -- (7).

3. Urinary catheters (UC)

Every year, millions of UCs are used in the different hospital services: Intensive Care Units (ICU), rehabilitation, neurology, neurosurgery and internal medicine, also in nursing homes for the elderly. Approximately, 25% patients in hospitals use UCs, considering the following criteria for its use:

1. Surgery
2. Urine output measure
3. Urine voiding when urine retention; generally caused by processes of urinary tract obstruction.
4. Urinary incontinence (8).

The majority of urinary tract complications are second to bacteriuria production. Trauma and urethritis are other less frequent complications.

A urinary catheter is a device which has been used since 1927, when Frederick E.B. Foley introduced it to control post-surgical bleeding in prostatectomy (9). From 1927 until 1950, UCs were used as open drainage system, i.e., urine made contact with air when drained, this led to 100% of the patients with open drainage system to develop bacteriuria at the fourth day of use (10). From 1950 to 1960, another system was implemented. This system used a drainage tube connected to a bag which collected urine, thus leading to the origin of closed drainage system. In this case, 100% of the patients developed bacteriuria at the thirtieth day of use. (9, 11)

Urinary catheters are classified as per:

1. Place of insertion.
2. Period of catheterization.
3. Material

Regarding the first, they can be urethral, suprapubic or nephrostomy catheters. As for the period of catheterization, there are two kinds, one for long-term catheterization, usually with indwelling Foley catheters, and for short-term catheterization, nelaton intermittent catheters are commonly used. And finally, catheters can be made in latex, silicone or Teflon, they can be latex or silicone-covered and some are coated with an antiseptic or antibiotic. They also have different diameters.

The majority of nosocomial CAUTIs are produced by bacteria which come from patient's own colon, which is known as endemic infection, whereas epidemic or secondary infection can be explained by different causes: incorrect aseptic techniques for equipment such as cystoscopes, contaminated irrigation solutions or contaminated disinfectants used for cleaning before catheter insertion, and the most recurrent: cross -transmission through hospital personnel hands.

4. Pathogenesis

NUTI production is often multifactorial, the main mechanisms to describe the process are:

4.1 Defense process and urinary infection

An average urinary tract has defense mechanisms to prevent or minimize interaction between epithelial cells and bacteria. Though a large amount of infectious agents that cause UTI previously colonize the periurethral area, the urethra represents the first obstacle for these agents to reach the bladder. Had the microorganism gone through the urethra and entered the bladder, micturition will purify 99.9% of these bacteria with the help of uromodulin and oligosaccharide -which are present in urine-, by a neutralizing action. However, a biofilm may remain adhered to the vesical mucosa, in which case, glycosaminoglycan inhibits bacterial adherence to epithelial cells. Still, in the case that these cells become infected; an acute inflammatory response is produced as a result of cytokine liberation of the infected epithelial cells. The last protecting instance of epithelial cells is an exfoliation process through which microorganisms are removed from the host. Antibody production and host cellular response contribute to a slower reaction, thus helping in the last states of acute infection.

4.2 Biofilms and urinary catheters

UC use can interfere with some of these natural defense mechanisms. Catheters increase urethral colonization by uropathogens, especially in women. Both, inner and outer catheter surfaces are niches where bacteria adhere to creating a biofilm which covers and protects bacteria from urinary flow and polymorphonuclear action.

A biofilm is a microorganism community that permanently adheres to biological or inert surfaces and it is embedded in a matrix of extracellular polymeric substances modifying growing and genetic transcription phenotypes. Bacteria constitute biofilms in especially high-stress environments, e.g. fast and turbulent flow milieus, which in return increases adhesion of floating cells on surfaces. Once a biofilm is formed and the exopolysaccharide matrix has been secreted by cells, the resultant structure is highly viscoelastic and resistant to mechanical breaking. Hence, the nature in structure and physiological attributes of biofilm's constituent organisms provide an inherent resistance to antimicrobial agents. (12)

4.3 Handling and care precautions of urinary catheters

Another factor encouraging CAUTIs in health care institutions is a failure in the draining system, therefore, large amounts of bacteria remain in the bladder and catheter presence interrupts interaction between glycosaminoglycan and epithelial cells. (11)

4.4 Hematogenous or lymphatic dissemination

It is important to remember that certain microorganism reach the kidney through bloodstream dissemination from a distant organ. The most common microorganisms in this particular scenario are: *S. aureus*, Candida, *Salmonella* and some species of *Pseudomonas*, for this reason, isolation of any of these in urine always suggests two possible sources: urinary tract or a source different from the kidney compromising it through hematogenous dissemination.

To summarize, CAUTIs at health care institutions can be present in four ways (13):

1. Early extraluminal: By direct inoculation of microorganisms in the bladder at the moment of UC insertion.
2. Late extraluminal: By microorganisms ascending from perineum to urethra and to catheter's outer surface.
3. Intraluminal: Due to closed-drainage system failure or when collected bag is contaminated.
4. In rare opportunities by hematogenous dissemination as a consequence of a systemic disease with kidney as target organ.

The final consequence of the interaction between host's defense mechanism and colonizing microorganisms in patients with UC is the presence of bacteria in urine or bacteriuria.

The majority of infectious agents causing catheter-associated bacteriuria originate in patient's own intestinal flora, which at the same time can be regular inhabitants of the colon, or exogenous, as in healthcare-associated infections (HAIs). As in UTI's pathogenesis, enterobactericeae can colonize periurethral areas of non-catheterized patients, especially women. Exogenous microorganisms can colonize UC through means of care personnel manipulation or less frequent circumstances, as in polluted products.

5. Risk factor for bacteriuria development

Asymptomatic bacteriuria is common but its prevalence among general public varies significantly with age, gender, and the presence of genitourinary tract alterations. Bacteriuria risk for catheterized patients is approximately 25% and its significance in relation to provide or not antimicrobial treatment in the asymptomatic patient is debatable considering that 80% of short-term catheterized patients receive antimicrobial treatment for a different purpose than that of a UTI. (14)

In a multivariate analysis and observations of 1474 catheterized patients, Platt et al., found nine independent risk factors for catheter-associated bacteriuria development. (15)

1. Period of catheterization
2. Lack of urinometer usage
3. Collector bag colonized by microorganisms
4. Diabetes mellitus
5. Lack of antibiotic usage
6. Mishandling in UC procedures
7. Female gender
8. Abnormal creatinine
9. Incorrect catheter care

5.1 Period of catheterization

According to UC usage standards, catheterization periods vary:

1. Surgery: 1-7 days

2. Cardiac output measure: 7-30 days
3. Urinary retention: 1-30 days
4. Urinary incontinence: >30 days

Period of catheterization is the main risk factor for associated bacteriuria development. Once UC is inserted, bacteriuria increases at the rate of 3 to 10% per day of UC permanence (catheter day) and, it is estimated that by the thirtieth catheter day, 100% of catheterized patients will present bacteriuria. For this reason, it is important to divide the period of catheterization in: (i) Short-term, for less than 30 days; and (ii) Long-term, for more than 30 days. In addition, bacteriuria may be asymptomatic or some symptoms may be identified having a real UTI.

5.2 Short-term catheterization

Between 15 to 25% of inpatients might have a UC for an average period of 2-4 days and approximately 10 to 13% of them will develop bacteriuria in comparison to 1% of non-catheterized inpatients that develop bacteriuria. The most common infectious agent found in these patients is *E. coli*, besides *Pseudomonas aeruginosa, Klebsiella pneumoniae, Proteus mirabilis, Enterobacter sp., Staphylococcus epidermidis, Staphylococcus aureus* and *Candida* species. In general, only one microorganism is isolated in the urine culture but 15% can be polymicrobial. Colony count can show a meaningful bacteriuria of equal or more than 10^5 bacteria. In general, this bacteriuria, aside from the colony count, is accompanied with pyuria. Most short-term UC associated bacteriuria are asymptomatic, nonetheless, lower urinary symptoms and fever may be present even in 30% of these patients and less than 5% will develop bacteremia. The impact of short-term UC associated bacteriuria on mortality is not clear and results from studies have shown to be contradictory.

5.3 Long-term catheterization

Long-term catheterization is needed for urinary incontinence in women, lower urinary tract obstruction in men as a consequence of prostatic hyperplasia and prostate carcinoma, and to urinary obstruction in postrenal failure in women secondary to cervical carcinoma, aside from neurogenic bladder related to spinal cord trauma both in men and women.

Bacteriuria incidence tends to be similar to that observed in hospitals (3 to 10% per day), hence, most patients will have bacteriuria at the end of 30 catheter days. Bacteriuria prevalence is a consequence of:

1. Bacteriuria incidence which is similar to that observed in short-term catheterization, by gram-negative and gram-positive bacteria, with an average permanence of a different infectious agent every two weeks.
2. Some bacteria residing for weeks and months in the urinary tract, like *E. coli* and *Providencia stuartii*.

Colony count is generally meaningful with 10^5 colonies or more and more than two infectious agents are present in more than 95% of long-term catheterization patients.

The most common infectious agents identified in these patients are *E. coli, P. aeruginosa, P. mirabilis, Providencia stuartii y Morganella morganii,* the latter two in less frequency. Most frequent complications are symptomatic bacteriuria, obstruction, urinary stones, periurethral infection, chronic kidney disease, renal failure and cancer when catheter is used over several years.

5.4 Therapy of asymtomatic bacteriuria

There is no need for rutinary microbiological studies in catheterized patients presenting asymptomatic bacteriuria or funguria, or those who have had treatment for that condition. Recommendation A-1 from CDC's (Control Diseases Centers) guidelines for bacteriuria prevention (16).

Antimicrobial treatment can be considered for women who have persistent asymptomatic bacteriuria after catheter removal. Recommendation B-1 (17).

6. Nosocomial urinary tract infection (NUTI) diagnosis

Besides presenting symptoms or not, a urine test and a urine culture are necessary to confirm either bacteriuria or NUTI. In table 3, CDC and NHSN diagnosis criteria for UTIs are shown (26).

7. Bacteriuria complications treatment

Several clinical manifestations can be present in patients with asymptomatic bacteriuria associated with UC usage.

- Cystitis is manifested through changes in the macroscopic characteristics of urine and it is combined with suprapubic pain, polakiuria, dysuria, urinary urgency, and vesical tenesmus, these latter symptoms are present when patients do not have sequelae of spinal shock. In the case a patient is catheterized due to spinal shock sequelae, the most recurrent symptom is associated with the change of macroscopic characteristics of urine (odor, color, and transparency). Urine culture and bacteria's in vitro susceptibility to certain antibiotics should be considered for the choice of antibiotherapy, which can range from 7 to 10 days.
- If the patient presents with fever, it is strongly recommended to exclude any other plausible cause for this symptom; if fever seems to be secondary to pyelonephritis caused by UC, then a 14-21 day treatment is implemented depending on the severity of the infectious process and on the susceptibility of the infectious agent.
- Candiduria is present in long-term catheterization patients that have had antibiotics previously. *Candida* presence in urine should be taken as possible hematogenous dissemination to kidney or other different organs. When candiduria is a result of candidemia or a disseminated candidiasis, it is recommended to exclude a systemic infection to determine the period of antimycotic treatment (18). Most of the times, candiduria is asymptomatic, but it can include complications such as a bladder or renal pelvis fungal bezoar, perinephric abscess and disseminated candidiasis. Treatment for asymptomatic candidiasis associated to UC is not clear, however, 40% of candiduria ends after UC removal and 20% does when UC is changed; this is a B-III recommendation (18). For asymptomatic patients who persist with candiduria and require catheter, several therapeutic strategies have been proposed. Bladder irrigation with 50 to 200 μg/mL of amphotericine B can clear funguria temporarily and it is not a frequent recommendation (recommendation C-III) (18); systemic use of fluconazole 200 mg/d for 14 days has demonstrated microbiological cure. Antimycotic treatment in patients with asymptomatic candiduria is not totally defined, but treatment is recommended when undergoing genitourinary surgical procedures. Even with apparent microbiological cure by UC removal or with systemic treatment, relapse is common, even more when there is still UC use.

Urinary tract infection	Clinical criteria	Laboratory criteria
Symptomatic NUTI At least one of the following:	1. At least one of the following signs or symptoms, without any other cause; fever >38°C, urinary urgency, frequency, dysuria or suprapubic pain and criteria 1 from laboratory 2. At least one of the following signs or symptoms, without any other cause; fever >38°C, urinary urgency, frequency, dysuria or suprapubic pain, and from laboratory criteria 2, one of the given criteria. 3. For children under 1, at least one of the following signs or symptoms, without any other cause; fever >38°C or rectal hypothermia <37°C, apnea, bradycardia, dysuria, lethargy or vomit, and the same 1 and 2 laboratory criteria respectively.	1. Urine culture with less than two microorganisms and colony count of $\geq 10^5$ 2. Positive leukocyte esterase; pyuria >10 leukocytes per hogh magnification field; >3 erythrocytes per hight magnification field; positive urine Gram in a non-cytospinned sample; two urine cultures with the same microorganism and a colony count of $\geq 10^2$ in a patient with previous effective antibiotherapy and a count of $\leq 10^5$; medical diagnosis or proper medical treatment for UTI.
Asymptomatic bacteriuria At least one of the following:	1. Patient with previous case of catheterization within the last 7 days and who has not fever, urinary urgency, dysuria or suprapubic pain, and laboratory criteria 1. 2. Patient who has not had UC in the previous 7 days to the first urine cultura, and that has not presented fever, urinary urgency, frequency, dysuria or suprapubic pain, and laboratory criteria 3.	3. Two positive urine cultures of $\geq 10^5$ with less than 2 microorganisms and showing the same microorganisms.

Urinary tract infection	Clinical criteria	Laboratory criteria
Other UTIs (kidney, urether, bladder, urethra, or retroperitoneum) At least one of the following:	1. Abscess or evidence of infection at direct, intraoperative or histological examination. 2. At least two of the following signs or symptoms, without any other cause; fever >38ºC, focused pain or pain in the implicated place, and at least one of the following; purulent drainage, or any of the laboratory criteria 2-5. 3. For children under 1, at least one of the following signs or symptoms, without any other cause; fever >38ºC or rectal hypothermia <37ºC, apnea, bradycardia, dysuria, lethargy or vomit, and at least one of the following; purulent drainage, or any of the laboratory criteria 5-8.	4. Positive culture from any fluid different from urine. 5. Positive blood culture from suspected infection site. 6. Compatible image with infection (CT scan, NMR, Scintigraphy) 7. Medical diagnosis of infection 8. Adequate medical treatment for infection.
Comments: The culture taken from the tip of a UC is not laboratory criteria for NUTI diagnosis. Urine samples should be obtained using the proper technique, i.e. clean technique or catheterization. With children, samples must be taken from catheterization or suprapubic puncture; urine collected from perineal bag is not accepted. Circumcision-associated infections should be informed as such.		

Source: Bibliographic reference 26.

Table 3. NUTI diagnosis criteria.

8. Prevention guidelines

Even though not all CAUTIs can be prevented, a great number can be avoided by proper catheter use. The following care recommendations should be implemented for short-term catheterization patients:

Prevention is directed to three sources:

1. Catheter colonization precautions.
2. Once UC is inserted, bacteriuria prevention.
3. Had bacteriuria developed, its complications should be avoided.

8.1 Urinary catheter colonization precautions

The most successful approach to prevent catheter-associated bacteriuria is to implement catheter colonization safety measures.

1. Use UC only when necessary.
2. Use external devices: external urinary collectors such as condom catheters for men with urinary incontinence is a good alternative, these condoms have devices to connect them to a closed drainage system. Even though this system decreases UC use, the urine that remains in the condom can induce high bacteria concentration growth in penis skin and favor bacteriuria. Further complications can include penis skin maceration, penis ulcers and even penis gangrene when condom makes inadequate pressure in penis' body.
3. Intermittent catheterization: it is used in patients with sequelae of spinal shock or with spinal cord injury. UC insertion for urine voiding and its immediate removal every 4 to 6 hours only increases bacteriuria in 1 to 3% per catheterization. For intermittent catheterization, clean are sterile techniques have been compared. In clean technique, catheter can be used again if sterilized at high temperatures before each use, and in sterile technique, catheter is new and sterile. There were no differences regarding UTI development in any of the two techniques, however, clean technique reduced costs. The most common complications are: bleeding, urethritis, fistula, stones, and hydronephrosis.
4. Suprapubic catheter (cystostomy): many factors explain the frequency in its use.
   - Abdomen skin has lower bacteria concentration than periurethral area.
   - External obstruction of suprapubic catheters favor urine voiding through the urethra.
   - Urethral structures are not injured.

   Besides hematoma in catheter insertion site (abdominal wall), its infection and fistula, there are no other important complications.
5. Gold-coated urethral catheter, polyurethane catheter or antimicrobial catheters have been used for long presurgical periods in patients with prostatic hyperplasia diagnosis and they have shown interesting results regarding less UTIs, but it cannot be proposed as universal recommendation since cost-effectiveness and superinfection evaluation has not been fully assessed. (19-22)
6. Surgical recommendations: Especially in patients with cancer or intractable incontinence, bladder reconstruction procedures using colon or ileum segments, like in an ileal conduit diversion, bacteriuria is common, producing complications such as: acute and chronic pyelonephritis and renal failure secondary to vesicoureteral reflux.

8.2 Bacteriuria prevention (23-25)

Once UC is inserted, two strategies are recommended to prevent bacteriuria.

- Use closed drainage systems: closed drainage systems in permanent catheterized patients must always remain closed. Junctures between catheters and collecting bag drainage tube must never be opened. Urine samples must be taken through syringe puncture and all aseptic measures should be observed during sample collection.
- Remove catheter as soon as possible. Short-term catheterization has less risk of bacteriuria development.

8.3 Bacteriuria complications prevention

Several clinical trials have demonstrated that despite catheterization period, asymptomatic bacteriuria need not antibiotic therapy. Nevertheless, some situations need a particular evaluation.

1. In the case that isolated microorganisms might have high bacteremia incidence, e.g. *Serratia marcescens*
2. Patients with high risk of serious complications: pregnant women, and neutropenic and transplanted patients
3. Patients pending for urologic surgery
4. Patients with prosthesis.

In these situations, antibiotic therapy is recommended for asymptomatic bacteriuria since complication risks are greatly avoided by this means.

Antibiotherapy after catheter removal has not proven to be successful either as to prevent UTI development or to favor microbiological cure. Likewise, it has been observed that catheterized patients with untreated asymptomatic bacteriuria clear it by just catheter removal. From prevention guidelines for CAUTIs, the following summary presents the main recommendations (16).

8.4 Main recommendations for catheter-associated urinary tract infection prevention – Summary—

Category I. Strongly recommended to adopt

- Personnel should be given training emphasizing on correct insertion techniques and catheter care measures.
- Urinary catheters should be used only when necessary and left in place only for as long as necessary.
- Promote handwashing and disinfection.
- Insertion should be done by persons who know the correct aseptic technique using only sterile equipment.
- Catheters should be appropriately assured to avoid urethral traction.
- Closed drainage system should always remain sterile.
- Use aseptic techniques for urine sample collection.
- Urine flow drainage should be kept free.

Category II. Moderately recommended to adopt

- Periodic training should be provided to people in charge of catheters.
- Small catheters should be chosen over catheters with larger diameters.
- Avoid irrigation unless needed to prevent or control obstruction.
- Daily meatal care with povidone-iodine should be avoided.
- Catheters should not be changed at fixed intervals

Category III. Weakly moderated to adopt

- Alternative draining techniques should be considered before resorting to catheterization.
- Substitute collecting system when sterile closed drainage has been violated.
- Separate infected and uninfected catheterized patients.
- Routine bacteriologic surveillance should be avoided.

9. Summary

Urinary infection is the main nosocomial infection and is it associated to urinary catheter use. Urinary catheters favor bacteriuria development, which is more frequent when catheterization period exceeds 30 days. The most effective solution to decrease bacteriuria appearance is to use catheters only when strictly necessary. By reducing catheterization time and implementing closed drainage systems, bacteriuria risk can be highly controlled when catheterization is needed. Bacteriuria can be asymptomatic, thus not needing antibiotherapy. Should bacteriuria complications arise with urinary tract infection symptoms, antibiotherapy will highly depend on cystitis and pyelonephritis diagnosis, in either event, length of treatment will range between 10 and 21 days. Other strategies aimed to bacteriuria prevention have been implemented and they are mainly intended to provide education and training to all medical personnel, paramedics and family or people in charge of catheterized patient's care.

10. Annex – prevention guidelines for catheter-associated urinary tract infection- CAUTI (16)

- Recommendations

1. PERSONNEL
    - Only persons (hospital team, family or patients) who know the correct insertion technique and catheter aseptic maintenance should handle catheters. Category I
    - Periodic training should be provided to hospital personnel taking care of catheters focusing on correct techniques and possible complications during catheterization. Category II
2. CATHETER USE
    - Urinary catheters should only be used when strictly necessary and removed as soon as possible. They should not be used for patient-care personnel convinience. Category I.
    - For selected patients, alternative urinary draining methods can be used, e.g. condom catheter, suprapubic catheter and intermittent catheterization. Category III.
3. HANDWASHING
    - Handwashing is imperative just before and after catheter manipulation. Category I
4. CATHETER INSERTION
    - Catheters must be inserted using proper aseptic technique and sterile equipment Category I.
    - Gloves, gauze, periurethral cleansing antiseptic solution, and single-use packet of lubricant should be used for insertion purposes. Category II.
    - Use as small a catheter as possible with good drainage consistency to avoid urethral trauma. Category II.
    - Urethral catheters should be properly secured after insertion to prevent movement and urethral traction. Category I.
5. CLOSED STERILE DRAINAGE
    - A closed sterile drainage system should always be mantained. Category I.
    - Catheter and drainage tube should never be disconnected. Category I

- If aseptic technique breaks, catheter disconnects from collecting bag or draining tube breaks, collecting system should be replaced using aseptic technique after disinfecting catheter and tube juncture. Category III.

6. IRRIGATION
   - Irrigation should be avoided unless obstruction anticipates. Category II
   - Catheter-tube juncture should be disinfected before disconnection. Category II
   - Irrigation solution and siringe must be disposable. Category I
7. SAMPLE COLLECTION
   - Use sterile syringe Category I
   - Large urine volumes for special analysis can be obtained aseptically from drainage bag. Category I
8. URINARY FLOW
   - Urine flow should be kept free. Category I
   - For unobstructed flow drainage Category I
   a. Disconnection between catheter and draining tube should be avoided.
   b. Draining bag should be cleared regularly using a separate collecting container for each patient.
   c. Poorly functioning or obstructed catheters need to be irrigated or replaced if necessary.
   d. Draining bag must be kept below patient's bladder.
9. MEATAL CARE WITH SOAP AND WATER OR WITH POVIDONE-IODINE
   - Daily cleansing with antiseptic solutions or soap and water do not reduce NUTI probability. Category II
10. CATHETER CHANGE INTERVAL
    - Catheters should not be changed at fixed intervals. Category II
11. SPATIAL SEPARATION OF CATHETERIZED PATIENTS
    - To diminish cross infection among uninfected and infected patients, they should be separarated Category III
12. BACTERIOLOGIC SURVEILLANCE
    - Routine bacteriologic surveillance is not recommended for catheterized patients. Category III

11. References

[1] Siegel JD, Rhinehart E, Jackson M, Chiallero L, and the Healthcare Infection Control Practices Advisory Committee, 2007. Guideline for isolation precautions: Preventing tranmission of infection agents in healthcare settings, June 2007 Consulta 24 de agosto de 2007. Available at: http://www.cdc.gov/incidod/dhqp/pdf/isolation 2007.pdf

[2] Platt R, Polk BF, Murdock B, Rosner B: Risk factors for nosocomial urinary tract infection. Am J Epidemiol 1986;124:977-85

[3] Warren JH. Catheter Associated Urinary Tract Infections. Inf Dis Clín N Am. 1997; 11(3): 609 - 622

[4] Kunin CM, McCormack RC. Prevention of catheter induced urinary tract infections by sterile closed drainage. N Engl J Med 1966;274:1155-62

[5] Richards MJ, Edwards JR, Culver DH, Gaynes RP. Nosocomial infections in medical intensive care units in the United States. National Nosocomial Infections Surveillance System. Crit Care Med. 1999;27: 887-92

[6] Rosenthal VD, Maki DG, Mehta A, Alvarez-Moreno C, Leblebicioglu H, Higuera F, et al. International Nosocomial Infection Control Consortium report, data summary for 2002-2007, issued January 2008. Am J Infect Control. 2008;36: 627-37

[7] Johnson JR, Kuskowski MA, Wilt TJ. Systematic review: antimicrobial urinary catheters to prevent catheter associated urinary tract infection in hospitalized patients. Ann Intern Med 2006 Jan 17;144(2):116-26

[8] Gariballdi RA, Burke JP, Dickman ML,SmithCB. Factors predisposing to bacteriuria during indwelling urethral catheterization. N Engl J Med 1974; 291:215-8

[9] Foley FEB. A hemostatic bag catheter. A one piece latex rubber structure for control of bleeding and constant drainage following prostatic resection. J Urol 1936;35:134-139

[10] Clec´h Ch, Schwebel C, Français A. Does catheter associated urinary tract infection increase mortality in critical ill patients? Infec Cont Hosp Epidemiol 2007; 28: 1367-73

[11] Slade N, Gillespie WA. The urinary tract and the catheter. Infection and other problems. New York: Weiley, 1985:63

[12] Tambyah PA, Halvorson Kt, Maki DG. A prospective study of pathogenesis of catheter associated urinary tract infections. Mayo clín Proc 1999; 74: 131 – 136

[13] Desautels RF, Walter CW, Graves RC, Harrison JH. Technical advances in the prevention of urinary tract infection. J Urol 1962;87:487-90

[14] Mooney BS, Garibaldi RA, Britt MR. Natural history ogf catheter-associated bacteriuria(colonization, infection, bacteremia): implication for protection. In: Proceedings of the 11th International Congress of Chemotherapy and the 19th Interscience Conference on Antimicrobial Agents and Chemotherapy. Boston. October 8-12, 1979. Washington DC, American Society of Microbiology 1980:1083-85

[15] Platt R, Polk BF, Murdock B, Rosner B: Risk factors for nosocomial urinary tract infection. Am J Epidemiol 1986;124:977-85

[16] Wong ES, Hooton Th. Guidelines for prevention of catheter associated urinary tract infections. Consulta 24 de agosto de 2002. Disponibe en: www.cdc.org

[17] Nicolle LE, Bradley S, Colgan R, Rice JC, Schaeffer A, Hooton Th. Infectious Disease Society of America Guidelines for the diagnosis and treatment of asymptomatic bacteriuria in adults CID 2005;40(5): 643-654

[18] Pappas P, Rex JH, Sobel JD, Filler SG, Dismukes WE, Walsh ThJ, Edwards JE. Guidelines for treatment of Candidiasis. CID 2004; 38(2): 161-89

[19] Trautner BW, Hull RA, Darouiche RO. Prevention of catheter associated urinary tract infection. Curr Opin Infect Dis 2005 Feb; 18(1):37-41

[20] Jahn P, Preuss M, Kernig A, Seifer-Hahmer A, Langer G. Types of indwelling urinary catheters for long term bladder drainage in adults. Cochrane Database Syst Rev 2007July 18; (3):CD 004997

[21] Crouzet J, Bertrand X, Venier AG, Badoz M, Husson C, Talon D. Control of the duration of urinary catheterization: impact on catheter associated urinary tract infection. J Hosp Infect 2007 Nov; 67(3):253-7

[22] Madigan E, Neff DF. Care of patients with long term indwelling urinary catheters. Online J Issues Nurs 2003;8(3):7

[23] Kass EH. Asymptomatic infections of the urinary tract. Trans Assoc Am Physicians 1956;69:56-63

[24] Saint S, Lipsky BA. Preventing Catheter related bacteriuria. ¿Should We? ¿Can We? ¿How? Arch Intern Med, 1999; 159: 800 – 806

[25] Donlan R, Costerton J. Biofilms: Survival mechanisms of clinically relevant microorganisms. Clin Microbiol Rev. 2002; 15 (2): 167-193

[26] Horan T, Andrus M, RN, BA, CIC, Dudeck Margaret. CDC/NHSN surveillance definition of health care associated infection and criteria for specific types of infections in the acute care setting. Am J Infec Cont 2008;36(5): 310-313

16

The Prevention and Treatment of Penile Prosthesis Infections

Bela Koves, Peter Tenke and Karoly Nagy
Department of Urology, South-Pest Hospital, Budapest, Hungary

1. Introduction

Since they introduction in the treatment of erectile dysfunction (ED), phosphodiesterase type 5 (PDE-5) inhibitors have achieved widespread acceptance. Today PDE-5 inhibitors are considered as first-line oral pharmacotherapy in the management of ED (Hatzimouratidis et al., 2010). However, penile implants are still a popular choice, especially in patients who have failed to achieve erections by chemical enhancement, who prefer a permanent solution to their condition or in those who have considerable scar tissue in the penis resulting in erection deformalities (Mulcahy 1999). Despite its invasiveness, penile prostheses provide high satisfaction rates (Montague & Angermeier 2001).

The types of prosthesis most commonly implanted are the two-piece and the three-piece inflatable device, and the soft and malleable prosthesis. In the last few years the three-piece inflatable device has been used for preference, as it improves the erection with the most acceptable functional and cosmetical results (Minervini et al., 2006; Bettocchi et al., 2008).

Engineering changes and designs revisions have reduced the mechanical malfunctions associated with inflatable penis prostheses to less than 5 % (Carson et al., 2000; Carson 2004). As penile prostheses are now expected to function for an average of 8-12 years post implantation, infection has become a more significant problem. The incidence of infection has been reported to range from 0.5 to 17.7% (Quesada & Light, 1993; Wilson & Delk, 1995) usually about 1-3 % in case of primary implantation, and about 10-13 % in case of revision or reimplantation (Abouassaly et al., 2004).

The traditional treatment of penile prosthesis infection is systematic and local antibiotics application with the complete removal of the device followed by reinsertion within 2–12 months. However, removal of the device can lead to corporeal fibrosis, making dilation of the corporeal bodies difficult and reinsertion of a new device more complicated (Brant et al., 1996; Mulcahy, 1999).

To reduce the risk of device associated infections and to avoid the difficulties associated with late reinsertions many modifications have been developed such as antibiotic or hydrophilic coated devices and immediate replacement of the infected prosthesis (salvage techniques).

The aim of this chapter is to summarize the different methods of prevention and treatment of penile prosthesis infections.

2. Pathogenesis/epidemiology

Staphylococcus species, especially *Staphylococcus epidermidis* are the most common infecting pathogens, isolated from 35 to 56% of infected penile prostheses patients (Carson , 2003). Gram-negative enteric bacteria including *Proteus mirabilis, Pseudomonas aeruginosa, Escherichia coli* and *Serratia marcenses* may also be pathogens, accounting for 20 % of infections (Abouassaly et al., 2004). Gram-negative bacteria can combine with anaerobic organisms in severe infections, such as *Bacteroides species*, and lead to gangrene of the penis. Fungi, mycobacteria and *Neisseria gonorrhea* have also been reported as etiological agents in penile prosthesis infections (Carson, 1989; Abouassaly et al., 2004).

Penile prostheses get infected predominantly secondary to bacterial seeding at the time of surgery. Prosthetic materials attract bacteria and support subsequent biofilm formation. In a multicenter study culture positive bacteria were found in 70% of patients with clinically uninfected penile prostheses during revision surgery for mechanical malfunction. *Saphylococcus species* were cultured in 90 % of the cases (Henry et al., 2004), which have an enhanced ability to produce glycocalyx biofilm.

Penile prosthesis infections can be divided into clinically apparent and subclinical infections. Clinical infections present with, penile pain, induration, erythema, fever, purulent drainage from the wound and extrusion. Subclinical infections most often manifest by chronic prosthesis-associated pain.

3. Risk factors

Known risk factors for penile prosthesis infection include urinary tract infection, infections elsewhere in the body and hematogenous spread (Carson & Robertson, 1988; Little & Rhodus, 1992). There is an increased incidence of infection among patients undergoing primary implantation with penile reconstruction or secondary prosthesis revision compared to primary implantation alone, probably due to the increased duration of surgery (Quesada & Light, 1993; Jarow, 1996). The role of diabetes mellitus and spinal chord injury, as risk factors of penile prosthesis infection are contradictory (Jarow, 1996; Cakan et al., 2003).

4. Prevention

4.1 General aspects

Because in most cases bacterial contamination occurs at the time of surgery, it is essential to use appropriate preoperative preparations. Short preoperative hospital stays have been documented to maintain low virulence (Carson, 2003). It is important to eliminate skin infections and to have sterile urine prior to surgery. Washing the genital region with strong soap in the days before the procedure, preoperative shaving and an aggressive scrub of the operating area is recommended to decrease the risk of infection (Mulcahy, 1999; Gomelsky & Dmochowski, 2003).

During surgery adequate sterile technique, short operating time, minimal tissue devitalization along with effective wound closure can all decrease the rate of perioperative infections (Scott, 1987).

4.2 Perioperative antibiotic prophylaxis

Athough the effectiveness of prophylactic perioperative antibiotics for implantation of penile prosthesis has never been proven by prospective studies, their use has become established and favored by most urologists. Antibiotics should be administered 1-2 hours prior to surgery and continued for 36-48 hours postoperative. Most common pathogenic organisms most likely to produce infections must be targeted when choosing prophylactic antibiotics. Therefore traditional prophylaxis include a parenteral aminoglycoside for Gram-negative and a first- or second generation cephalosporin or vancomycin for Gram-positive organisms coverage (Schwartz et al., 1996; Naber et al., 2001). Schwarz et al found in a randomized prospective trial of 20 patients that oral fluoroquinolone (ofloxacin) administered 2 hours before surgery achieved significantly higher intracavernosal levels and was more cost-effective than the combination of gentamicin and cefazolin (Schwartz et al., 1996). To estimate the safety and efficacy of this prophylaxis modality, further studies with similar settings, but bigger sample size should be performed.

4.3 Antibiotic impregnation

Early efforts in device impregnation focused on coating catheters with antibiotics. In 1995 Raad et al reported that in *in vitro* studies catheters coated with a combination of rifampin and minocycline provided significantly better inhibitory activities against *S. epidermidis, S. aureus* and *E. faecalis* than catheters coated with either drug alone or vancomycin (Raad et al., 1995). After additional *in vitro* and *in vivo* studies in 2001 the US Food and Drug Administration approved the use of penile prosthesis coated with a combination of rifampin and minocycline called InhibiZone. The concentrations of the antibiotics, while adequate for decreasing colonization, provided only minimal serum levels of the agents. Coated inflatable penile prostheses are implanted in a fashion similar to those without antibiotic treatment except that the devices are not soaked prior to implantation (Carson, 2004).

In a retrospective study Carson et al reported 61,7% decrease in perioperative infection with InhibiZone compared to controls at 1 year post infection (Carson, 2004). The same group recently published their long-term clinical outcomes of almost 40,000 implants. There were significantly less revisions due to infections in the impregnated compared to the non-impregnated group at up to 7.7 years of follow-up (1.1% vs 2.5%, respectively)(Carson et al., 2011). In a subset of diabetic patients in the same series, the rate of infection-related revisions was significantly lower in the impregnated group compared to the controls at 7 years (1,62 % vs 4,24 %)(Mulcahy & Carson, 2011).

In 2007 Wilson et al. began a prospective randomized study comparing the infection rate of rifampin and minocycline coated implants with implants without impregnation (Wilson et al., 2007). After it became evident that the infection rate was less with the impregnated group they abandoned the other arm because of ethical considerations and compared they results with the previously published series of the same surgical team with noncoated implants (Wilson & Delk, 1995; Wilson et al. 1998). The use of antibiotic coated inflatable penile prosthesis resulted in a statistically significant reduction in the infection rates compared with the historical data in nondiabetic virgin implant patients (*p=0,0024*), diabetic virgin implant patients (*p=0,0141*) and in revision patients in whom washout with antiseptic solutions was used (*p= 0,0095*). Revision without washout had the same infection rate (10%) as with noncoated implants.

4.4 Hydrophilic coating

In 2002 a hydrophilic penile prosthesis coating was developed which has been shown to decrease bacterial adherence *in vitro* and in animal models (Rajpurkar et al., 2004). This coating absorbs surgeon chosen intraoperative antibiotics that can elute into surrounding tissues over 24-72 h to further decrease infection (Hellstrom et al., 2003).

Mansouri and colleagues compared the spectrum and durability, both in vitro and in vivo of the hydrophilic coated prosthesis dipped in vancomycin and the InhibiZone implants, and found that the antibiotic pre-impregnated prosthesis had a broader spectrum in vitro and a more durable antimicrobial activity in vitro and in an animal model than implants dipped in vancomycin (Mansouri et al. 2009).

Clinical data on the hydrophilic coated inflatable penile prosthesis is limited. Wolter et *al.* presented their one-year experience with the device (Titan, Mentor Corporation, Santa Barbara, CA) (Wolter & Hellstrom 2004), the infection rate for 2357 coated penile prostheses was 1,06 % compared to 2,07 % in 482 uncoated penile prostheses implanted over the same time period. Although preliminary data using this device shows promise, long-term follow-up and prospective studies are not yet available.

5. Treatment

Subclinical infections may be more common than clinically apparent infections. These infections are difficult to diagnose and even more challenging to treat. Parsons *et al.* recommend initial trial of oral antibiotic therapy using long-term antibiotics (ciprofloxacin 500mg twice daily) (Parsons et al., 1993). Following initiation of antibiotics, pain suppression should suggest continuing antibiotics for 10–12 weeks. The authors reported a 60% success rate with conservative treatment of subclinical penile prosthesis infections. The use of oral cephalosporins (cefalexin and cephradine) has also been suggested for 10-12 weeks, although success rates are lower at 25-30% (Choong & Whitfield, 2000; Carson, 2003). If pain fails to resolve or rapidly returns after antibiotics, however, surgical intervention is appropriate. Parsons *et al.* have reported 90% success rate in treating these prostheses with an exchange protocol including systemic antibiotics for 24–48 h using vancomycin. The suspected infected prosthesis is then removed and a combination of vancomycin and protamine was used for antibiotic irrigation prior to reimplantation of a new prosthesis. Patients are maintained on vancomycin and parental antibiotics for 1 week (Parsons et al., 1993; Carson, 2003).

In case of clinically apparent infection surgical intervention along with antibiotics is of critical importance. The traditional treatment consists of the immediate removal of all the components followed by delayed reimplantation 2-12 months later (Gomelsky & Dmochowski, 2003; Mulcahy, 2003). The advantage of this solution is that the new implant is scheduled only when the infection has completely cleared. However, removal of the device along with inflammation from the infectious process leads to corporeal fibrosis and scarring, which almost always results in penile shortening and may make dilation of the corporeal bodies very difficult, resulting reinsertion of a new device more complicated and sometimes impossible (Brant et al., 1996; Mulcahy, 1999).

A salvage protocol was instituted in 1991 to avoid difficult reinsertion and maintain as much penile length as possible. The salvage procedure involves removing all parts of the infected prosthesis, washing the wound, and replacing the device at the same procedure. Mulcahy *et al.* recommend a sequence of irrigating solutions including kanamycin and bacitracin in normal saline followed by half-strength hydrogen peroxide, half-strength povidone-iodine solution, pressurized normal saline containing vancomycin and gentamicin, half-strength povidone-iodine, half-strength hydrogen peroxide, and finally another kanamycin/bacitracin solution (Mulcahy et al., 1995). Gloves, instruments, gowns, and drapes are changed and a new inflatable penile prosthesis is immediately implanted. Postoperatively, patients are treated with antibiotics (2x500 mg ciprofloxacin) for 4-6 weeks. Antibiotics can be modified based on culture and sensitivity results. The reported success rate of the salvage procedure is 84-91% (Brant et al., 1996; Mulcahy, 2003). To avoid complications of late reinsertion the salvage protocol is a treatment alternative of traditional delayed reimplantation, although in patients with life-threatening systemic conditions such as septicemia, or diabetic ketoacidosis, or in whom necrotizing infections with death of penile skin is occurring salvage procedure is not recommended (Brant et al., 1996; Mulcahy, 1999).

The delayed salvage procedure consists of placement of a drainage tube after removal of the prosthesis; antibiotic solution is irrigated through the drain and a new prosthesis is placed about 3 days later. However, Knoll et al could not find a statistically significant difference between immediate and delayed salvage procedure (Knoll, 1998), while there are the additional cost of the second surgical procedure.

6. Further research

Prospective studies and long-term follow up are needed to make stronger recommendations about the different methods in the prevention or treatment of penile prostheses infections, especially about the hydrophilic coated penile prosthesis.

7. Conclusion

The efforts to apply more effective methods of prevention and the new developments of prosthesis coatings resulted a significant reduction of the infectious complications of penile prosthesis implantation. Further improvements of surgical procedures and prosthesis materials and coatings can lead to further decrease of the infection rates in the future.

8. References

Abouassaly, R., D. K. Montague, et al. (2004). "Antibiotic-coated medical devices: with an emphasis on inflatable penile prosthesis." Asian J Androl 6(3): 249-57.

Bettocchi, C., P. Ditonno, et al. (2008). "Penile Prosthesis: What Should We Do about Complications?" Adv Urol: 573560.

Brant, M. D., J. K. Ludlow, et al. (1996). "The prosthesis salvage operation: immediate replacement of the infected penile prosthesis." J Urol 155(1): 155-7.

Cakan, M., F. Demirel, et al. (2003). "Risk factors for penile prosthetic infection." Int Urol Nephrol 35(2): 209-13.

Carson, C. (2004). "Antibiotic impregnation of inflatable penile prostheses: effect on perioperative infection." Expert Rev Med Devices 1(2): 165-7.

Carson, C. C. (1989). "Infections in genitourinary prostheses." Urol Clin North Am 16(1): 139-47.

Carson, C. C. (2003). "Diagnosis, treatment and prevention of penile prosthesis infection." Int J Impot Res 15 Suppl 5: S139-46.

Carson, C. C., 3rd (2004). "Efficacy of antibiotic impregnation of inflatable penile prostheses in decreasing infection in original implants." J Urol 171(4): 1611-4.

Carson, C. C., 3rd, J. J. Mulcahy, et al. (2011). "Long-term infection outcomes after original antibiotic impregnated inflatable penile prosthesis implants: up to 7.7 years of followup." J Urol 185(2): 614-8.

Carson, C. C., J. J. Mulcahy, et al. (2000). "Efficacy, safety and patient satisfaction outcomes of the AMS 700CX inflatable penile prosthesis: results of a long-term multicenter study. AMS 700CX Study Group." J Urol 164(2): 376-80.

Carson, C. C. and C. N. Robertson (1988). "Late hematogenous infection of penile prostheses." J Urol 139(1): 50-2.

Choong, S. and H. Whitfield (2000). "Biofilms and their role in infections in urology." BJU Int. 86((8)): 935-41.

Gomelsky, A. and R. R. Dmochowski (2003). "Antibiotic prophylaxis in urologic prosthetic surgery." Curr Pharm Des 9(12): 989-96.

Hatzimouratidis, K., E. Amar, et al. "Guidelines on male sexual dysfunction: erectile dysfunction and premature ejaculation." Eur Urol 57(5): 804-14.

Hellstrom, W. J., J. S. Hyun, et al. (2003). "Antimicrobial activity of antibiotic-soaked, Resist-coated Bioflex." Int J Impot Res 15(1): 18-21.

Henry, G. D., S. K. Wilson, et al. (2004). "Penile prosthesis cultures during revision surgery: a multicenter study." J Urol 172(1): 153-6.

Jarow, J. P. (1996). "Risk factors for penile prosthetic infection." J Urol 156(2 Pt 1): 402-4.

Knoll, L. D. (1998). "Penile prosthetic infection: management by delayed and immediate salvage techniques." Urology 52(2): 287-90.

Little, J. W. and N. L. Rhodus (1992). "The need for antibiotic prophylaxis of patients with penile implants during invasive dental procedures: a national survey of urologists." J Urol 148(6): 1801-4.

Mansouri, M. D., T. B. Boone, et al. (2009). "Comparative assessment of antimicrobial activities of antibiotic-treated penile prostheses." Eur Urol 56(6): 1039-45.

Minervini, A., D. J. Ralph, et al. (2006). "Outcome of penile prosthesis implantation for treating erectile dysfunction: experience with 504 procedures." BJU Int 97(1): 129-33.

Montague, D. K. and K. W. Angermeier (2001). "Penile prosthesis implantation." Urol Clin North Am 28(2): 355-61, x.

Mulcahy, J. J. (1999). "Management of the infected penile implant--concepts on salvage techniques." Int J Impot Res 11 Suppl 1: S58-9.

Mulcahy, J. J. (2003). "Treatment alternatives for the infected penile implant." Int J Impot Res 15 Suppl 5: S147-9.

Mulcahy, J. J., M. D. Brant, et al. (1995). "Management of infected penile implants." Tech Urol 1(3): 115-9.

Mulcahy, J. J. and C. C. Carson, 3rd (2011). "Long-Term Infection Rates in Diabetic Patients Implanted With Antibiotic-Impregnated Versus Nonimpregnated Inflatable Penile Prostheses: 7-Year Outcomes." Eur Urol.

Naber, K. G., A. G. Hofstetter, et al. (2001). "Guidelines for the perioperative prophylaxis in urological interventions of the urinary and male genital tract." Int J Antimicrob Agents 17(4): 321-6.

Parsons, C. L., P. C. Stein, et al. (1993). "Diagnosis and therapy of subclinically infected prostheses." Surg Gynecol Obstet 177(5): 504-6.

Quesada, E. T. and J. K. Light (1993). "The AMS 700 inflatable penile prosthesis: long-term experience with the controlled expansion cylinders." J Urol 149(1): 46-8.

Raad, I., R. Darouiche, et al. (1995). "Antibiotics and prevention of microbial colonization of catheters." Antimicrob Agents Chemother 39(11): 2397-400.

Rajpurkar, A., M. Fairfax, et al. (2004). "Antibiotic soaked hydrophilic coated bioflex: a new strategy in the prevention of penile prosthesis infection." J Sex Med 1(2): 215-20.

Schwartz, B. F., S. Swanzy, et al. (1996). "A randomized prospective comparison of antibiotic tissue levels in the corpora cavernosa of patients undergoing penile prosthesis implantation using gentamicin plus cefazolin versus an oral fluoroquinolone for prophylaxis." J Urol 156(3): 991-4.

Scott, F. B. (1987). "Prosthetic infections." J Urol 138(1): 113.

Wilson, S. K., C. C. Carson, et al. (1998). "Quantifying risk of penile prosthesis infection with elevated glycosylated hemoglobin." J Urol 159(5): 1537-9; discussion 1539-40.

Wilson, S. K. and J. R. Delk, 2nd (1995). "Inflatable penile implant infection: predisposing factors and treatment suggestions." J Urol 153(3 Pt 1): 659-61.

Wilson, S. K., J. Zumbe, et al. (2007). "Infection reduction using antibiotic-coated inflatable penile prosthesis." Urology 70(2): 337-40.

Wolter, C. E. and W. J. Hellstrom (2004). "The hydrophilic-coated inflatable penile prosthesis: 1-year experience." J Sex Med 1(2): 221-4.

Part 6

Treatment of Urinary Tract Infection

17

The Role of Calgranulins in Urinary Tract Infection

Leticia Reyes, Ayman B. Allam,
Benjamin K. Canales and Mary B. Brown
*University of Florida, Gainesville, Florida,
United States of America*

1. Introduction

Calgranulins A (S100A8), B (S100A9) and C (S100A12) are members of the superfamily of EF-hand calcium binding proteins. The term calprotectin specifically refers to the Calgranulin A and B heterodimer that is formed by a non-covalent interaction. A distinguishing feature of calgranulins is their involvement in innate immunity and inflammation. As secreted proteins, calgranulins can directly inhibit microbial growth in the extracellular milieu, presumably through their ability to chelate zinc. Cells that actively express calgranulins are more resistant to bacterial adherence and invasion. Calgranulins also support optimal functioning of the cells that comprise the innate immune system. For example, granulocytes depend on the intracellular calgranulin A/B complex to adequately participate in cell adhesion, cytokinesis, cytokine secretion, and activation of the respiratory burst. Calgranulin A/B can down-regulate immune responses through inhibition of immunoglobulin production by lymphocytes and induction of myeloid derived suppressor cells. In addition, calgranulin induces apoptosis in cells that stimulate the inflammatory cascade. Calgranulin A expression may also be important in promoting the induction of a regulatory macrophage phenotype that down-regulates inflammation and facilitates a healing response.

Under normal conditions, calgranulins support an optimal immune response, leading to resolution of infection and inflammation. When normal expression and/or secretion of calgranulins are perturbed, inflammation is exacerbated with adverse implications for host tissues. As an example, dysregulation in the expression or secretion of calgranulins can have detrimental effects by promoting chronic active inflammation that leads to collateral tissue damage. Excessive amounts of calgranulin A/B in extracellular compartments of tissues correlates with a variety of inflammatory disorders. Expression and release of calgranulin A/B in the extracellular milieu can be triggered by IL-1α. Extracellular calgranulin A/B can then bind to and activate toll like receptor 4 (TLR 4), which in turn initiates further expression of pro-inflammatory mediators such as IL-1, IL-6, and IL-8. The interaction of these cytokines and chemokines with calgranulin A can create an autocrine / paracine mediated pro-inflammatory feedback loop that does not necessarily resolve infection. In the urinary tract, over expression of calgranulin A is not specific for infection. Over expression of calgranulins has been reported in a variety of inflammatory disorders of the urinary tract, including interstitial cystitis, interstitial nephritis, glomerulonephritis and neoplasia. This suggests that while calgranulin A may be a useful biomarker for chronic active inflammation, in general it may not be important in the defence against bacterial pathogens. Recent studies in rodent models of urinary tract infection (UTI) suggest that calgranulins are not required for innate defence against urogenital pathogens. Moreover, the exaggerated expression of these proteins during infection may be contributing to complicated urinary tract diseases such as struvite urolithiasis.

This review will focus on the role of calgranulin A and B in innate immune responses with particular attention to diseases of the urinary tract. The interaction of calgranulins with various host cell signal transduction pathways important in innate immunity and inflammation of the urinary tract will be reviewed. Further, potential consequences of aberrant signalling that may contribute to perturbations of regulation of calgranulins will also be discussed.

2. Classification and general function of calgranulins

Calgranulins are members of the superfamily of EF-hand calcium binding proteins that are involved in innate immune and pro-inflammatory processes. In the literature, these proteins have been given a variety of names including S100A8, myeloid related protein 8 (MRP), and L1 light chain for calgranulin A. Calgranulin B is also known as MRP-14 and S100A9. Calgranulin C may be referred to as S100A12 and EN-RAGE (Nacken et al., 2003). The name calprotectin specifically refers to the Calgranulin A and B heterodimer that is formed by a non-covalent interaction. Calgranulin C does not appear to form a heterodimer complex with either Calgranulin A or B (Foell et al., 2007).

Calgranulin C appears to be exclusively expressed in granulocytes (Vogl et al., 1999). However, calgranulins A and B are constitutively expressed in a variety of cells including granulocytes, monocytes, dendritic cells, epithelial cells, and keratinocytes (Foell et al., 2007; Frosch et al., 2004; Nacken et al., 2003). In healthy individuals, low concentrations of calprotectin can be detected in plasma, saliva, cerebrospinal fluid, urine and feces (Johne et al., 1997). Typically calgranulin gene expression is tightly regulated. However, during inflammation, expression is induced in cells such as macrophages and fibroblasts that do not normally produce calgranulins (Foell et al., 2007; Frosch et al.., 2004; Hsu et al., 2005; Nacken et al., 2003). Further, cells that constitutively express calgranulins are induced to secrete calprotectin into the extracellular milieu when stimulated (Kido et al., 2003). Therefore, calprotectin is considered a biomarker of inflammatory conditions such as rheumatoid arthritis, Crohn's disease, and chorioamnionitis (Kostakis et al., 2010; Perere et al., 2010).

Calprotectin deficiency has never been reported in humans, suggesting that this protein is essential for life. The need for calgranulin A was confirmed with a null mutation in mice, which resulted in early resorption of mouse embryos (Passey et al., 1999a). Null mutation of the S100A9 gene (calgranulin B) was not lethal in the mouse (Hobb et al., 2003). Interestingly, although the S100A9 -/- mouse expresses S100A8 (calgranulin A) mRNA, the protein is not detected in peripheral tissues.. Consequently, this mouse strain does not produce calprotectin, making it convenient for use in studying the role of calprotectin in various disease processes. Although the calgranulin genes are conserved among higher vertebrates, there are structural and functional differences among the various species (Nacken et al., 2003). For example, in rodents, calgranulin A is chemotactic for granulocytes but this is not the case in humans (Foell et al., 2007). Calgranulin C, which is not present in rodents, is the potent granulocyte chemoattractant in humans (Yang et al., 2001) and is highly expressed in activated tissue macrophages localized within sites of inflammation (Perera et al., 2010). Calgranulin C also serves as a ligand for RAGE (Perera et al., 2010). Although, rodents possess RAGE, there is no evidence that either calgranulin A, B, or calprotectin act as a ligand for this receptor. To date, there are no published studies demonstrating a role for calgranulin C in urinary tract infection. Therefore, this review will focus on calgranulins A and B.

2.1 The contribution of calgranulins to defense against infection

The innate immune system comprises the first attack against invading microorganisms. Both intracellular and extracellular calgranulins play an integral role in modulating leukocyte activation, trafficking, and amplification of immune responses during infection. Intracellular calgranulins regulate cell adhesion, migration, phagocytosis, and bacterial killing through direct interactions with the cell cytoskeleton and plasma membrane components. Calprotectin and calgranulin B facilitate phagocyte transmigration by coordinating microtubule dynamics (Vogl, et al., 2004). Specifically, the calprotectin complex induces polymerization of microtubules that can be disrupted by phosphorylation of calgranulin B by p38 mitogen-activated protein kinase. With disruption of the calprotectin complex the microtubule depolymerizes. A similar mechanism in squamous epithelial cells increases their resistance to intracellular invasion by mucosal pathogens such as *Porphyromonas gingivalis, Listeria monocytogenes,* and *Salmonella enterica* serovar *Typhimurium* (Nisapakultorn et al., 2001a, 2001b; Zaia et al., 2009). In neutrophils, calgranulin B is a selective stimulator of MAC-1 mediated adhesion (Newton & Hogg, et al., 1995). Calgranulin B does not directly bind to MAC-1 but its stimulatory effects on β2 integrin / MAC-1 appear to be mediated through a G protein coupled receptor. Calgranulin A can inhibit MAC-1 affinity activation by dimerizing with calgranulin B. In addition to modulating leukocyte trafficking, calgranulins also enhance microbial killing through enhancing the generation of reactive oxygen species in phagocytes. In neutrophils, calgranulin A and the calprotectin complex activate NADPH oxidase by facilitating enzyme complex assembly at the plasma membrane (Kerkoff, et al., 2005). The calprotectin complex transfers arachidonic acid, an essential cofactor, to the enzyme complex while the calgranulin A subunit contributes to NADPH enzyme assembly by directly binding to the $p67^{phox}$ subunit (Kerkoff, et al., 2005). In macrophages, calgranulins contribute to the generation of nitric oxide mediated killing through induction of nitric oxide synthase gene expression (Pouliot et al., 2008).

Active secretion of calgranulins from neutrophils can be induced through engagement of toll-like receptor/CD14 and nuclear factor κβ (Kido et al., 2003) or through protein kinase C in monocytes (Nacken et al., 2003). Calgranulins can be found in mucosal body fluids that are normally colonized with bacteria, such as the oral cavity. Moreover, calprotectin concentrations increase in mucosal fluids in response to certain infections such as *Helicobacter pylori* (Leach et al., 2008). It has been suggested that the increased expression of calprotectin at these sites confers resistance to bacterial invasion or dissemination into deeper tissues (Hsu et al., 2009). Increased expression of calprotectin in humans with chronic sinusitis directly correlates with resistance to bacterial infection (Hsu et al., 2009). In our rodent model of ureaplasmal induced urinary tract infection, some animals with asymptomatic bladder infection and baseline levels of calprotectin developed ascending renal infections. However, animals with bladder infections accompanied by high amounts of calprotectin did not develop ascending renal infection (Reyes et al., 2008, 2009). Therefore, suggesting that calprotectin may be somewhat protective in the urinary tract.

Calprotectin microbicidal activity towards *Candida albicans, Staphylococcus aureus, Straphylococcus epidermis, Escherichia coli, and Klebisiella species* has been demonstrated *in vito* (Brandtzaeg, et al., 1995). Further, calprotectin has been shown to be effective in inhibiting the growth of *S. aureus* within liver abscesses of mice (Corbin et al., 2008). The mechanism of action by calprotectin appears to be chelation of magnesium, manganese, and zinc, which are required for growth by bacteria (Corbin et al., 2008, Hsu et al., 2009).

Extracellular calgranulins also augment immune defense mechanisms in a cytokine like manner. Calgranulin B enhances neutrophil microbial killing by stimulating degranulation of matrix metalloproteinase through p38 mitogen activated protein kinase (Simard et al., 2010). Calprotectin stimulates production of interleukin-8 in airway epithelial cells (Ahmad et al, 2003). Calprotectin binding to microvascular endothelial cells promotes chemokine secretions, up regulation of cell adhesion molecules, and disruption of the endothelial barrier (Viemman et al., 2005, Eue et al., 2000), facilitating leukocyte migration into sites of infection. Calprotectin may also contribute to bacterial clearance from uroepithelium through its ability to enhance activation of toll-like receptor (TLR) 4 (Ehrchen, et al., 2009). Song et al. identified an additional alternative pathway in uroepithelium in which activation of TLR 4 by uropathogenic type 1 fimbriated *E. coli* or *Klebsiella pneumoniae* results in rapid activation of adenylate cyclase 3. The increased intracellular cAMP causes rapid expression and secretion of interleukin-6 that precedes cytokine production through the classical NF-κβ mediated pathway (Song et al., 2007). This pathway may be critical for early defense against invading microbes. More importantly, cAMP blocks intracellular invasion of bacteria into uroepithelium and promotes expulsion of bacteria through inhibition of Rac-1 mediated mobilization of the cytoskeleton (Song et al., 2007). This is an intriguing concept, but it appears that calprotectin may not be contributing to this unique defense mechanism. Dessing et al., compared the ability of uropathogenic *E. coli* to establish acute ascending infection in wild type and calprotectin deficient mice (S100A9 -/-). In this study animals received an intraurethral inoculation of 10^8 organisms and were examined at 24 and 48 hours post-inoculation. Despite significant increases in calprotectin in both the bladder and kidney tissues of wild type mice, they did not exhibit any difference in microbial load or lesion severity when compared S100A9 -/- mice. Therefore, suggesting that calprotectin is not critical for early clearance of bacteria from the urinary tract.

2.2 Regulation of immunity by calgranulins

Successful defense against infection depends on a well controlled inflammatory response that is able to remove the pathogen without extensive collateral damage of the surrounding host tissues. During an effective immune response the signal transduction pathways trigger production and /or release of pro-inflammatory mediators that potentiate removal of the pathogen, and simultaneously or sequentially activate anti-inflammatory factors and protect surrounding tissues from proteases and reactive oxygen species. Calgranulins participate in several of these processes most of which have been identified in macrophages (Lim et al. 2009; Passey et al., 1999b; Xu et al., 2001). For example, bacterial lipopolysaccaride, IFN-γ, TNF-α, and interleukin-10 all induce calgranulin gene expression in murine macrophages (Xu et al., 2001). Glucocorticoids also amplify calgranulin expression in macrophages that have been primed with lipopolysacarride (Hsu et al., 2005). Methylprednisolone treatment in rheumatoid arthritis patients significantly increases the number of calgranulin A and B expressing macrophages in synovium (Hsu et al., 2005).

Secreted calgranulins also exhibit anti-inflammatory properties in neutrophils. Sroussi et al., have shown that both calgranulin A and B can repel human neutrophils *in vitro*, and that calgranulin A can inhibit the recruitment of neutrophils *in vivo* (Sroussi et al., 2006, 2007). Recently, they have demonstrated that calgranulin A and B also inhibit neutrophil oxidative metabolism (Sroussi et al., 2010). Although the mechanism of action has not been elucidated, adenosine metabolites are known to be involved.

Calgranulins that have undergone post-translational modifications can down-regulate inflammation or provide protection from granulocyte secreted products such as reactive oxygen species. Calgranulin A, in particular, is highly susceptible to oxidation by hydroxyapatite, hydrogen peroxide, and hypochlorite (Lim et al., 2009; Harrison et al, 1999). Calgranulins therefore act as sinks for reactive oxygen species, providing protection of the microenvironment from collateral damage. Both calgranulins A and B can be nitrosylated (addition of nitric oxide molecule) (Lim et al., 2008, 2009). Nitrosylated calgranulin A suppresses mast cell mediated activation, leukocyte adhesion, and extravasation into the microcirculation (Lim et al., 2008).

Calgranulins A and B modulate various aspects of adaptive immunity. Calgranulin A has been reported to inhibit immunoglobulin G production in lymphocytes (Brun et al., 1995). Calgranulin B may down regulate responsiveness to toll-like receptor mediated stimulation in dendritic cells (Averill et al., 2011). During murine myeloid differentiation, increased expression of calgranulin B in embryonic stem cells favors development into myeloid derived suppressor cells over dendritic cells (Lim et al. 2009). Myeloid derived suppressor cells promote immune tolerance during infection and inflammation by suppression of T cell activation and promotion of a T helper type 2 cytokine phenotype involving expression of interleukin-4 and interleukin-13 (Delano et al., 2007; Ezernitchi et al., 2006; Haile et al., 2008). Moreover, calprotectin secreted by myeloid derived suppressor cells prolongs their immunosuppressive effects through an autocrine positive feedback loop (Lim et al., 2009).

2.3 Pro-inflammatory effects of calgranulins

Increases in extracellular calgranulin concentrations are associated with several inflammatory and auto-immune disorders including cystic fibrosis, chronic bronchitis, sepsis, pyelonephritis, oral candidiasis, periodontitis, *Helicobacter pyloris* infections, rheumatoid arthritis, systemic lupus erythematosus, Crohn's disease, Sjogren's syndrome, and atherosclerosis (Foell et al., 2007; Johne et al., 1997; Perera et al., 2010). In the urinary tract calgranulins are found to be a major component of calcium oxalate, calcium phosphate, (Canales et al, 2008, 2010) and struvite uroliths (Bennett et al., 1994), all of which are associated with inflammation (Mushtaq et al., 2007; Reyes et al., 2009). In the case of calcium phosphate and calcium oxalate stones, renal injury with inflammation contributes to urolith formation (Khan, 2005). Struvite stones are sequela to severe inflammatory urinary tract infection caused by urease producing bacteria (Reyes et al., 2009). Due to their close association with inflammation, calgranulins are often used as diagnostic biomarkers for inflammatory disorders (Altwegg et al., 2007; Healy et al., 2006). There is a growing body of evidence that calgranulins play more than a passive role in at least some of these disorders. For example, Croce et al. showed that the inflammatory response to vascular injury is attenuated in calprotectin deficient animals. Further, deletion of calprotectin in atherosclerosis prone ApoE-/- mice reduces their susceptibility to the disease (Croce et al, 2009). Similar effects have been observed in CD40L over-expressing mice that spontaneously develop dermatitis, nephritis, auto-antibodies in serum, and auto-reactive $CD8^+$ T cells (Loser et al., 2010). In these animals, genetic deletion of S100A9 alleviates the progression of the disease.

One mechanism by which calprotectin amplifies inflammation is through direct activation of TLR 4. In the CD40L over-expressing mouse, calgranulin mediated activation of TLR 4 increases expression of interleukin-17, which activates autoreactive CD8+ T cells (Loser et al., 2010). In experimentally induced sepsis, calprotectin enhancement of TLR 4 activation induces exaggerated secretion of TNF-α with endotoxic shock, which is not observed in S100A9 -/- mice. However, septic S100A9 -/- mice treated with recombinant calprotectin exhibit the same degree of endotoxic shock and mortality as their wild type counterparts. It is important to note that calprotectin mediated enhancement of TLR 4 pathway only occurs in systems that have already been immunologically activated. For example, in the case of the sepsis model, the initial activation of TLR 4 occurred by bacterial lipopolysaccaride. These results prompted us to re-evaluate our rat model of inflammation induced struvite urolithiasis secondary to experimental infection with *Ureaplasma parvum* (Reyes et al., 2008, 2009). In this model, expression of calprotectin is only observed in animals with inflammation secondary to urinary tract infection. Therefore, we wondered if activation of TLR 4 may also be a aspect in this disease. An important feature of *Ureaplasma parvum* is that this pathogen does not activate TLR 4, but does activate TLRs 1, 2, and 6 in macrophages (Shimizu et al., 2008). Moreover, ureaplasmas do not induce pro-inflammatory cytokine expression in uroepithelium as shown in Figure 1.

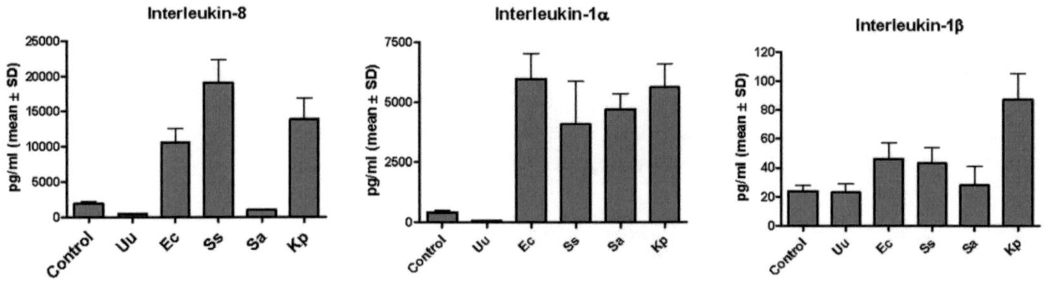

Fig. 1. Chemokine/cytokine profile of RT4 cell culture supernatants.

In an unpublished study of women with first time urinary tract infection, we identified the predominant pathogens present. *Escherichia coli* was isolated from 59.8% of 82 samples that had high numbers (>300,000 CFU/ml clean catch urine), and from 64.8% of 54 urines with medium microbial loads (100,000 to 300,000 CFU/ml clean catch urine). The next most common isolates present in high numbers were *Ureaplasma Spp* (20.7%), *Staphylococcus saprophyticus* (7.3%), and *Proteus mirabilis* (7.3%). *Escherichia fergusonii, Klebsiella pneumoniae,* and *Proteus vulgaris* each accounted for 1.2% of remaining urines with >300,000 CFU/ml. At CFU 100,000 to 300,000/ml urine, *S. saprophyticus* was isolated from 7.4% of urines. *K. pneumoniae, P. mirabilis, Staphylococcus aureus, S. epidermidis, S. haemolyticus, and Streptococcus agalactiae* were isolated from 3.7% of urines, with *Citrobacter koseri, Enterobacter aerogenes,* and *K. oxytoca* each accounting for 2% of urine samples. We determined the cytokine/chemokine profile of RT4 cells. Test pathogens were chosen on the basis of predominance in our study patients. RT4 cells were sham inoculated with sterile carrier (control) or, *U. urealyticum* (Uu), *E. coli* (Ec), *S. saprophyticus* (Ss), *S. agalactiae* (Sa), or *K. pneumoniae* (Kp) at a multiplicity of infection of 100. At 24 hours post-inoculation, cell culture supernatants were harvested and evaluated for the presence of interleukin-8, interleukin-1α, and interleukin-1β. Values in the graph represent the mean ± sd (n = 4) of 2 independent experiments. Chemokine and cytokine concentrations were measured with a multiplex antibody assay as previously described (Reyes, et al. 2006).

Ureaplasmal infections are asymptomatic as long as their colonization is restricted to the urogenital mucosa. However, if these bacteria invade the deeper stromal layers, they induce an exaggerated host immune response that does not eliminate infection, but rather causes tremendous tissue damage at sites of colonization. In our rodent model of infection, invasion of bacteria into the submucosa triggered a smoldering inflammation within the submucosa that persisted. By two weeks post-inoculation, animals with ongoing submucosal infection developed struvite uroliths and an exaggerated pro-inflammatory cytokine profile in their urine. Since *U. parvum* is not capable of eliciting these responses in uroepithelium, we surmised that the initiator of uroepithelial cytokine production (see Figure 2) is a paracine factor originating from the inflamed submucosa. On the other hand, animals in which the microbe is found only on the mucosal layer exhibited asymptomatic infection. In these animals, bladder uroepithelium appears quiescent and urine cytokine concentrations are comparable to uninfected controls as shown in Figure 2. This is similar to what is observed in human RT4 cell study.

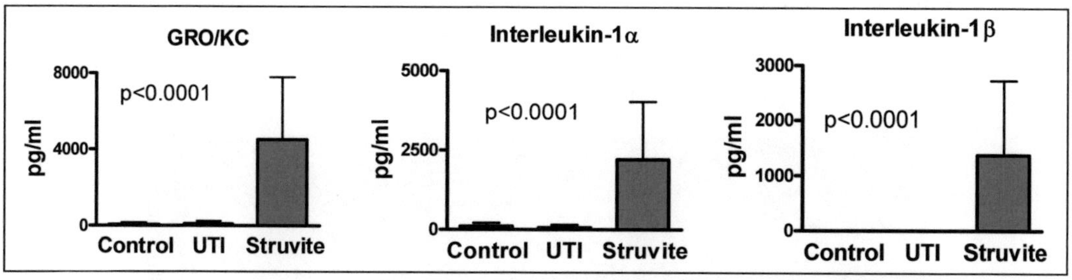

Fig. 2. Chemokine/cytokine profile in urine obtained from uninfected rats (Control), rats with asymptomatic urinary tract infection (UTI), or rats with struvite urolithiasis (Struvite). Values represent the mean ± sd of 5 biological replicates. Data was analyzed by ANOVA followed by Fishers PLSD test.

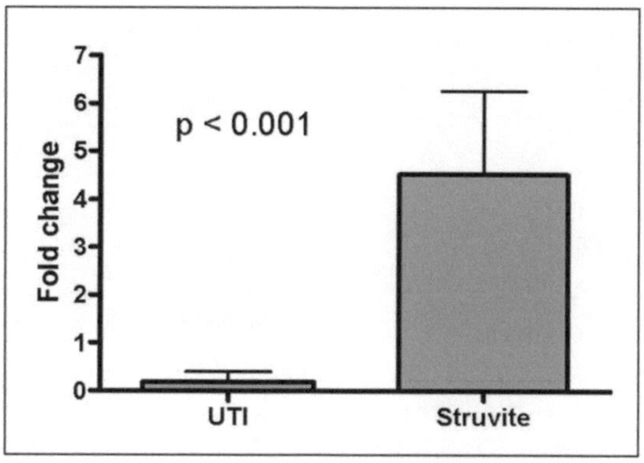

Fig. 3. Induction of calgranulin A in *U. parvum* infected rat bladder tissues. Calgranulin concentrations in rat bladder tissue homogenates from sham inoculated controls, animals with asymptomatic (UTI), and complicated (Struvite) urinary tract infection were measured by ELISA (Reyes et al., 2009). Absorbance values obtained by ELISA were normalized to total protein concentration of tissue homogenates. Values represent the mean ± sd fold change (infected/control) in the calgranulin concentration from 5 biological replicates. Data were analyzed by unpaired student's t test.

In our rodent model of *U. parvum* induced urinary tract infection, proteome analysis of bladder tissues revealed that concentrations of calgranulins A and B were seven fold higher in tissues from struvite positive animals (Reyes et al., 2009). Calgranulin A concentrations were confirmed by ELISA as shown in Figure 3. Moreover, the calgranulin A concentrations in bladder tissue homogenates directly correlated with urine pro-inflammatory cytokine concentrations, suggesting a link between calgranulin A, GRO/KC, IL-1α,and IL-1β.
We also evaluated the distribution of calprotectin within the bladder tissues of animals infected with *U. parvum* for 72 hours and 2 weeks post-inoculation. Calprotectin within uroepithelium was detected in bladder tissues obtained from struvite positive animals at 2 weeks post-inoculation (as shown in Figure 4). In these animals, calprotectin was also detected within endothelial cells that were surrounded by leukocyte infiltrates (Figure 4D). Despite the fact the uroepithelium of animals with asymptomatic urinary tract infection was colonized with *U. parvum*, these animals did not exhibit bladder inflammation or expression of calprotectin by uroepithelium (Figure 4B). We did not observe uroepithelial expression of calprotectin in the 72 hour group, even in animals with ongoing inflammation within the submucosa. Since calprotectin staining could be observed within neutrophils present in these tissues, we were confident that the lack of staining was not an artifact.

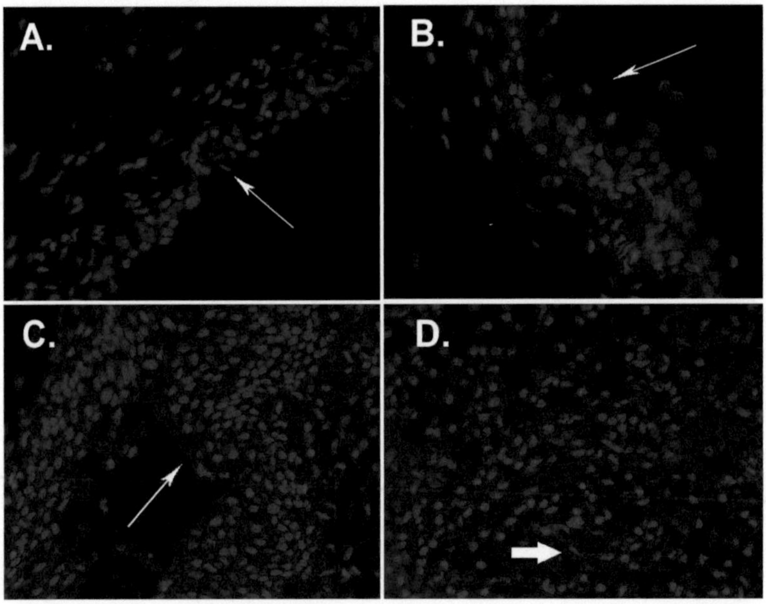

Fig. 4. Distribution of calprotectin in bladder tissues of Fisher rats. Images are 400x magnification of representative bladder tissue sections obtained from sham inoculated control (A), asymptomatic urinary tract infection (B), and struvite positive animals (C and D). Thin white arrows are placed within the lumen and point to the uroepithelial surface in panels A, B, and C. Panel D shows the distribution of calprotectin (red) detected within the submucosa that was infiltrated with, some of which are concentrated around the blood vessel (identified by the block arrow). Bladder tissue sections were processed as previously described (Reyes et al., 2009). Calprotectin was detected with monoclonal antibody (clone MAC 387, from Thermo Scientific, Fremont, CA., USA) followed by goat anti-rabbit conjugated to Alexa-660. Cell nuclei (blue) were labeled with DAPI stain. Images were captured with Olympus IX81 Spinning disk confocal microscope.

Danger-associated pattern molecules (DAMP) are endogenous ligands of toll like receptors. These molecules are often by-products of inflammation such as reactive oxygen species (Frantz et al., 2001) or tissue degradation products from the extracellular matrix (Okamura et al., 2001). Calprotectin is now considered a DAMP because of its ability to activate TLR4 (Ehrchen et al., 2009). Since we observed a correlation between uroepithelial calprotectin expression and pro-inflammatory cytokines in the urine of struvite positive animals, we measured the amount and distribution of TLR 4 in the bladder tissues of rats infected for 72 hours and 2 weeks post-inoculation.There were no appreciable differences in the amount of TLR 4 detected in bladder tissues from sham inoculated controls, or *U. parvum* infected animals at 72 hours post-inoculation. However, at 2 weeks post-inoculation, struvite positive animals exhibited more intense staining of TLR 4 in uroepithelium than uninfected controls or animals with asymptomatic urinary tract infection (see Figure 5).
Since *Ureaplasma* does not directly activate TLR 4, the increased expression observed in struvite positive animals is most likely mediated by DAMPS. Our current study cannot confirm if this activation was initiated by calprotectin or other DAMPS that were detected in our proteome studies such as heat shock protein 60 (Chen et al., 2007) and a variety of extracellular matrix proteins. Nevertheless, the lack of TLR 4 activation in inflamed tissues from the 72 hour time point, coupled with the direct association of uroepithelial calprotectin expression and TLR 4 expression suggests that calprotectin is contributing to an adverse inflammatory response in the struvite group.

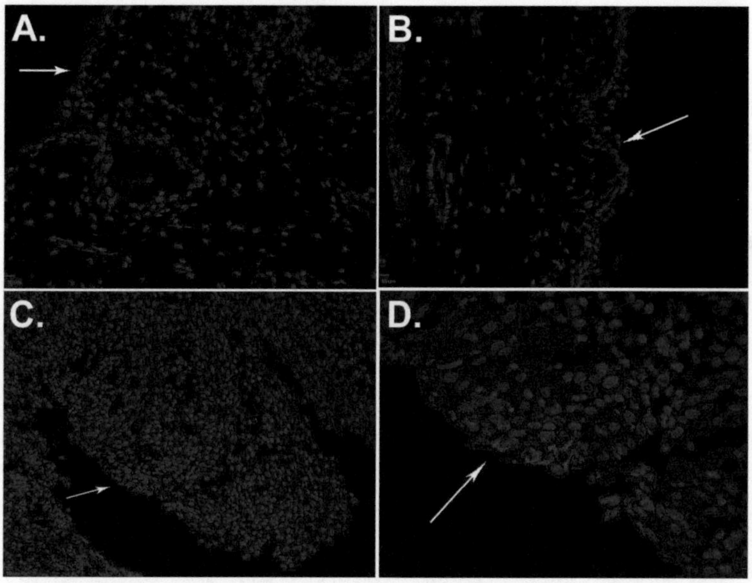

Fig. 5. Distribution of TLR 4 in rat bladder tissues of Fisher rats. Images in panels A, B, and C are 200x magnification of representative bladder tissue sections obtained from sham inoculated control (A), asymptomatic urinary tract infection (B), and struvite positive animals (C and D). Thin white arrows are placed within the lumen and point to the uroepithelial surface. Panel D is a 400x magnification of panel C. Tissues were processed as previously described (Reyes et al., 2009). TLR 4 (red) was detected with rabbit polyclonal antibody (Abbiotec, LLC, San Diego, CA) followed by goat anti-rabbit conjugated to Alexa-594. Cell nuclei (blue) were labeled with DAPI stain. Images were captured with Olympus IX81 Spinning disk confocal microscope.

2.4 Regulation of calgranulin gene expression in different cell populations

In addition to participating in immune defence, calgranulins are involved in embryogenesis, growth, and differentiation. Therefore, it is not surprising that the expression of these proteins is tightly regulated in a cell and tissue specific manner, which can change in response to environmental cues. For example, most mucosal epithelial cells have a basal level of calgranulin expression that changes in response to the appropriate stimulus (Ross & Hertzberg, 2001, Hsu et al., 2005, 2009). The appropriate stimulus for one tissue type is not necessarily the same for another. For example, calgranulin expression in oral squamous epithelial cells increases in response to interleukin-1α, but bacterial lipopolysaccaride does not induce an effect (Ross & Hertzberg, 2001). This may pertain to the fact that the oral cavity is heavily colonized with bacteria. On the other hand, bronchiolar epithelium increases its calgranulin expression in response to lipopolysaccaride mediated activation of TLR4 (Henke et al., 2006). Uroepithelium has a low basal expression of calgranulins A and B, which is significantly up regulated in cancer and inflammation (Yao et al., 2007; Tyagi et al., 2008). It is not known what specific cytokines or factors induce up regulation of calgranulin gene expression in these cells, but the studies performed by our laboratory and Dressing et al., imply that uroepithelium would respond to both interleukin-1α and toll like receptor activation.

Varieties of cell types that reside within bladder submucosa either repress or express calgranulins in response to changes within the tissue microenvironment. Cells pertinent to urinary tract infection are fibroblasts, dendritic cells, macrophages, and neutrophils (Cresswell, et al., 2001; Shafik, et al., 2004; Christmas & Botazzo, 1992; Shimizu et al., 2011). Fibroblasts do not participate in antimicrobial processes during urinary tract infection, but their response to mediators released by uroepithelial cells exposed to *E. coli* can influence their ability to migrate and remodel the extracellular matrix, which is particularly important in renal interstitial scarring (Kapoor et al., 2001). Furthermore, calgranulin expressing fibroblasts can be detected during the early stages of wound healing (Rahimi et al., 2005). Fibroblast growth factor-2 or interleukin-1β increases expression of calgranulins by fibroblasts. However, transforming growth factor-β, which promotes fibroblast migration in response to bacterial/urothelial products, can block calgranulin expression in these cells (Kapoor et al., 2001).

Dendritic cells are important in immune surveillance and can express calgranulins in varying intensity depending on their level of maturation (Kumar et al., 2003; Koga et al., 2008). Immature dendritic cells express higher amounts of calgranulins A and B than mature cells (Koga et al., 2008). Interleukin-10 promotes induction of tolerogenic dendritic cells, which then exhibit increased expression of calgranulins (Kumar et al., 2003). Further, calgranulin B may down regulate cytokine release in dendritic cells after toll-like receptor stimulation (Averill et al., 2011).

Macrophages represent differentiated monocytes that have migrated into tissues in response to pro-inflammatory signals or part of a homeostatic process. When differentiation is complete these cells cease to express calgranulins unless they become activated (Nacken et al., 2003). It is important to note that not all activated macrophages express calgranulins. Presently, three macrophage phenotypes with distinctly different functions have been identified (Benoit et al., 2008; Mosser & Edwards, 2008). The phenotype is determined by the type of stimulus the cell receives during the process of activation. For example, macrophages exposed to interferon-γ in combination with TNF-α, and induction of TLR transforms them into the classically activated or microbicidal macrophage (Benoit et al., 2008; Mosser & Edwards, 2008). Classically activated macrophages are known for their enhanced microbial killing through induction of nitric oxide synthase, secretion of pro-inflammatory cytokines (TNF, interleukin-1β, interleukin-6, and interleukin-12) and secretion of chemokines (CCL2, CCL5, and CXCL8) (Benoit et al., 2008). Resident macrophages that are exposed to interleukin-4 and/or interleukin-13 transform into a wound healing phenotype. Instead of participating in pro-inflammatory events, these cells primarily secrete extracellular matrix proteins and contribute to tissue remodelling. The third activated phenotype is referred to as the regulatory macrophage because these cells express high amounts of co-regulatory molecules that bind to T cell receptors. In addition, regulatory macrophages secrete high amounts of interleukin-10, and these cells are primarily involved in down-regulation of the inflammatory response (Mosser & Edwards, 2008). Of the three phenotypes, only regulatory macrophages express calgranulins, in particular calgranulin A (Benoit et al., 2008; Hsu et al., 2009). Therefore, calgranulin A may be a useful molecular marker for the *in situ* identification of these cells.

A common feature of regulatory macrophages is that they develop from simultaneous exposure to two stimuli (Mosser & Edwards, 2008). The first signal has little to no stimulatory function. Weak agonists known to induce a regulatory phenotype include immunoglobulin complexes, prostaglandins, apoptotic cells, glucocorticoids, interleukin-10, or G-protein coupled receptor ligands. The second signal involves TLR activation. It has been postulated that calgranulin expression by regulatory macrophages contributes to their immunosuppressive function (Hsu et al., 2009). Support for this argument is that regulatory macrophages exclusively express calgranulin A, which can reduce the damaging effects of inflammation by acting as a scavenger for reactive oxygen species. Furthermore, secreted calgranulin A also repels or inhibits recruitment of neutrophils (Hsu et al., 2009; Sroussi et al., 2010; Xu et al., 2001). Although regulatory macrophages may be highly beneficial during sterile inflammation, their presence at sites of infection may be potentially detrimental. Regulatory macrophages can be exploited by bacterial, parasitic, and viral pathogens. For example, during invasion of macrophages, *Leishmania* species can utilize immunoglobulin complexes to promote the induction of a regulatory phenotype (Moser & Edwards, 2008). Regulatory macrophages may also be inadvertently assisting microbial persistence in the urogenital tract. For example, *Ureaplasmas* are chronic and persistent colonizers of the human urogenital tract, and infections are often asymptomatic (Reyes et al., 2008, 2009; Volgmann et al., 2005). However, these organisms are also associated with pro-inflammatory disorders including interstitial nephritis, urethritis, and overactive bladder (Latthe et al., 2008; Lee et al., 2010). As urease producers, *Ureaplasmas* promote development of struvite uroliths (Grenabo et al., 1988). During infection these microbes induce secretion of prostaglandin E_2 and interleukin-10 in host cells (Aaltonen et al., 2007; Estrada-Gutierrez et al., 2010; Moser et al., 2009), which are recognized promoters of the regulatory macrophage phenotype (Moser & Edwards, 2008). Although this connection has yet to be demonstrated with this organism, it is an intriguing notion that *Ureaplasmas* may be benefiting from such a mechanism.

3. Conclusion

The biological function of calgranulins is complex, diverse and paradoxical. Therefore, extrapolations from studies outside of the context of urinary tract infection must be made with caution. To date, there are only two published reports that refer to calgranulins during urinary tract infection. Based on these reports, we can only conclude that the antimicrobial properties of calgranulins are minimally effective in the urinary tract. More than likely, the pro-inflammatory properties of calgranulins contribute to complicated inflammatory diseases such as struvite urolithiasis, pyelonephritis, and possibly interstitial cystitis. The positive correlation between increased calgranulin expression and inflammation in tissues, support the argument that these proteins may serve as biomarkers for chronic complicated urinary tract infections. However, additional studies are required in order to determine which clinical settings would benefit from monitoring calgranulin concentrations during urinary tract infections. Of more immediate benefit may be the use of calgranulins as molecular markers in basic science research. For example, monitoring these proteins during maturation and activation of different cell types that comprise innate defense may provide new insights into mechanisms of immune dysregulation induced by various microbial pathogens of the urinary tract.

4. Acknowledgments

Portions of this work were supported by award number K08DK075651 from the National Institute of Diabetes And Digestive And Kidney Diseases (NIDDK), and award number RO1 AI45875 from the National Institute of Allergy and Infectious Disease (NIAID). The content is solely the responsibility of the authors and does not necessarily represent the official views of the NIDDK, NIAID or the National Institutes of Health.

5. References

Aaltonen, R., Heikkinen, J., Vahlberg, T., Jensen, J.S., Alanen, A. (2007) Local inflammatory response in choriodecidua induced by Ureaplasma urealyticum. *Bjog* 114, 1432-5.

Ahmad, A., Bayley, D.L., He, S., Stockley, R.A. (2003) Myeloid related protein-8/14 stimulates interleukin-8 production in airway epithelial cells. *Am J Respir Cell Mol Biol* 29, 523-30.

Altwegg, L.A., Neidhart, M., Hersberger, M., Muller, S., Eberli, F.R., Corti, R., Roffi, M., Sutsch, G., Gay, S., von Eckardstein, A., Wischnewsky, M.B., Luscher, T.F., Maier, W. (2007) Myeloid-related protein 8/14 complex is released by monocytes and granulocytes at the site of coronary occlusion: a novel, early, and sensitive marker of acute coronary syndromes. *Eur Heart J* 28, 941-8.

Anumanthan, G., Tanaka, S.T., Adams, C.M., Thomas, J.C., Wills, M.L., Adams, M.C., Hayward, S.W., Matusik, R.J., Bhowmick, N.A., Brock, J.W., 3rd, Pope, J.C.t. (2009) Bladder stromal loss of transforming growth factor receptor II decreases fibrosis after bladder obstruction. *J Urol* 182, 1775-80.

Averill, M.M., Barnhart, S., Becker, L., Li, X., Heinecke, J.W., Leboeuf, R.C., Hamerman, J.A., Sorg, C., Kerkhoff, C., Bornfeldt, K.E. S100A9 Differentially Modifies Phenotypic States of Neutrophils, Macrophages, and Dendritic Cells: Implications for Atherosclerosis and Adipose Tissue Inflammation. *Circulation* 123, 1216-26.

Bennett, J., Dretler, S.P., Selengut, J., Orme-Johnson, W.H. (1994) Identification of the calcium-binding protein calgranulin in the matrix of struvite stones. *J Endourol* 8, 95-8.

Benoit, M., Desnues, B., Mege, J.L. (2008) Macrophage polarization in bacterial infections. *J Immunol* 181, 3733-9.

Brandtzaeg, P., Gabrielsen, T.O., Dale, I., Muller, F., Steinbakk, M., Fagerhol, M.K. (1995) The leucocyte protein L1 (calprotectin): a putative nonspecific defence factor at epithelial surfaces. *Adv Exp Med Biol* 371A, 201-6.

Brun, J.G., Ulvestad, E., Fagerhol, M.K., Jonsson, R. (1994) Effects of human calprotectin (L1) on in vitro immunoglobulin synthesis. *Scand J Immunol* 40, 675-80.

Canales, B.K., Anderson, L., Higgins, L., Ensrud-Bowlin, K., Roberts, K.P., Wu, B., Kim, I.W., Monga, M. (2010) Proteome of human calcium kidney stones. *Urology* 76, 1017 e13-20.

Canales, B.K., Anderson, L., Higgins, L., Slaton, J., Roberts, K.P., Liu, N., Monga, M. (2008) Second prize: Comprehensive proteomic analysis of human calcium oxalate monohydrate kidney stone matrix. *J Endourol* 22, 1161-7.

Chen, K., Huang, J., Gong, W., Iribarren, P., Dunlop, N.M., Wang, J.M. (2007) Toll-like receptors in inflammation, infection and cancer. *Int Immunopharmacol* 7, 1271-85.

Christmas, T.J., Bottazzo, G.F. (1992) Abnormal urothelial HLA-DR expression in interstitial cystitis. *Clin Exp Immunol* 87, 450-4.

Corbin, B.D., Seeley, E.H., Raab, A., Feldmann, J., Miller, M.R., Torres, V.J., Anderson, K.L., Dattilo, B.M., Dunman, P.M., Gerads, R., Caprioli, R.M., Nacken, W., Chazin, W.J., Skaar, E.P. (2008) Metal chelation and inhibition of bacterial growth in tissue abscesses. *Science* 319, 962-5.

Cresswell, J., Robertson, H., Neal, D.E., Griffiths, T.R., Kirby, J.A. (2001) Distribution of lymphocytes of the alpha(E)beta(7) phenotype and E-cadherin in normal human urothelium and bladder carcinomas. *Clin Exp Immunol* 126, 397-402.

Croce, K., Gao, H., Wang, Y., Mooroka, T., Sakuma, M., Shi, C., Sukhova, G.K., Packard, R.R., Hogg, N., Libby, P., Simon, D.I. (2009) Myeloid-related protein-8/14 is critical for the biological response to vascular injury. *Circulation* 120, 427-36.

Delano, M.J., Scumpia, P.O., Weinstein, J.S., Coco, D., Nagaraj, S., Kelly-Scumpia, K.M., O'Malley, K.A., Wynn, J.L., Antonenko, S., Al-Quran, S.Z., Swan, R., Chung, C.S., Atkinson, M.A., Ramphal, R., Gabrilovich, D.I., Reeves, W.H., Ayala, A., Phillips, J., Laface, D., Heyworth, P.G., Clare-Salzler, M., Moldawer, L.L. (2007) MyD88-dependent expansion of an immature GR-1(+)CD11b(+) population induces T cell suppression and Th2 polarization in sepsis. *J Exp Med* 204, 1463-74.

Dessing, M.C., Butter, L.M., Teske, G.J., Claessen, N., van der Loos, C.M., Vogl, T., Roth, J., van der Poll, T., Florquin, S., Leemans, J.C. (2010) S100A8/A9 is not involved in host defense against murine urinary tract infection. *PLoS One* 5, e13394.

Ehrchen, J.M., Sunderkotter, C., Foell, D., Vogl, T., Roth, J. (2009) The endogenous Toll-like receptor 4 agonist S100A8/S100A9 (calprotectin) as innate amplifier of infection, autoimmunity, and cancer. *J Leukoc Biol* 86, 557-66.

Estrada-Gutierrez, G., Gomez-Lopez, N., Zaga-Clavellina, V., Giono-Cerezo, S., Espejel-Nunez, A., Gonzalez-Jimenez, M.A., Espino y Sosa, S., Olson, D.M., Vadillo-Ortega,

F. (2010) Interaction between pathogenic bacteria and intrauterine leukocytes triggers alternative molecular signaling cascades leading to labor in women. *Infect Immun* 78, 4792-9.

Eue, I., Pietz, B., Storck, J., Klempt, M., Sorg, C. (2000) Transendothelial migration of 27E10+ human monocytes. *Int Immunol* 12, 1593-604.

Ezernitchi, A.V., Vaknin, I., Cohen-Daniel, L., Levy, O., Manaster, E., Halabi, A., Pikarsky, E., Shapira, L., Baniyash, M. (2006) TCR zeta down-regulation under chronic inflammation is mediated by myeloid suppressor cells differentially distributed between various lymphatic organs. *J Immunol* 177, 4763-72.

Foell, D., Wittkowski, H., Vogl, T., Roth, J. (2007) S100 proteins expressed in phagocytes: a novel group of damage-associated molecular pattern molecules. *J Leukoc Biol* 81, 28-37.

Frantz, S., Kelly, R.A., Bourcier, T. (2001) Role of TLR-2 in the activation of nuclear factor kappaB by oxidative stress in cardiac myocytes. *J Biol Chem* 276, 5197-203.

Frosch, M., Vogl, T., Waldherr, R., Sorg, C., Sunderkotter, C., Roth, J. (2004) Expression of MRP8 and MRP14 by macrophages is a marker for severe forms of glomerulonephritis. *J Leukoc Biol* 75, 198-206.

Grenabo, L., Hedelin, H., Pettersson, S. (1988) Urinary infection stones caused by Ureaplasma urealyticum: a review. Scand J Infect Dis Suppl 53, 46-9.

Haile, L.A., von Wasielewski, R., Gamrekelashvili, J., Kruger, C., Bachmann, O., Westendorf, A.M., Buer, J., Liblau, R., Manns, M.P., Korangy, F., Greten, T.F. (2008) Myeloid-derived suppressor cells in inflammatory bowel disease: a new immunoregulatory pathway. *Gastroenterology* 135, 871-81, 881 e1-5.

Harrison, C.A., Raftery, M.J., Walsh, J., Alewood, P., Iismaa, S.E., Thliveris, S., Geczy, C.L. (1999) Oxidation regulates the inflammatory properties of the murine S100 protein S100A8. *J Biol Chem* 274, 8561-9.

Healy, A.M., Pickard, M.D., Pradhan, A.D., Wang, Y., Chen, Z., Croce, K., Sakuma, M., Shi, C., Zago, A.C., Garasic, J., Damokosh, A.I., Dowie, T.L., Poisson, L., Lillie, J., Libby, P., Ridker, P.M., Simon, D.I. (2006) Platelet expression profiling and clinical validation of myeloid-related protein-14 as a novel determinant of cardiovascular events. *Circulation* 113, 2278-84.

Henke, M.O., Renner, A., Rubin, B.K., Gyves, J.I., Lorenz, E., Koo, J.S. (2006) Up-regulation of S100A8 and S100A9 protein in bronchial epithelial cells by lipopolysaccharide. *Exp Lung Res* 32, 331-47.

Hobbs, J.A., May, R., Tanousis, K., McNeill, E., Mathies, M., Gebhardt, C., Henderson, R., Robinson, M.J., Hogg, N. (2003) Myeloid cell function in MRP-14 (S100A9) null mice. *Mol Cell Biol* 23, 2564-76.

Holt, J., Fagerhol, M.K., Dale, I. (1983) Quantitation of a leukocyte protein (L1) in urine. *Acta Paediatr Scand* 72, 615-6.

Hsu, K., Champaiboon, C., Guenther, B.D., Sorenson, B.S., Khammanivong, A., Ross, K.F., Geczy, C.L., Herzberg, M.C. (2009) Anti-Infective Protective Properties of S100 Calgranulins. *Antiinflamm Antiallergy Agents Med Chem* 8, 290-305.

Hsu, K., Passey, R.J., Endoh, Y., Rahimi, F., Youssef, P., Yen, T., Geczy, C.L. (2005) Regulation of S100A8 by glucocorticoids. *J Immunol* 174, 2318-26.

Johne, B., Fagerhol, M.K., Lyberg, T., Prydz, H., Brandtzaeg, P., Naess-Andresen, C.F., Dale, I. (1997) Functional and clinical aspects of the myelomonocyte protein calprotectin. *Mol Pathol* 50, 113-23.

Kapoor, R., Reddy, K., Liatsikos, E.N., Smith, A.D., Singhal, P.C. (2001) Escherichia coli-human uroepithelial cell interaction products enhance fibroblast migration and matrix accumulation. *J Endourol* 15, 155-9.

Kerkhoff, C., Nacken, W., Benedyk, M., Dagher, M.C., Sopalla, C., Doussiere, J. (2005) The arachidonic acid-binding protein S100A8/A9 promotes NADPH oxidase activation by interaction with p67phox and Rac-2. *Faseb J* 19, 467-9.

Khan, S.R. (2005) Hyperoxaluria-induced oxidative stress and antioxidants for renal protection. *Urol Res* 33, 349-57.

Kido, J., Hayashi, N., Kataoka, M., Nagata, T. (2005) Calprotectin expression in human monocytes: induction by porphyromonas gingivalis lipopolysaccharide, tumor necrosis factor-alpha, and interleukin-1beta. *J Periodontol* 76, 437-42.

Koga, Y., Matsuzaki, A., Suminoe, A., Hattori, H., Hara, T. (2008) Expression of cytokine-associated genes in dendritic cells (DCs): comparison between adult peripheral blood- and umbilical cord blood-derived DCs by cDNA microarray. *Immunol Lett* 116, 55-63.

Kostakis, I.D., Cholidou, K.G., Kallianidis, K., Perrea, D., Antsaklis, A. The role of calprotectin in obstetrics and gynecology. *Eur J Obstet Gynecol Reprod Biol* 151, 3-9.

Kumar, A., Steinkasserer, A., Berchtold, S. (2003) Interleukin-10 influences the expression of MRP8 and MRP14 in human dendritic cells. *Int Arch Allergy Immunol* 132, 40-7.

Latthe, P.M., Toozs-Hobson, P., Gray, J. (2008) Mycoplasma and ureaplasma colonisation in women with lower urinary tract symptoms. J Obstet Gynaecol 28, 519-21.

Leach, S.T., Mitchell, H.M., Geczy, C.L., Sherman, P.M., Day, A.S. (2008) S100 calgranulin proteins S100A8, S100A9 and S100A12 are expressed in the inflamed gastric mucosa of Helicobacter pylori-infected children. *Can J Gastroenterol* 22, 461-4.

Lee, Y.S., Kim, J.Y., Kim, J.C., Park, W.H., Choo, M.S., Lee, K.S. (2010) Prevalence and treatment efficacy of genitourinary mycoplasmas in women with overactive bladder symptoms. *Korean J Urol* 51, 625-30.

Lim, S.Y., Raftery, M., Cai, H., Hsu, K., Yan, W.X., Hseih, H.L., Watts, R.N., Richardson, D., Thomas, S., Perry, M., Geczy, C.L. (2008) S-nitrosylated S100A8: novel anti-inflammatory properties. *J Immunol* 181, 5627-36.

Lim, S.Y., Raftery, M.J., Goyette, J., Hsu, K., Geczy, C.L. (2009) Oxidative modifications of S100 proteins: functional regulation by redox. *J Leukoc Biol* 86, 577-87.

Loser, K., Vogl, T., Voskort, M., Lueken, A., Kupas, V., Nacken, W., Klenner, L., Kuhn, A., Foell, D., Sorokin, L., Luger, T.A., Roth, J., Beissert, S. The Toll-like receptor 4 ligands Mrp8 and Mrp14 are crucial in the development of autoreactive CD8+ T cells. *Nat Med* 16, 713-7.

Mosser, D.M., Edwards, J.P. (2008) Exploring the full spectrum of macrophage activation. *Nat Rev Immunol* 8, 958-69.

Mushtaq, S., Siddiqui, A.A., Naqvi, Z.A., Rattani, A., Talati, J., Palmberg, C., Shafqat, J. (2007) Identification of myeloperoxidase, alpha-defensin and calgranulin in calcium oxalate renal stones. *Clin Chim Acta* 384, 41-7.

Nacken, W., Roth, J., Sorg, C., Kerkhoff, C. (2003) S100A9/S100A8: Myeloid representatives of the S100 protein family as prominent players in innate immunity. *Microsc Res Tech* 60, 569-80.

Newton, R.A., Hogg, N. (1998) The human S100 protein MRP-14 is a novel activator of the beta 2 integrin Mac-1 on neutrophils. *J Immunol* 160, 1427-35.

Nisapakultorn, K., Ross, K.F., Herzberg, M.C. (2001a) Calprotectin expression in vitro by oral epithelial cells confers resistance to infection by Porphyromonas gingivalis. *Infect Immun* 69, 4242-7.

Nisapakultorn, K., Ross, K.F., Herzberg, M.C. (2001b) Calprotectin expression inhibits bacterial binding to mucosal epithelial cells. *Infect Immun* 69, 3692-6.

Okamura, Y., Watari, M., Jerud, E.S., Young, D.W., Ishizaka, S.T., Rose, J., Chow, J.C., Strauss, J.F., 3rd (2001) The extra domain A of fibronectin activates Toll-like receptor 4. *J Biol Chem* 276, 10229-33.

Passey, R.J., Williams, E., Lichanska, A.M., Wells, C., Hu, S., Geczy, C.L., Little, M.H., Hume, D.A. (1999a) A null mutation in the inflammation-associated S100 protein S100A8 causes early resorption of the mouse embryo. *J Immunol* 163, 2209-16.

Passey, R.J., Xu, K., Hume, D.A., Geczy, C.L. (1999b) S100A8: emerging functions and regulation. *J Leukoc Biol* 66, 549-56.

Perera, C., McNeil, H.P., Geczy, C.L. S100 Calgranulins in inflammatory arthritis. *Immunol Cell Biol* 88, 41-9.

Pouliot, P., Plante, I., Raquil, M.A., Tessier, P.A., Olivier, M. (2008) Myeloid-related proteins rapidly modulate macrophage nitric oxide production during innate immune response. *J Immunol* 181, 3595-601.

Rahimi, F., Hsu, K., Endoh, Y., Geczy, C.L. (2005) FGF-2, IL-1beta and TGF-beta regulate fibroblast expression of S100A8. *Febs J* 272, 2811-27.

Reyes, L., Alvarez, S., Allam, A., Reinhard, M., Brown, M.B. (2009) Complicated urinary tract infection is associated with uroepithelial expression of proinflammatory protein S100A8. *Infect Immun* 77, 4265-74.

Reyes, L., Reinhard, M., Brown, M.B. (2009) Different inflammatory responses are associated with Ureaplasma parvum-induced UTI and urolith formation. *BMC Infect Dis* 9, 9.

Reyes, L., Reinhard, M., O'Donell L, J., Stevens, J., Brown, M.B. (2006) Rat strains differ in susceptibility to Ureaplasma parvum-induced urinary tract infection and struvite stone formation. *Infect Immun* 74, 6656-64.

Ross, K.F., Herzberg, M.C. (2001) Calprotectin expression by gingival epithelial cells. *Infect Immun* 69, 3248-54.

Shafik, A., El-Sibai, O., Shafik, A.A., Shafik, I. (2004) Identification of interstitial cells of Cajal in human urinary bladder: concept of vesical pacemaker. *Urology* 64, 809-13.

Shimizu, T., Kida, Y., Kuwano, K. (2008) Ureaplasma parvum lipoproteins, including MB antigen, activate NF-{kappa}B through TLR1, TLR2 and TLR6. *Microbiology* 154, 1318-25.

Simard, J.C., Girard, D., Tessier, P.A. (2010) Induction of neutrophil degranulation by S100A9 via a MAPK-dependent mechanism. *J Leukoc Biol* 87, 905-14.

Song, J., Duncan, M.J., Li, G., Chan, C., Grady, R., Stapleton, A., Abraham, S.N. (2007a) A novel TLR4-mediated signaling pathway leading to IL-6 responses in human bladder epithelial cells. *PLoS Pathog* 3, e60.

Song, J., Bishop, B.L., Li, G., Duncan, M.J., Abraham, S.N. (2007b) TLR4-initiated and cAMP-mediated abrogation of bacterial invasion of the bladder. *Cell Host Microbe* 1, 287-98.

Sroussi, H.Y., Berline, J., Dazin, P., Green, P., Palefsky, J.M. (2006) S100A8 triggers oxidation-sensitive repulsion of neutrophils. *J Dent Res* 85, 829-33.

Sroussi, H.Y., Berline, J., Palefsky, J.M. (2007) Oxidation of methionine 63 and 83 regulates the effect of S100A9 on the migration of neutrophils in vitro. *J Leukoc Biol* 81, 818-24.

Sroussi, H.Y., Lu, Y., Zhang, Q.L., Villines, D., Marucha, P.T. (2010) S100A8 and S100A9 inhibit neutrophil oxidative metabolism in-vitro: involvement of adenosine metabolites. *Free Radic Res* 44, 389-96.

Tyagi, P., Chen, X., Hayashi, Y., Yoshimura, N., Chancellor, M.B., de Miguel, F. (2008) Proteomic investigation on chronic bladder irritation in the rat. *Urology* 71, 536-40.

Viemann, D., Strey, A., Janning, A., Jurk, K., Klimmek, K., Vogl, T., Hirono, K., Ichida, F., Foell, D., Kehrel, B., Gerke, V., Sorg, C., Roth, J. (2005) Myeloid-related proteins 8 and 14 induce a specific inflammatory response in human microvascular endothelial cells. *Blood* 105, 2955-62.

Vogl, T., Ludwig, S., Goebeler, M., Strey, A., Thorey, I.S., Reichelt, R., Foell, D., Gerke, V., Manitz, M.P., Nacken, W., Werner, S., Sorg, C., Roth, J. (2004) MRP8 and MRP14 control microtubule reorganization during transendothelial migration of phagocytes. *Blood* 104, 4260-8.

Vogl, T., Propper, C., Hartmann, M., Strey, A., Strupat, K., van den Bos, C., Sorg, C., Roth, J. (1999) S100A12 is expressed exclusively by granulocytes and acts independently from MRP8 and MRP14. *J Biol Chem* 274, 25291-6.

Vogl, T., Tenbrock, K., Ludwig, S., Leukert, N., Ehrhardt, C., van Zoelen, M.A., Nacken, W., Foell, D., van der Poll, T., Sorg, C., Roth, J. (2007) Mrp8 and Mrp14 are endogenous activators of Toll-like receptor 4, promoting lethal, endotoxin-induced shock. *Nat Med* 13, 1042-9.

Volgmann T, Ohlinger R, Panzig B. (2005) Ureaplasma urealyticum-harmless commensal or underestimated enemy of human reproduction? A review. *Archives of gynecology and obstetrics* 273,133-139.

Xu, K., Yen, T., Geczy, C.L. (2001) Il-10 up-regulates macrophage expression of the S100 protein S100A8. *J Immunol* 166, 6358-66.

Yang, Z., Tao, T., Raftery, M.J., Youssef, P., Di Girolamo, N., Geczy, C.L. (2001) Proinflammatory properties of the human S100 protein S100A12. *J Leukoc Biol* 69, 986-94.

Yao, R., Lopez-Beltran, A., Maclennan, G.T., Montironi, R., Eble, J.N., Cheng, L. (2007) Expression of S100 protein family members in the pathogenesis of bladder tumors. *Anticancer Res* 27, 3051-8.

Zaia, A.A., Sappington, K.J., Nisapakultorn, K., Chazin, W.J., Dietrich, E.A., Ross, K.F., Herzberg, M.C. (2009) Subversion of antimicrobial calprotectin (S100A8/S100A9 complex) in the cytoplasm of TR146 epithelial cells after invasion by Listeria monocytogenes. *Mucosal Immunol* 2, 43-53.

18

Effect Investigation of Aqueous Cranberry (*Vaccinium arctostaphylos* L.) Extract in Accompanied with Antibiotics on Urinary Tract Infections (UTI) Created by *Escherichia coli in Vitro*

Avat (Arman) Taherpour[1] and Arezou Taherpour[2]
[1]*Faculty of Science, Islamic Azad University, Arak Branch, Arak,*
[2]*Microbiology and Immunology Department,*
Kurdistan University of Medicinal Sciences, Pasdaran Ave.,
Sanandaj, Kurdistan Province,
Iran

1. Introduction

The bladder wall is coated with various mannosylated proteins which interfere with the binding of bacteria to the uroepithelium. As binding is an important factor in establishing pathogenicity for these organisms, its disruption results in reduced capacity for invasion of the tissues.[1a,b] Moreover, the unbound bacteria are more easily removed when voiding. The use of urinary catheters (or other physical trauma) may physically disturb this protective lining, thereby allowing bacteria to invade the exposed epithelium.[1a,b]Over ninety percent of all UTIs are ascending and starting with colonization of periuretheral area.[1c-d] The most common organism implicated in Urinary tract infections UTIs (80–85%) is *E. coli*,[1a,b] while *Staphylococcus saprophyticus* is the cause in 5–10%. [1a,b] The genus *Escherichia coli* (*E.coli*) with five species is a member of Entrobacteriaceae family. This gram negative bacilli is associated with a variety of diseases, such as urinary tract nfections(UTIs), meningitis and so on. *E.coli* can produce adhesins (P pili, AAF/I,AAF/III,..) which bind to cells lining the bladder and upper urinary tract.[1c-d] During cystitis, uropathogenic *Escherichia coli* (UPEC) subvert innate defenses by invading superficial umbrella cells and rapidly increasing in numbers to form intracellular bacterial communities (IBCs).[1,2] By working together, bacteria in biofilms build themselves into structures that are more firmly anchored in infected cells and are more resistant to immune-system assaults and antibiotic treatments.[2a,b] This is often the cause of chronic urinary tract infections.
Bacteruria can be symptomatic or asymptomatic. There are no signs in asymptomatic Bacteruria but bacteria are isolated; in these cases treatment is necessary for pregnant women and patients who have instrument in genitourinary tract. Therefore, infection is defined by clinical parameters and special situations, no by identification of microbe solely.[1c-d] In complicated or questionable cases, confirmation via urinalysis, looking for the presence of nitrites, leukocytes, or leukocyte esterase, or via urine microscopy, looking

for the presence of red blood cells, white blood cells, and bacteria, may be useful.[1a,b] Urine culture shows a quantitative count of greater than or equal to 10^3 colony-forming units (CFU) per mL of a typical urinary tract organism along with antibiotic sensitivity is useful to select appropriate antibiotic .[1a,b] On the whole, diagnosis is based on symptoms and urine culture.[1c-d]

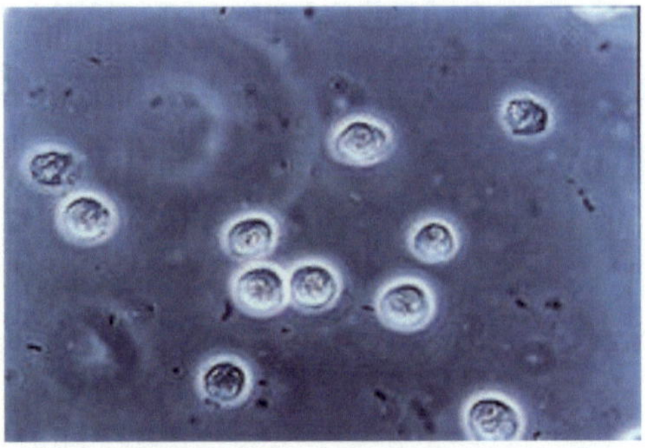

Fig. 1. Multiple bacilli (rod-shaped bacteria have shown as black and bean-shaped) shown between white cells at urinary microscopy. This is called bacteriuria and pyuria, respectively. These changes are indicative of a UTI. See [1a,b]

Accurately, estimate of its incidence is difficult because many cases have not been reported. According to the 1997 National Ambulatory Medical Care Survey and National Hospital Ambulatory Medical Care Survey, urinary tract infection accounted for nearly 7 million office visits and 1 million emergency department visits, resulting in 100,000 hospitalizations.[1,3] The other investigate reported over 1.7 million emergency department visits and more than 8.8 million office visits between 1999 and 2000.[1d]

UTIs are frequently seen among women than men. Assessments show 50 percent of all women have an episode of UTI during their lifetime. Others are at risk for UTIs due to elderly, pregnancy, catheters, genitourinary tract abnormalities, underlying diseases (i.e. diabetes), renal stones and so on. Uncomplicated UTIs occur in young women in sexually active age, but complicated UTIs occur in individuals who have one or more structural abnormalities in genitourinary tract or have catheters indwelling. .[1a-d,4] Some of agents (abnormalities in urinary tract, renal stones, diabetes, genetic factors like receptors for bacterial pili, spinal cord injuries and etc.) which promote women for UTIs, also are common in men, and could add prostatitis and spermicides agents as other promoting factors in men. Albeit, the incidence of UTIs in men <65 year old is very low; but incidence of UTIs in men older than 65 increases dramatically, as UTIs ratio in female-to- male declines.[1a-d]

Pediatrics UTIs create great morbidity and long standing problems, including impaired renal function and hypertension. Bacteria have been seen in approximately 1% of all babies' and more in boys' bladder, and bacteremia often is present. Risk of UTIs in non-circumcised males younger than 6 months is 12 times more than circumcised control group. According to statistics from 1990, the prevalence of urinary tract infections in pre-school and school girls was 1% to 3%, nearly 30-fold higher than that in boys.[1a,4] Also, the statistics from the same year show that approximately 5% of girls will develop at least one urinary tract infection in their school years.[1a] Children with recurrent UTIs may be treated with preventative antibiotics that decrease the rate of microbiological recurrence but not symptomatic recurrence.[1a,5] These infections are often asymptomatic and it can be cause of most renal damages.[1a-d]

Cranberries have enormous medical value. This was known to man from a very long time ago. The name cranberry derives from "craneberry", first named by early European settlers in America who felt the expanding flower, stem, calyx, and petals resembled the neck, head, and bill of a crane. Another name used in northeastern Canada is mossberry. The traditional English name for Vaccinium oxycoccos, fenberry, originated from plants found growing in fen (marsh) lands. In 17th century New England cranberries were sometimes called "bearberries" as bears were often seen feeding on them.[6]

In North America, Native Americans were the first to use cranberries as food. Native Americans used cranberries in a variety of foods, especially for pemmican, wound medicine and dye. Calling the red berries Sassamanash, natives may have introduced cranberries to starving English settlers in Massachusetts who incorporated the berries into traditional Thanksgiving feasts. In the 1820s cranberries were shipped to Europe.[6,7] Cranberries became popular for wild harvesting in the Nordic countries and Russia. In Scotland, the berries were originally wild-harvested but with the loss of suitable habitat, the plants have become so scarce that this is no longer done. Cranberries are a group of evergreen dwarf shrubs or trailing vines in the genus *Vaccinium* subgenus *Oxycoccos*, or in some treatments, in the distinct genus *Oxycoccos*. They can be found in acidic bogs throughout the cooler regions of the Northern Hemisphere.[6]

Vaccinium arctostaphylos L. genus that is relevant to the *Ericaceae* family has over 450 species which are found mostly in the cooler areas. A deciduous shrub grows to 3m by 2m. It is in flower from May to July, and the seeds ripen in September. The flowers are hermaphrodite (have both male and female organs) and are pollinated by Insects.[8,9] The plant prefers light (sandy) and medium (loamy) soils and requires well-drained soil. The plant prefers acid soils and can grow in very acid soil (pH 4-5). It can grow in semi-shade (light woodland) or no shade. It requires moist soil.[8,9] This kind of Cranberry (*Vaccinium arctostaphylos L.*) is growing in north and the parts of west of Iran. The local name of this herb is Qare-Qat (QΛre-QΛt).[8,9]

Historically, cranberry beds were constructed in wetlands. Currently cranberry beds are constructed in upland areas that have a shallow water table. The topsoil is scraped off to form dykes around the bed perimeter.[6a] Clean sand is hauled in to a depth of four to eight inches. The surface is laser leveled flat to provide even drainage. Beds are frequently drained with socked tile in addition to the perimeter ditch. In addition to making it possible to hold water, the dykes allow equipment to service the beds without driving on the vines. Irrigation equipment is installed in the bed to provide irrigation for vine growth and for spring and autumn frost protection.[6a]

Cranberries are related to bilberries, blueberries, and huckleberries, all in *Vaccinium* subgenus *Vaccinium*. These differ in having stouter, woodier stems forming taller shrubs, and in the bell-shaped flowers, the petals not being reflexed. Cranberries are susceptible to false blossom, a harmful but controllable phytoplasma disease common in the eastern production areas of Massachusetts and New Jersey. [6a]

2. Urinary tract infections (UTI)

UTIs are a serious health problem affecting millions of people each year. Infections of the urinary tract are the second most common type of infection in the body. The urinary tract includes the kidneys, ureters, bladder and urethra. Any part of the urinary tract can become infected, but bladder and urethra infections are the most common. Women are especially prone to UTIs for reasons that are not yet well understood. One woman in five develops a UTI during her lifetime. A UTI is a bacterial infection that affects any part of the urinary tract.[10] The main causal agent is *Escherichia coli*. When bacteria get into the bladder or kidney and multiply in the urine, they may cause a UTI. The most common type of UTI is acute cystitis often referred to as a bladder infection. An infection of the upper urinary tract or kidney is known as pyelonephritis, and is potentially more serious. Although, they cause discomfort, urinary tract infections can usually be easily treated with a short course of antibiotics with all no significant difference between the classes of antibiotics commonly used.[10] UTIs are common in women and children and it causes some permanent side effect on kidneys. Since many years, peoples to treatment UTI utilize this herb and sometimes with appropriate antibiotics.[10]

3. Chemistry of cranberry

The chemical compositions of the different genius of *Cranberry* were studied widely. In the most genius of *Cranberry* some chemical compounds such as flavonoids, sugar, protein, total fat and some important fatty acids were identified. Raw cranberries have moderate levels of dietary fiber, Ca, Mg, Mn, P, K, Na, Vitamins C, A, K, Carotene, Lutein, Zeaxanthin and the essential dietary mineral, manganese, as well as a balanced profile of other essential micronutrients.[8] Cranberries also contain malic acid. By measure of the Oxygen Radical Absorbance Capacity with an ORAC score of 9,584 units per 100 g, cranberry ranks near the top of 277 commonly consumed foods.[6a,11,12] Raw cranberries are a source of polyphenol antioxidants, phytochemicals under active research for possible benefits to the cardiovascular system and immune system, and as anti-cancer agents.[6a,13,14]

Cranberry juice contains a chemical component, a high molecular weight non-dialyzable material (NDM), as noted above, that is able to inhibit and even reverse the formation of plaque by *Streptococcus mutans* pathogens that cause tooth decay.[6a,15,16] Cranberry juice components also show efficacy against formation of kidney stones.[6a,17,18] Raw cranberries and cranberry juice are abundant food sources of flavonoids such as proanthocyanidins, flavonols and anthocyanidins (cyanidin, peonidin and quercetin). [6a,19,20] These compounds have shown promise as anti-cancer agents in in vitro studies. However, their effectiveness in humans has not been established, and may be limited by poor absorption into cells and rapid elimination from the blood.[6a] Since 2002, there has been an increasing focus on the potential role of cranberry polyphenolic constituents in preventing several types of cancer.[6a,21-26] In a 2001 University of Maine study that compared cranberries with twenty other fruits demonstrated that cranberries had the largest amount of both free and total phenols, with red grapes at a distant second place. [6a-27] Cranberry tannins have anti-clotting properties and may reduce urinary tract infections [6a-28] and the amount of dental plaque-causing oral bacteria, thus being a prophylaxis for gingivitis.[6a-29]

The main chemical compositions that extracted from *Cranberry* contain mineral compounds, flavonoids, benzoic acid, triterpenoids, anthocyanins, catechin, β-hydroxybutiric acid, citric acid, glucuronic acid, quinic acids, ellagic acid, sugar(fructose, *D*-mannose), protein, total fat and some important fatty acids. In one study, the chemical composition of *Vaccinium arctostaphylos L.* essential oil were determined by utilize GC and GC/MS methods.[9,30] The major determined volatiles in this type of Cranberry, are: hexadecanoic acid(27%), vitispirane(6.5%), β-ionone(5.9%) and sandaracopimaradiene(4.8%).[9,30] L. Y. Foo et al. in 2000 reported the proanthocyanidin fraction of Cranberry, isolated from the ethyl acetate extract that was investigated for ability to prevent adherence of *E. coli* to mannose-resistance adhesion by determining the ability to prevent agglutination of both isolated P-receptor resin-coated beads and human erythrocytes.[9,31] The characterization of Flavonols in Cranberry (*Vaccinium macrocarpon*) were investigated by N. Vorsa et al.[4]. In this report, the main Flavonols were extracted by acetone and ethylacetate and identified in this herb, such as: myricetin-3-β-xylopyranoside, quercetin-3-β-galactoside, quercetin-3-β-glucoside, quercetin-3-α-arabinopyranoside, quercetin-3-α-arabinofuranoside, 3′-methoxyquercetin-3-α-xylopyranoside, quercetin-3-O-(6″-p-coumaroyl)β-galactoside and quercetin-3-O-(6″-benzoyl)β-galactoside.[9,32]

In 2004, two species, *Vaccinium membranaceum* and *Vaccinium ovatum*, native to Pacific Northwestern North America, were evaluated for their total, and individual, anthocyanin and polyphenolic compositions by Lee et al..[33,34] *Vaccinium ovatum* had greater total anthocyanin (ACY), total phenolics (TP), oxygen radical absorbing capacity (ORAC), and ferric reducing antioxidant potential (FRAP) than did *V. membranaceum*. The pH were also higher in *V. ovatum*. Berry extracts from each species were separated into three different fractions anthocyanin, polyphenolic, and sugar/ acids by solid-phase extraction.[33] The anthocyanin fractions of each species had the highest amount of ACY, TP, and antioxidant activity. Each species contained 15 anthocyanins (galactoside, glucoside, and arabinoside of delphinidin, cyanidin, petunidin, peonidin, and malvidin) but in different proportions. Their anthocyanin profiles were similar by high-performance liquid chromatography (HPLC) with photodiode array detection (LC-DAD) and high-performance liquid chromatography with photodiode array and mass spectrometry detections (LC-DAD-MS).[33] Each species had a different polyphenolic profile. The polyphenolics of both species were mainly composed of cinnamic acid derivatives and flavonol glycosides. The major polyphenolic compound in *V. membranaceum* was neochlorogenic acid, and in *V. ovatum*, chlorogenic acid.[33] Some of the main compounds achieved, are: gallic acid, protocatechuic acid; neochlorogenic acid; cinnamic acid dervatives; catechin; chlorogenic acid; vanillic acid; caffeic acid; epicatechin; flavonol glycosides; delphinidin 3-galactoside; delphinidin 3-glucoside; delphinidin 3-arabinoside; cyanidin 3-galactoside; cyanidin 3-glucoside; petunidin 3-galactoside; cyanidin 3-arabinoside; petunidin 3-glucoside; peonidin 3-galactoside; petunidin 3-arabinoside; malvidin 3-galactoside; peonidin 3-glucoside; peonidin 3-arabinoside; malvidin 3-glucoside; malvidin 3-arabinoside.[33,34]

In 2006, the chemical composition of the *Qare-Qat* or Iranian *Vaccinium (V.arctostaphylos L.)* had been investigated by Sedaghathoor etal.[30] It is a shrub that grows in the north of Iran. The fruits of *Qare-Qat* were collected from natural habitats and examined for chemical composition such as minerals. The results showed that the ripe fruit of *V.arctostaphylos L.* had 30.6% sugars, 15.5% protein, 1.5% total fat and 2% soluble solids. Dry matter, nitrogen and calcium contents of fruits were 22.3%, 2.5% and 1.4%, respectively.[30] Furthermore, about twelve compounds were identified as essential oil components of shoots of this plant. The major volatiles present in *Vaccinium arctostaphylos L.* shoots were hexadecanoic acid (27.0%), vitispirane (6.5%), *Beta*-ionone (5.9%) and sandaracopimaradiene (4.8%). Some of the essential oil components of this type of cranberry are: 2-Cyclopenten-1-one, 4-acetyl - 2,3,5,5-pentamethyl; Acetic acid 1-hydroxy-3,7-dimethyl-oct-6-enyl ester; Delta-3-Carene; Vitispirane; Naphthalene-1,2-dihydro-5,8-trimethyl; 1,3-Diacetylbenzene; *β*-Ionone; 2-

Pentadecanone; Sandaracopimaradiene; Hexadecanoic acid; Eicosane-2,6,10,14,18-pentamethyl and Isopimaradiene.[30]
Some of the physicochemical properties, like the logarithm of calculated Octanol-Water partitioning coefficients ($logK_{ow}$), total biodegradation and (TB_d in mol/h) and median lethal concentration 50 (LC_{50}) were calculated for some of the chemicals of the cranberry speciesby the EPI-suit v4.00 package.[35] See Table 1.
The octanol-water partition coefficient (K_{ow}) is a measure of the equilibrium concentration of a compound between octanol and water that indicates the potential for partitioning in to soil organic matter (i.e., a high K_{ow} indicates a compound which will preferentially partition into soil organic matter rather than water). This coefficient is inversely related to the solubility of a compound in water. The $logK_{ow}$ is used in models to estimate plant and soil invertebrate bioaccumulation factors. This parameter is also used in many environmental studies to help determine the environmental fate of chemicals.[9,35-38]
Biodegradation is usually quantified by incubating a chemical compound in presence of a degrader, and measuring some factors like oxygen or production of CO_2. The biodegradation studies demonstrate that microbial biosensors are a viable alternative means of reporting on potential biotransformation. However, a few chemicals are tested and large data sets for different chemicals need for quantitative structural relationship studies.[9,39]
An LC_{50} value is the concentration of a material in air that will kill 50% of the test subjects (animals, typically mice or rats) when administered as a single exposure (typically 1 or 4 hours). Also called the median lethal concentration and lethal concentration 50, this value gives an idea of the relative acute toxicity of an inhalant material. Typical units for LC_{50} values are parts per million (ppm) of material in air, micrograms (10^{-6} = 0.000001 g) per liter of air and milligrams (10^{-3} = 0.001 gr) per cubic meter of air.[9,40]
In accordance with the calculated data of the components 1-21 in cranberries, by EPI-suit v4.00 package (see Table-1), hexadecanoic acid (6.962), sandaracopimaradiene, isopimaradiene (6.445), 2-pentadecanone (5.658), δ-3-carene (4.611), β-ionone (4,424), naphthalene-1,2-dihydro-5,8-trimethyl (3.303) and acetic acid 1-hydroxy-3,7-dimethyl-oct-6-enyl ester (3.023) have the highest logarithm of octanol-water partition coefficient ($logK_{ow}$), respectively. Accordingly, the compounds have the lowest water solubility (S_w, mg.L^{-1}/25ºC). Neochlorogenic acid and Chlorogenic acid with -1.014 have the lowest amount of $logK_{ow}$. The compound with the highest lethal concentration (LC_{50}, mg/L) was gallic acid. Meanwhile, sandaracopimaradiene, isopimaradiene had the lowest LC_{50} (0.04). The total biodegradation (TB_d) of naphthalene-1,2-dihydro-5,8-trimethyl among and δ-3-carene among 1-21 were the highest and for β-ionone was the lowest (in mol/h×10^{-5}).

5. Urinary tract infections (UTI) and cranberry

As discussed Cranberries have enormous medicinal value. These berries are not just good to eat; they also contain different kinds of chemicals that are nutritious. While the people in the 17th century and there about knew generally the basic medicinal values of cranberries (the East Europeans even believed it to have the ability to cure cancer), research today has discovered other medicinal benefits that we can derive from cranberries.[41a-c] Cranberries have been found to be effective in battling urinary tract inflammation, oral disease, as well as even heart ailments. Here we will see how cranberries help prevent Urinary Tract Infection (UTI).[41a-c] While different food products or plants work in different ways, cranberries have their own way of reducing the risk of illness in the human body.[41a-c]

No.	Compounds in Cranberries	Calculated concerns		
		$logK_{ow}$	LC_{50} [b] (in mg/L or ppm)	Total Biodegradation (in mol/h ×10^{-5})
1	2-Cyclopenten-1-one, 4-acetyl -2,3,5,5-pentamethyl	1.531	344.87	5.2
2	Acetic acid 1-hydroxy-3,7-dimethyl-oct-6-enyl ester	3.023	22.52	5.8
3	δ-3-Carene	4.611	0.53	7.9
5	Naphthalene-1,2-dihydro-5,8-trimethyl	3.303	11.44	8.1
6	1,3-Diacetylbenzene	1.354	462.55	5.7
7	β-Ionone	4.424	1.32	1.3
8	2-Pentadecanone	5.658	0.11	3.1
9	Sandaracopimaradiene	6.445	0.04	2.6
10	Hexadecanoic acid	6.962	0.09	3.0
12	Isopimaradiene	6.445	0.04	2.6
13	Gallic acid	0.855	1218.82	5.4
14	Protocatechuic acid	0.914	985.24	6.0
15	Neochlorogenic acid	-1.014	272.80	2.6
16	Cinnamic acid	2.071	989.53	6.5
17	Catechin	1.175	1115.68	3.2
18	Chlorogenic acid	-1.014	272.80	2.6
19	Vanillic acid	1.219	593.19	5.5
20	Caffeic acid	1.110	785.65	5.1
21	Epicatechin	1.175	1115.68	3.2

[a]The values were calculated by EPI-suit v4.00 package.[35] [b] Asterisk designates, Chemical may not be soluble.

Table 1. The calculated logarithm of calculated Octanol-Water partitioning coefficients ($logK_{ow}$), water solubility at 25°C (mg/L), median lethal concentration 50 (LC_{50}) and total biodegradation and (TB_d in mol/h) of some of the chemical components of some species of Cranberries.[35]

One of the biggest and most widely health benefits of eating cranberries, in whatever form, either as whole fruit or juice or cocktail, is that it helps prevent urinary tract infection (UTI). While this was what our elders passed on to us as traditional oral medicinal knowledge, it is now recognized as official medical fact.[41a-c]

Kidney stones are most often caused by high levels of ionized calcium (as in calcium salts) in the urine. Cranberries can help prevent this condition because they are rich in quinic acid, which increases the acidity of the urine. As a result, the levels of ionized calcium in the urine are lowered. The infection is basically caused by bacteria.[41a-c, 42] The bacteria latch on to the surface or lining of the cells of different body parts. Once they are attached to the lining of the specific body part in question, they feed off the cells or the surface or the lining they are attached to, and increase their numbers by reproducing, and in the process cause infections. In the case of UTI, this process happens in the lining of the urinary tract.[41a-c,

42] Initially, researchers went off-track when they figured that the cranberries' ability to prevent UTI was because of its acidity. It has reported that cranberries prevent UTI by preventing the bacteria causing UTI from attaching itself to the surface of the urinary tract lining. Amy Howell published this discovery in the New England Journal of Medicine in 1998.[41a-c-50] The research shows that cranberries are basically rich in proanthocyanidins. Proanthocyanidins are tannins, a type of organic chemical compound, that have been condensed. This is how it works. The proanthocyanidins have their own specific way of functioning - they are blockers that block the bacteria from attaching themselves to the surface of the lining of the specific body part in question. In the case of UTI, the proanthocyanidins prevent the bacteria from getting glued to the lining of the urinary tract.[42-50] The most common side effects associated with excessive cranberry consumption are diarrhea and an increased risk of developing kidney stones. Regular cranberry consumption by women trying to prevent UTIs may result in *vulvovaginal candidiasis*. Alterations in the normal vaginal bacteria may lead to increased *fungal* growth.[42]

In 1984 was surveyed the anti adhering of Cranberry on 77 strains of *E. coli* that in 75% samples it was verified.[38] In 1994, was examined the extraction of this herb for treating 153 persons who involved to UTI.[39] In 1995, was showed that UTI in women is decreased for 52% by Craberry extract prophylaxy.[9,40,51] In 2006, was investigated the effect of Cranberry in prevention on urinary tract infection in children, and prevention of nonspecific bacterial cell adhesion in immunoassays by use of Cranberry juice.[9,52,53] Sometimes peoples to treatment UTIs, utilize this herb with appropriate antibiotics.

6. Experimental section

In this study, were examined 61 isolated *E. coli* from urine sample of the patients that they had referred to the hospitals and laboratories of Sanandaj city. Dried fruit of Cranberry (*Vaccinium arctostaphylos L.*) was altered to powder and then was acquired aqueous extraction (1%) from it. This concentration was based on Boland's study.[9] The most concentration of Cranberry in media was selected that had not any effect on bacteria on the media than media without plant extract. One control plate (Mueller-Hilton agar without Cranberry) was chosen for each strain.

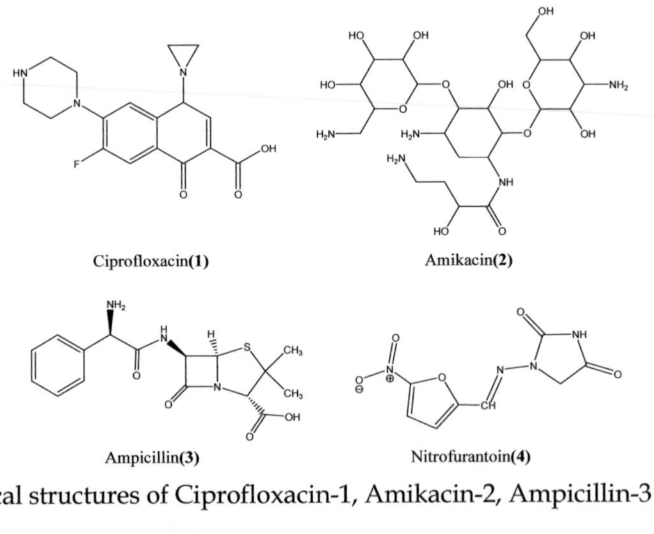

Fig. 2. The chemical structures of Ciprofloxacin-1, Amikacin-2, Ampicillin-3 and Nitrofurantoin-4.

The other plate contained Mueller-Hilton agar accompanied Cranberry 1% extraction. A certain number of bacterias (1.5x10^8 CFU/ml) based on 0.5 Macfarland scale was cultured on the media. After this stage, the antibiotic disks (Ciprofloxacin-1, Amikacin-2, Ampicillin-3, Tetracyclin, Co-trimoxazole, Nalidixic acid, Ceftazidime and Nitrofurantoin-4) were cultured. After 24 hours incubation in 37°C was measured the zone around of the each disks and compared with standard schedule.[9,54]

6.1 Results and discussions

The results of the investigation were demonstrated in Table-1. The results were analyzed based on Ki test. The most susceptibility belonged to Amikacin-2 in frequency of the control group with 93.45%. The lowest frequency was 9.8% for Ampicillin-3. The other type of antibiotics the susceptibilities in control group were: Co-trimoxazol 39.34%, Ceftazidime 51%, Nalidixic acid 54.1%, Nitrofurantoin 62.3%, Tetracyclin 72.13% and Ciprofloxacin-1 73.8%. In test group, Nitrofurantoin-4 shows the most susceptibility (72.13%) and the lowest belongs to Ampicilline(18%). In addition, percentage of susceptibility for other antibiotics as Amikacin, Co-trimoxazole, Nalidix acid, Ceftazidime and Tetracyclin were: 28.87%, 34.42%, 52.48%, 55% and 70.5%, respectively.[9] In accordance with the results, not only aqueous extract of Cranberry did not show any synergistic effect with any antibiotics, but also it showed sever antagonistic effect against Ciprofloxacine-1 and Amikacine-2 ($P=0.00$). See Table-2. However, in acidic pH Ampicillin-3 and Nitrofurantoin-4 had 10% increased in function, but in the whole statistical computation did not show any significant difference (see Table-2). Nitrofurantoin-4 shows better function in acidic pH. Ampicillin and Amoxicillin are resistant and absorbed much better in acidic pH. On the contrary, Co-trimoxazole is more effective in alkaline pH.[9] In neutral or acidic media it is changed to crystal form and precipitate.[9,54] In spite of the fact that there are no significant statistical difference between two plates (test plate and control plate), It was found that antagonistic effect between Cranberry and two antibiotic disks i.e. Ciprofloxacin-1 and Amikacin-2 ($P=0.00$). The results show that use Cranberry with some antibiotics that explained here can diminish the medicinal effects of the antibiotics in UTIs treatments. The awareness about interfere and the suppression of the appropriate medicinal effect of antibiotics by *Vaccinium arctostaphylos L.* can be useful for treating UTIs.[9]

Some of the physicochemical properties like: the logarithm of calculated Octanol-Water partitioning coefficients ($logK_{ow}$), total biodegradation and (TB_d in mol/h and gr./h), water solubility (S_w, mg.L^{-1}/25°C) and median lethal concentration 50 (LC_{50}) were calculated for the antibiotics (Ciprofloxacin, Amikacin, Ampicillin and Nitrofurantoin). The octanol-water partition coefficient (K_{ow}) is a measure of the equilibrium concentration of a compound between octanol and water that indicates the potential for partitioning in to soil organic matter (i.e., a high K_{ow} indicates a compound which will preferentially partition into soil organic matter rather than water).[35-40] The TB_d is another useful and important factors in chemical and biochemical studies. It needs to use the effective and useful mathematical methods for making good concern between several data in chemistry and biochemistry. An LC_{50} value is the concentration of a material in air that will kill 50% of the test subjects (animals, typically mice or rats) when administered as a single exposure (typically 1 or 4 hours). One of the other important physicochemical factors of compounds is water solubility (S_w, mg.L^{-1}/25°C). Some of the other calculated physicochemical properties of the antibiotics (Ciprofloxacin, Amikacin, Ampicillin and Nitrofurantoin) on UTIs that is created by *Escherichia coli* in Vitro and some of the chemical components of *Cranberry* were calculated.

Concerns		Ciprofloxacin(1)			Amikacin(2)			Ampicillin(3)			Nitrofurantoin(4)		
		Blank	Cranberry	Total	Blank	Cranberry	Total	Blank	Cranberry	Total	Blank	Cranberry	Total
Susceptibility	No.	45	11	56	57	17	74	6	11	17	38	44	82
	%	73.8	18	-	93.45	28.87	-	9.8	18	-	62.3	72.13	-
Stability	No	16	50	66	4	44	48	55	50	105	23	17	40
	%	26.2	82	-	6.55	72.13	-	90.2	82	-	73.7	27.87	-

*The P-value for the samples was 0.00.

Table 2. The comparison of the sensitivity of *Escherichia coli* to the antibiotics (1-4).[9]

Antibiotics 1-4	Calculated concerns			
	$logK_{ow}$ [a]	Water Solubility at 25°C (mg/L)	LC_{50} [b] (in mg/L or ppm)	Total Biodegradation (in mol/h $\times 10^{-5}$)
Ciprofloxacin(1)	-8×10^{-4}	11480	9303.95	2.8
Amikacin(2)	-8.7807	1×10^{6}	3.15×10^{8}	1.6
Ampicillin(3)	1.4538	439.3	780.24	2.7
Nitrofurantoin(4)	-0.1675	1382.0	12523.00	3.9

[a]The values were calculated by EPI-suit v4.00 package.[35] [b] Asterisk designates, Chemical may not be soluble.

Table 3. The calculated logarithm of calculated Octanol-Water partitioning coefficients ($logK_{ow}$), water solubility at 25°C (mg/L), median lethal concentration 50 (LC_{50}) and total biodegradation and (TB_d in mol/h) of the antibiotics Ciprofloxacin(1), Amikacin(2), Ampicillin(3) and Nitrofurantoin(4).[9,35]

[35-40] See Table-3. In accordance with the calculated data of the antibiotics (ciprofloxacin-1, Amikacin-2, Ampicillin-3 and Nitrofurantoin-4), by EPI-suit v4.00 package (see Table-3), ampicillin-3 (1.4538) has the highest logarithm of octanol-water partition coefficient ($logK_{ow}$). Accordingly, the compound has the lowest water solubility (S_w, mg.L^{-1}/25°C). Amikacin-2 with -8.7807 has the lowest amount of $logK_{ow}$ among selected antibiotics 1-4. The calculations show that the antibiotic with the highest lethal concentration (LC_{50}, mg/L) was amikacin-2. Meanwhile, ampicillin-3 had the lowest LC_{50}. The total biodegradation (TB_d) of Nitrofurantoin-4 among the selected antibiotics 1-4 was the highest and for amikacin-2 was the lowest (in mol/h$\times10^{-5}$).

7. Conclusion

The chemical compositions of the different types of Craberry were investigated. It was determined that this type of medicinal herb was utilized for UTI treatments. *Vaccinium arctostaphylos L.* genus was used to investigate the synergistic effect of aqueous Cranberry (*Vaccinium arctostaphylos L.*) extract in accompanied with antibiotics (Ciprofloxacin-1, Amikacin-2, Ampicillin-3 and Nitrofurantoin-4) on UTIs created by *Escherichia coli* in Vitro. The results show that use Cranberry with some antibiotics that explained here can show some interference effects with the antibiotics and diminish the medicinal effects of the antibiotics (antagonist effect) in Urinary tract infections (UTI) treatments.[9] Some of the physicochemical properties, like the logarithm of calculated Octanol-Water partitioning coefficients ($logK_{ow}$), total biodegradation and (TB_d in mol/h) and median lethal concentration 50 (LC_{50}) were calculated for some of the chemicals of the cranberry species and antibiotics (Ciprofloxacin-1, Amikacin-2, Ampicillin-3 and Nitrofurantoin-4).[9,35-40]

8. References

[1] a)Urinary tract infection ,Wikipedia:
http://en.wikipedia.org/wiki/Urinary_tract_infection.

b) Nicolle LE (February 2008). "Uncomplicated urinary tract infection in adults including uncomplicated pyelonephritis". *Urol. Clin. North Am.* 35 (1): 1–12.
c) Murray P., Rsental K., Pfaller M."Medical Microbiology", 2005, ; ElSEVIER MOSBY; 5th ed.
d) Mahon C., Lehman D.,Manuselis G. "Text Book of Diagnostic Microbiology"; 2007; ; ElSEVIER; 3rd ed.
e) "Bacteriology- TOPLEY and WILSON'S Microbiology and Microbial I nfections", 2005, , Edward Arnold, volume 2, Edward Arnold publisher,10th ed.
[2] a) Justice S, Hunstad D, Seed P, Hultgren S (2006). Filamentation by *Escherichia coli* subverts innate defenses during urinary tract infection. *Proc Natl Acad Sci USA* 103 (52): 19884–9.
b) http://www.biofilmsonline.com/cgi-bin/biofilmsonline/00448.html.
[3] Foxman, B (2003). "Epidemiology of urinary tract infections: incidence, morbidity, and economic costs.". *Disease-a-month* 49 (2): 53–70.
[4] Hooton, T. M. (1990). "The epidemiology of urinary tract infection and the concept of significant bacteriuria". *Infection* 18: S40–3.
[5] Dai, B; Liu, Y; Jia, J; Mei, C (2010). "Long-term antibiotics for the prevention of recurrent urinary tract infection in children: a systematic review and meta-analysis.". *Archives of disease in childhood* 95 (7): 499–508.
[6] a) http://en.wikipedia.org/wiki/Cranberry.
b) http://www.cranberryinstitute.org/about_cranberry.htm.
c) http://www.tcpalm.com/news/2009/nov/19/give-thanks-for-cranberries-grown-with-a-taste.
d) http://www.hortresearch.co.nz/index/news/493.
[7] http://www.cranberries.org/cranberries/history.html.
[8] a) Schonbeck-Temesy E., Wien, K. H. Rechinger K. H.(1992) *Flora Iranica*, Graz. b) Huxley A., (1992) *The New RHS Dictionary of Gardening,* MacMillan Press, New York. c)http://en.wikipedia.org/wiki/Vaccinium;http://www.ibiblio.org/pfaf/cgibin/arr_html?Vaccinium+arctostaphylos&CAN=LATIND .
[9] Taherpour A., Noorabadi P., Abedii F. and Taherpour A. A., (2008) Effect of Aqueous Cranberry(*Vaccinium arctostaphylos L.*)Extract Accompanied with Antibiotics on UTIs caused by Escherichia coli in vitro, *J. Pur. & Appl. Micro.,* 2(1), 135-138.
[10] a) http://kidney.niddk.nih.gov/kudiseases/pubs/utiadult/
b) http://familydoctor.org/online/famdocen/home/women/gen-health/190.html.
c) http://www.wrongdiagnosis.com/u/urinary_tract_infections/intro.htm.
d) http://www.patient.co.uk/doctor/Urinary-Tract-Infection-in-Adults.htm.
[11] Oxygen Radical Absorbance Capacity (ORAC) of Selected Foods (2007). Prepared by Nutrient Data Laboratory Beltsville Human Nutrition Research Center (BHNRC) Agricultural Research Service (ARS) U.S. Department of Agriculture (USDA). http://www.ars.usda.gov/nutrientdata.
[12] http://www.nal.usda.gov/fnic/foodcomp/search/.
[13] Seifried H.E., Anderson D.E., Fisher E.I., Milner J.A. (2007). A review of the interaction among dietary antioxidants and reactive oxygen species. *J Nutr Biochem.* 18 (9): 567–79.

[14] Halliwell B. (2007). Dietary polyphenols: good, bad, or indifferent for your health?. *Cardiovasc Res.* 73(2) 341–7.

[15] http://www.cranberryinstitute.org/health/dental.htm.

[16] http://www.webmd.com/food-recipes/news/20051123/cranberry-juice-cuts-cavities.

[17] McHarg T., Rodgers A., Charlton K. (2003) Influence of cranberry juice on the urinary risk factors for calcium oxalate kidney stone formation. *BJU Int.* 92(7) 765–8.

[18] Kessler T., Jansen B., Hesse A. (2002). Effect of blackcurrant-, cranberry- and plum juice consumption on risk factors associated with kidney stone formation. *Eur J Clin Nutr,* 56(10) 1020–3.

[19] Duthie S.J., Jenkinson A.M., Crozier A., *et al.* (2006) The effects of cranberry juice consumption on antioxidant status and biomarkers relating to heart disease and cancer in healthy human volunteers. *Eur J Nutr* 45 (2): 113–22.

[20] Zheng W., Wang S.Y. (2003) Oxygen radical absorbing capacity of phenolics in blueberries, cranberries, chokeberries, and lingonberries. *J Agric Food Chem.* 51 (2) 502-9.

[21] I.O. Vvedenskaya & N. Vorsa, Flavonoid composition over fruit development and maturation in American cranberry, Vaccinium macrocarpon *Ait. Plant Science,* 167(5), 2004, 1043-1054.

[22] http://newsletter.cancerresearchsociety.ca/bulletin/omni/articles/4190.aspx.

[23] Neto C.C. (2007). "Cranberry and blueberry: evidence for protective effects against cancer and vascular diseases". *Mol Nutr Food Res* 51 (6): 652–64.

[24] Ferguson P.J., Kurowska E.M., Freeman D.J., Chambers A.F., Koropatnick J. (2006). "In vivo inhibition of growth of human tumor lines by flavonoid fractions from cranberry extract". *Nutr Cancer* 56 (1): 86–94.

[25] Seeram N.P., Adams L.S., Zhang Y., *et al.* (December 2006). "Blackberry, black raspberry, blueberry, cranberry, red raspberry, and strawberry extracts inhibit growth and stimulate apoptosis of human cancer cells in vitro". *J Agric Food Chem.* 54 (25): 9329–39.

[26] Sun J., Chu Y.F., Wu X., Liu R.H. (2002). Antioxidant and antiproliferative activities of common fruits. *J Agric Food Chem.* 50 (25): 7449–54.

[27] Vinson J.A., Su X., Zubik L., Bose P. (2001). Phenol antioxidant quantity and quality in foods: fruits. *J Agric Food Chem.* 49 (11): 5315–21.

[28] Efros M., Bromberg W., Cossu L., Nakeleski E., Katz A.E. (2010), Novel concentrated cranberry liquid blend, UTI-STAT with Proantinox, might help prevent recurrent urinary tract infections in women. *Urology.* 76(4) 841-5.

[29] http://www.eurekalert.org/pub_releases/2008-07/wpi-cjc072108.php.

[30] Sedaghathoor S., Kashi A. K., Talaei A. R., Khalighi A. (2006), *In. J. Agr. Bio.,* 8(1), 45-46.

[31] Foo L. Y., Lu Y., Howell A. B. and Vorsa N. (2000) *Phytochemistry,* 54, 173-181.

[32] Vvedenskaya I. O., Rosen R. T., Guido J. E., Russell D. J., Mills K. A. and Vorsa N. (2004) *J. Agri. Food Chem.,* 52(2), 188-195.

[33] Lee J., Finn C. E. and Wrolstad R. E. (2004) *J. Agric. Food Chem.,* 2004, 52, 7039-7044.

[34] Lee, J.; Finn, C. E.; Wrolstad, R. E. (2003) Anthocyanin pigment and total phenolic content of three *Vaccinium* species native to the Pacific Northwest of North America. *HortScience, 5,* 959-964.

[35] Foo L. Y., Lu Y., Howell A. B. and Vorsa N. (2000),, *Phytochemistry,* 54, 173-181.

[36] Vvedenskaya I. O., Rosen R. T., Guido J. E., Russell D. J., Mills K. A. and Vorsa N. (2004) *J. Agri. Food Chem.*, 52(2), 188-195.

[37] Sobota A. (1984) *J. Urol.*, 131(5), 1013-1016.

[38] Ofek I., Goldhar G., Zafriri D., N. (1991) *Engl. J. Med.*, 324, 1599.

[39] Foxman B., Geiger A. M., Palin K. (1995) *Epidemiology*, 6(2), 162-168.

[40] a) http://www.furtherhealth.com/article/54_1_The-Cranberry/.
b) http://www.furtherhealth.com/article/54_2_Cranberry-Facts/.
c) http://www.furtherhealth.com/article/54_3_Benefits-of-Cranberries/.

[41] http://www.altmd.com/Articles/Cranberry--Encyclopedia-of-Alternative-Medicine

[42] Davies J.R. (2000), *Healing Herbs-In a Nutshell: CRAN BERRY*.Boston:Element Books, Inc.

[43] Fetrow C. W. and Juan R. A. (2000) *The Complete Guide to Herbal Medicines*. Springhouse, PA: Springhouse Corporation.

[44] McCaleb R., Evelyn L. and Krista M. (2000) *The Encyclopedia of Popular Herbs: Your Complete Guide to the Leading Medicinal Plants*. Rocklin, CA: Prima Health.

[45] Murray M. and Joseph P. (1998) *Encyclopedia of Natural Medicine*. Rocklin, CA: Prima Health.

[46] Avorn J., Monane M., Gurwitz J.H., et al. (1994) Reduction of Bacteriuria and Pyuria after Ingestion of Cranberry Juice. *J. of the American Medical Association*, 271, 751-4.

[47] Jepson R., Mihaljevic L. and Craig J.,(2004) Cranberries for preventing urinary tract infection. *Cochrane Database Syst Rev*.

[48] Patel, D.A., B. Gillespie, J.D. Sobel, et al. (2004) Risk factors for recurrent vulvovaginal candidiasis in women receiving maintenance antifungal therapy: Results of a prospective cohort study,*American Journal of Obstetrics and Gynecology*, 644–53.

[49] Weiss, E.I., A. Kozlovsky, D. Steinberg, R., et al. (2004) A high molecular mass cranberry constituent reduces mutans streptococci level in saliva and inhibits in vitro adhesion to hydroxyapatite. *FEMS Microbiol Lett*, 89–92.

[50] Schlager T. A., Anderson S., Trudell J. K. (1999) *J. Pediatric*, 135(6), 698-702.

[51] Fanos V., Atzei A., Zaffanello M., Piras A. and Cataldi L. (2006) *J. Chemoth.*,18(3), 21-24.

[52] Johnson-White B., Buquo L., Zeinali M., Ligler F. S. (2006) *Analy. Chem.*, 78(3), 853-857.

[53] Bertran G. (2001) *Basic & Clinical Pharmacology*, 8th Ed., pp. 771, 757, 765, 796, 798, 800, 808, 810 and 846.

Part 7

Urinary Tract Infection in Children

19

Urinary Tract Infection in Children

Hsiao-Wen Chen
Department of Pediatric Urology
Chang Gung Children Hospital
Chang Gung University
Taoyuan,
Taiwan

1. Introduction

Urinary tract infection(UTI) is not uncommon cause of bacterial illness in children,4-8% of children have had an UTI from a population based study (Sureshkumar, Jones et al. 2009). The prevalence of UTIs is quite different between two gender and age with high incidence in girls(1% in male and 3% in female), except the male infants with an incidence of 0.7% compared to the 0.1~0.4% of female infants (Foxman 2002),which is due to bacterias harbor in prepuce of youg infant,there was at least a tenfold increased risk for UTIs in noncircumcised compared with circumcised infant(Thomas, Wiswell et al.1986). The symptomatic UTIs raise a significant anxiety for parents and physician with concerning the potential of associated urinary tract disorders or abnormalities. Furthermore, UTIs recur more than 20% in young population, antimicrobial treatment and further investigation warrant in this circumstances. The most common cause of recurrent UTIs is related to the abnormal urinary tract, such as vesicoureteral reflux (VUR), duplex collecting system , spinal dysraphism with neurogenic bladder, Hinman's syndrome …etc. However, the modalities of clinical survey are still controversial regarding the invasiveness and discomfort of examination, it may be need anesthesia. In addition, imaging for UTIs is bearing risk of radiation exposure, the recent reports advocate that the invasive examination such as voiding cystourethrography(VCUG) should be reserved for those with likelihood of VUR with renal damage or dysplasia from the less invasive studies, such as ultrasoud (US) (Preda, Jodal et al. 2011). Meanwhile, additional subject of management for congenital urinary abnormalities associated with UTIs is ongoing debate. This chapter will review the relevant literatures and examine the practical scenarios to cover the top-down approach of urinary tract infection in children, including pathogenesis, host-defense mechanism of the urinary tract, the comprehension of relationship between UTIs and congenital abnormalities or dysfunction, as well as the up-to-date of treatment concept.

2. Pathogenesis of UTIs

The etiology of UTIs is not well understood, and though to be related to gender, bowel habit, urinary incontinence and congenital abnormalities of urinary tract. The most frequent organism is Escherichia (E. Coli),which is originally an harmless flora in human intestine and has some properties as virulence factors (VFs) to overcome the new environment, with bearing the ability to colonize and adhere to the uro-epithial cell through its fimbriase (P fimbriae, type-1 fimbria),the prevalence of P fimbriation from patients with severe UTIs such as urosepsis is high as 71% compared with 70% in pyelonephritis and 28% in other sources of infection (Brauner, Leissner et al.1987). The process of invasion acts as cytotoxic/endotoxic effect via lipopolysaccharide, aerobactin and enterochelin production, whereas the process of pyelonephritis occurring so call "Nephropathy" (Gally, Bogan et al. 1993; Olianti, Imperiale et al. 2004). Moreover,several gene polymorphisms such as toll-like receotor-2(TLR2) gene,TLR4 gene,heat shock protein 72(HSPA1B) gene are closely associated with the hosts who were vulnerable to UTIs(Karoly, Fekete et al.2006; Tabel, Berdeli et al.2007). In addition,the micro-organisms can alter the gene expression with changing their phenotype in order to adjust to host environment (Johnson 1991).At the point of host defence,urinary tract of human can fundamentally prevent ascending infection from micro-organisms. For instance, urine bolus excretes from renal calyces into bladder through the eccentric peristalsis of ureter, on the other hand, urine from bladder is not allow to reflux backward into ureter by the antireflux competence of submucosal tunnel subset between ureter and bladder. The regular empty of bladder can also prevent the pathogens stasis within lower urinary tract. For these reasons, most of UTIs in children are incidental and promptly recovery with appropriate antibiotics or correction of daily hygiene. However, a minority need to be paid attention on the risk of morbidities, including nephropathy from the chronic pyelonephritis, associated congenital abnormalities, or voiding disorders.

3. Clinical manifestations

Comparing to the adults the symptoms of UTIs in children are not specific owing to the limitation of the verbal expression, fever or chillness is the most general manifestation (National Collaborating Centre for Women's and Children's Health 2007) and followed with lethargic or irritable presentations. Low urinary tract syndrome such as dysuria, pain on micturiction, frequency, incontinence, suprapubic discomfort may be present.

3.1 Acute pyelonephritis

Acute pyelonephritis (APN) is considered if a febrile UTI associated with excess of CRP (Naber, Bergman et al. 2001; Huang, Huang et al. 2007).On the basis of Technetium-99m dimercaptosuccinic acid scintigraphy(DMSA), Nikfar et al. found procalcitonin concentration test could also be useful in the diagnosis of APN with 77% and 89% of sensitivity and specificity comparing to 80% and 65% of C-reative protein(CRP)(Nikfar, Khotaee et al. 2010). However, DMSA still remains the standard tool for diagnosis of APN (Levitchenko, Lahy et al. 2001). At 6 months after APN, 88% of scars were observed by Parex et al., the overall of scars persisted in 27% after 3 years of follow-up. Additionally, increased number of scars from APN was related to high grade VUR (Parrex, Willi et al 2008).

3.2 Acute lobar nephronia

The progression of APN may cause acute and nonsuppurative renal infection with focal tissue edema and leukocytic infiltration that affect one or more lobules of kidney, so call acute lobar nephronia (ALN), which represents a focal mass effect in US or CT, histology may present with acute pyelonephritis and micro-abscesses (Rosenfield, Glickman et al 1979). Klar et al. report 13 patients with 16 episodes of ALN in 210 hospitalized children with urinary tract infection, the most commen pathogen was *E.coli* (Klar, Hurvitz et al.

1996). It is crucial to differentiate ALN from renal abscess regard to their different pathogenesis and treatment, as the ALN needs antibiotics treated with duration at least 2-3 weeks, whereas renal abscess may recquire drainage in addition to antibiotic control (Mark, Zaontz et al. 1984; Rothore, Barton et al. 1991)

3.3 Cystitis

Cystitis is rare in children and usually present with acute symptoms including suprapubic pain, dysuria, frequency or incontinence, the differentiation to the non-infected lower urinary dysfunction (LUTD) should be made based on the urine finding.The uncommon inflammation of bladder caused by fungus, virus or allergy, sometimes masquerade as bladder tumor in US finding (Friedman, Friedman et al.1993; Rosenberg, Eggli et al.1994).

4. Diagnosis and management strategies

In addition to the clinical manifestations, the diagnosis of UTIs can be definitely based on the finding of urine sample either via clean mid-stream urine directly voided by child or collection of urine by sterile bag attached around the urethra in infants or young children who are unable to void voluntarily, otherwise, catheterization or suprapubic aspiration may be used. UTIs should be considered in an urine sample with pyuria or bacteria (National Collaborating Centre for Women's and Children's Health 2007). The threshold of diagnosis depends upon the access of urine sample collection, the less of false positive rate, the more invasive in the fashion of urine obtaining (Hellerstein 1982). As matter of fact, 80% of general pratitioners recommended the use of an urine bag reported by Kennedy et al., the remaining 20% recommended using a dean catch sample (Kennedy, Glynn et al. 2010).

UTIs should be identified as simple or complicated infection by localization of infectious nidus (Figure 1) and whether a recurrent or atypical UTI(Box 1). In order to facilitate the diagnosis and treatment decision, the differentiation of upper urinary tract infection including kidney or ureter between lower urinary tract including bladder or urethra should be conducted based on the clinical symptoms and signs.

Although the prediction rate of US for abnormalities has been questioned (Zamir, Sakran et al. 2004; Riccabona and Fotter 2009), notwithstanding, many congenital abnormalities of urinary tract have currently been detected by prenatal sonography. US is still considered an ideal tool to examine the urinary tract for children with first UTI for its noninvasiveness, reproducibility and lack of radiation exposure. The subtle architecture of kidney can be investigated in the context of APN including acute focal bacterial nephritis (ALN), renal abscess, pyohydronephrosis or stone associated infection (Klar, Hurvitz et al. 1996; Sureshkumar, Jones et al. 2009). Additionally, US can investigate the children with lower urinary tract dysfunction with estimation of residual urine, bladder outline and capacity (Uehling, Hahnfeld et al. 2000; Dacher and Savoye-Collet 2004).

DMSA scintigraphy remains the important examination in the diagnosis of APN,defects in renal outline without any loss of renal volume can be found, whereas in scarring, the defect is associated with focal loss of renal mass (Piepsz A, Colarinha P et al. 2001). However, a 100% of high negative diagnostic value for detection of renal scarring during the acute stage of infection was reported by Hitzel et al., therefore, the follow-up should be ongoing after 6 months of acute pylonephritis to avoid the negative diagnostic value (Hitzel, Liard et al. 2002).

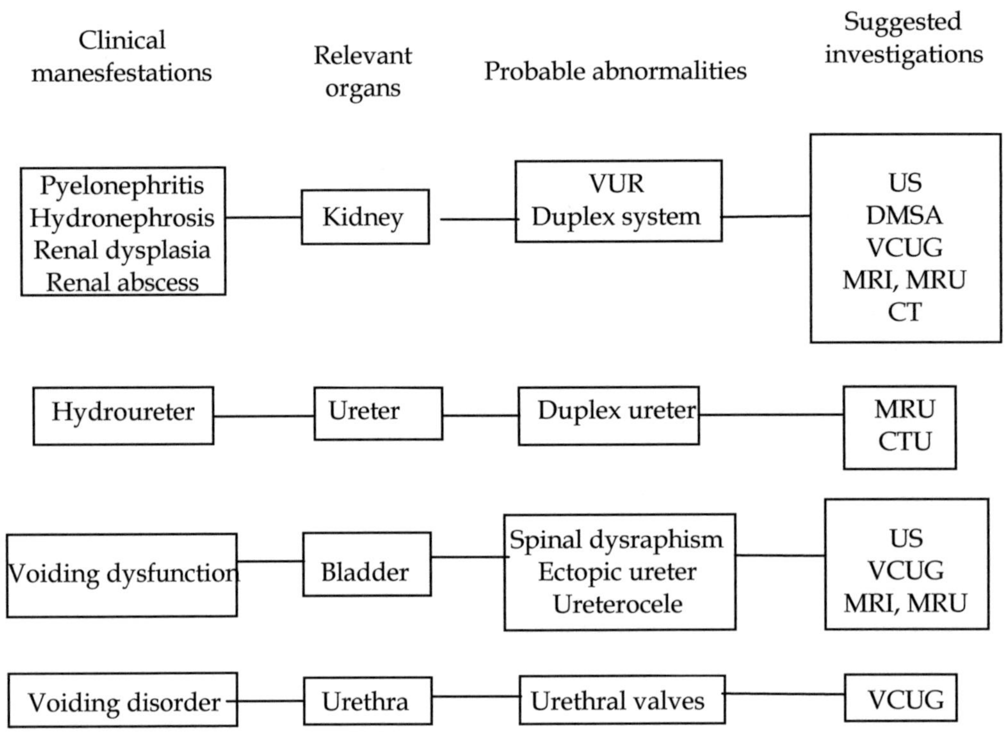

Fig. 1. Algorithm for Investigation of Associated Abnormalities in Children with UTIs.

Atypical (any of the following)

- Septicaemia or patients who looks seriously ill (see NICE guideline [2])
- Poor urine flow
- Abdominal or bladder mass
- Raised creatinine concentration
- Failure to respond to treatment with suitable antibiotics within 48 hours
- Infection with non-Escherichia coli organisms

Recurrent(any of the following)

- Two or more episodes of urinary tract infection with acute pyelonephritis or upper urinary tract infection
- One episode of urinary tract infection with acute pyelonephritis or upper urinary tract infection plus one or more episode of urinary tract infection with cystitis or lower urinary tract infection
- Three or more episodes of urinary tract infection with cystitis or lower urinary tract infection

Box 1. Main characteristics of patients with atypical or recurrent tract infection. Adapted from Rintaro et al.(2007).BJM 25:335:395-396; http://guidance.nice.org.uk/CG54

Magnetic resonance imaging (MRI, MRU) and enhanced CT are recently applied for depiction of APN and renal scarring. As the detection rate is questioning and availability is limited for requirement of sedation and injection of a potentially nephrotoxic medium while performaning the examination, which is reserved for children with doubtful diagnosis or suspicion of congenital abnormalities (Lonergan, Pennington et al. 1998; Kavanagh, Ryan et al. 2005). However, in UTIs with voiding dysfunction, MRI is practical to evaluate the spinal cord and facilitate the diagnosis of abnormalities associated with neurogenic bladder,such as spinal dysraphism with tethered cord (Siomou, Giapros et al. 2009).
VCUG remains a reference examination for VUR, which requires urethral catheterization and radiation exposure, many parents are reluctant to the performance and it is reserved on an individual with likehood of VUR from otherwise noninvasive access, such as DMSA scan or US examination (Herz, Merguerian et al. 2010, Preda , Jodal et al. 2011). However, VCUG permits the effective grading of VUR when the treatment strategy is demanding. Moreover, in case with suspicion of urethral valves or VURD syndrome, VCUG is indispensable to search the urethra, bladder and even voiding function.

5. Nosocomial infection of urinary tract

Urinary tract infection in nosocomial infection is less common in children compared with adults, it encountered the 3rd to 5th most common infection in hospitalized children with incidence varied from 6-42% according to the different denominators (Ford-Jones, Mindorff et al. 1989; Weber, Sheridan et al. 1997; Orrett, Brook et al. 1999). *E. coli* is still the predominant pathogen followed by *Candida* species, *Enterococcus, Pseudomonas* species and *Klebsiella* species (Langley, Hanakowski et al. 2001; Prelog, Schieficker et al. 2007). Several risk factors include immunocompromise, broadly antibiotics use, or obstruction of urinary tract can cause nosocomial infection. However, instrustment of the urinary tract is still the most frequent risk for nosocomial urinary tract infection. Therefore, the surveillance of the use of urinary catheter is the main focus for the infection control in hospitalized children.

6. Complex UTIs

Most UTIs are simple and easy to be controlled by antibiotic treatment. Sureshkumar et al. reported female gender,encopresis,daytime urinary incontinence and renal anatomical problems are risk factors associated with UTIs(Sureshkumar,Jones et al.2009).Nonetheless, infants with febrile UTIs or children younger than 2 years of age are highly associated with congenital urinary tract abnormalities.Therefore, many different factors and scenario should be considered when children with recurrent or atypical UTIs,then anatomic or neurological evaluations warrant ongoing.

6.1 VUR and associated abnormalities

VUR encountered the most abnormalities with 25%to 50% of children with UTIs (Smellie, Normand et al. 1981; Downs 1999) which are also related to the hydronephrosis, renal dysplasia, duplex collecting system, or voiding dysfunction. Reflux nephropathy is the main concerning as 13~25% of patients develop end-stage renal disease from the inflammatory and immunological processes(Askari and Belman 1982; Craig, Irwig et al. 2000; Ardissino, Avolio et al. 2004). The risk of developing "Reflux nephropathy" is multiprediposing and related to the host susceptibility and virulence of bacteria(Matsuoka, Nakashima et al. 2006;

Cendron 2008; Coulthard 2008). Although the management of VUR remains controversial, the ultimate goal is to prevent the further renal injury from reflux and repeat UTIs. Not more than 30% of spontaneous resolution rate for mild to moderate grade of VUR and less for high grade (Green field and Wan 1996; Kundson, Austin et al. 2007). Series of literatures reported no significant benefits in control of renal scarring or recurrent UTIs with antibiotic use (Garin, Olavarria et al. 2006). Comparing with antibiotics alone, there is no any additional benefit of surgery except for a reduction of UTIs from a meta-analyses data(Wheeler, Vimalachandra et al. 2003). Surgical correction may at least mitigate the UTIs and process of nephropathy. In addition, several new antireflux techniques have been introduced with less invasiveness or high success rate from 70~98% (Lakshmanan and Fung 2000; Chen, Yuan et al. 2004; Routh, Inman et al. 2010).

Otherwise, the abnormalities associated with VUR such as duplex ureters with an obstruction of one renal moiety, ureterocele, ectopic opening of ureteral orifice that causes incontinence, or reflux associated with urethral valves, then surgical correction should be considered to prevent repeat UTIs and further renal damage.

6.2 Voiding disorders

Children with voiding dysfunction may present with UTIs or VUR as the consequence of urinary stasis and high bladder pressure (Whelan and McKenna 2004; Chen, Mao et al. 2004; Feldman and Bauer 2006). Twenty percent of children with high grade of VUR had lower urinary tract dysfunction by high bladder capacity and increased post-void residual urine(Sillén, Bradström et al. 2010)). Disorder of voiding can be categorized into the sequence of neurogenic abnormalities including spinal dysraphism with tethered cord syndrome, or cerebral palsy(Houle, Vernet et al. 1998; Rendeli, Ausili et al. 2007). In a series reported that urologic symptoms included VUR and renal failure were shown in 33% and 14% of children with spinal dysraphism after a long term follow-up (Silveri, Capitanucci et al. 1997). The non-neurogenic disorders affect the voiding function in children including posterior urethral valves, Hinmain's syndrome, prune belly syndrome(Chaichanamong Kol, Ikeda et al. 2008; Youssif, Dawood et al. 2009; Routh, Huang et al. 2010), which are highly associated with febrile UTI and chronic renal failure (Őborn and Herthelius 2010). The management of UTIs in children associated with voiding dysfunction is complex, the underlying disorders should be appraised when the symptoms are initially presented. The neurologic abnormalities or the urinary tract disorder required accurate evaluations and correction at different times in order to prevent irreversible damage of neurological and renal function.

6.3 Renal abscess

Perirenal or renal abscess and pyonephrosis are not common in UTIs of children, most occur in the urinary tract with obstruction, treatments depend on the individual scenario, subcutaneous drainage of the infection nidus under ultrasound or CT guide to preserve the kidney and antibiotics treatment is the main principle.

6.4 Correction of bowel habit

Several studies showed the relationship between bladder voiding and defecation in constipated children, urinary incontinence and UTIs are caused from the urinary outflow obstruction by bowel distention. Twenty nine to thirty four percent of children with chronic constipation or encopresis were associated with daytime or nighttime urinary incontinence, moreover, 11% of these children were present with UTIs. Interestingly, treatment of the underlying bowel disorders resulted in improving of urinary incontinence in 63-89% of patients and disappearance of recurrent UTIs in children who had no urinary tract abnormalities (Loening-Baucke 1997;Sureshkumar, Jones 2009).

6.5 Antibiotics treatment

The empirical treatment with ampicilline and gentamycin may be provided once the UTIs were diagnosed and may switch to an appropriate antibiotics when the definitive results of urine culture and sensitivities are available. For upper urinary tract infection, oral antibiotics are not inferior to the parenteral antibiotics, low resisted antibiotics such as cephalosporin is recommended with course for 7-10 days. Parenteral antibiotics can be used in cases of oral antibiotics cannot be used, ceftriaxone or cefataxime for 4-7 days, depends upon the responding of infection control. For lower urinary tract infection, amxocillin, cephalosporin, trimethoprim or nitrofurantoin may be used for 3-7 days. Prophylasis of antibiotics is not recommended for prevention of recurrent UTIs ,which may increase the risk of drug resistance (Hsu, Tan et al. 2010; Nicolau 2011).

6.6 Probiotics

Many experimental and clinical use of probiotics for inflammatory bowel disease with promising results has been extensively reported (Alfaleh, Anabrees et al. 2008; Hedin, Mullard et al. 2010). The application for urinary tract infection is increasing. Certain strains isolated from lactic acid bacteria demonstrated major antimicrobial activity against most of uropathogens in the pediatric urinary tract infection (Lim, Lee et al. 2009). Currently, the benefits for inhibition of UTIs varied according to the types of strains(Abad and Safda 2009), further research on different strains and clinical administration are needed to be ongoing.

7. Conclusion

The prompt diagnosis and treatment of UTIs are considered importantly to prevent subsequent renal damage, particular in very young children. In order to avoid unnecessary examinations or delay in treatment, the abnormalities associated with UTIs should be evaluated under suggested treatment algorithm or guidelines when the clinical manifestations are initially occurred. Although many treatment guidelines or recommendations have been established and need to be adjusted based on the most evidence or consensus, however, the treatment of UTIs in children can be simple or complex according to the scenario of individual.

8. References

(2007). National Collaborating Centre for Women's and Children's Health. Feverish illness in Children. Assement and initial management in children younger than 5 years. London, UK: National Institute for Health and Clinical Excellence. http://guidance.nice.org.uk/CG47.

Askari A, and Belman AB. (1982). "Vesicoureteral reflux in black girls". J Urol 127:747-748.

Ardissino G. Avolio L, Dacco V, Testa S. Marra G, Vigano S, et al. (2004). "Long-term outcome of vesicoureteral reflux associated chronic renal failure in children. Itakid Project." J Urol 172:305-310.

Alfaleh K, Anabrees J, Bassler D, Al-Kharfi T.(2008). "Probiotics for prevention of necrotizing enterocolitis in preterm infants." Update of Cochrance Database Syst Rev. CD005496:PHID:1825081.

Abad CL, and Safda N. (2009). "The role of lactobacillas probiotics in the treatment or prevention of urogenital infection - a systemic review." J Chemotherapy 21(3):243-252.

Brauner A, Boeufgras JM, Jacobson SH, Kaijser B, Kallenius G, Svenson SB. (1987). "The use of biochemical markers, serotype and fimbriation in the detection of *Escherichia coli* clones." J Gen Microbiol 133:2825-2834.

Craig JC, Irwig LM, Knight JF, Roy LP. (2000). "Does treatment of vesicoureteric reflux in children prevent end-stage renal disease attributable to reflux nephropathy?" Pediatrics 105:6:1236-1241.

Cendron M. (2008). "Reflux nephropathy." J Pedatr Urol 4:414-421.

Coulthard MG. (2008). "Is reflux nephropathy preventable,and will the NICE childhood UTI guidelines help?" Arch Dis Child. 93:196-199.

Chen HW, Yuan SSF, Lin CJ. (2004). "Ureteral reimplantation for vesicoureteral reflux: comparison of minimally invasive extravesical with transvesical and conventional extravesical techniques." Urology 63:364-368.

Chen JJ, Mao W, Homayoon K, Steinhardt GF. (2004). "A multivariate analysis of dysfunctional elimination syndrome and its vesicoureteral reflux in children." J Urol 171:1907-1910.

Chaichanamongkol V, Ikeda M, Ishikura K, Hamasaki Y, Hataya H, Satoh H, et al. (2008). "An infantile case of Himman syndrome with severe acute renal failure." Clin Exp Nephrol 12:4:309-311.

Dacher JN, and Savoye-Collet C. (2004). "Urinary tract infection and functional bladder sphincter disorders in children." Eur Radial 14:L101-106.

Downs SM. (1999). "Technical report: urinary tract infections in febrile infants and young children." The urinary tract subcommittee of the American academy of pediatrics committee on quality improvement. Pediatrics 103:4:e54.

Ford-Jones E, Mindorff C, Langley J, Allen U, Návás L, Patrick ML, et al. (1989). "Epidemiologic study of 4684 hospital-acquired infections in pediatric patients." Pediatr Infect Dis J 8:668-675.

Feldman AS, and Bauer SB. (2006). "Diagnosis and management of dysfunctional voiding." Curr Opin Pediatr 18:139-147.

Foxman B. (2002). "Epidemiology of urinary tract infections: incidence, morbidity, and economic costs." Am J Med 113:1A:5S-13S.

Fridman EP, de Bryn R, Mather S. (1993)." Pseudotumoral cystitis in children: a review of the ultrasound features in four cases." British J Radiology 66:787:605-608.

Gally DL, Bogan JA, Eisenstein BI, Blomfield IC. (1993). "Environmental regulation of the fim switch controlling type I fimbrial phase variation in Escherichia coli K-12: effects of temperature and media." J Bacteriol 175:19:6186-6193.

Greenfield SP. and Wan J. (1996). "Vesicoureteral reflux: Practical aspects of evaluation and management." Pediatr Nephrol 10:789-794.

Garin EH, Olavarria F, Garcia Nieto V, Valenciano B, Campos A, Young L.(2006). "Clinical significance of primary vesicoureteral reflux and urinary antibiotics prophylaxis after acute pyelonephritis: a multicenter, randomized, controlled study." Pediatrics 117:626-632.

Hellerstein S.(1982). "Recurrent urinary tract infections in children." Pediatr Infect Dis 1:4: 271-281.

Huang DTN, Huang FY, Tsai TC, Tsai JD, Chiu NC, Lin CC. (2007). "Clinical differentiation of acute pyelonephritis from lower urinary tract infection in children." J Microbiol Immunol Infect 40:513-537.

Hitzel A, Liard A, Vera P, Manrique A, Menard JF, Dacher JN. (2002). "Color and power Doppler sonography versus DMSA scintigraphy in acute pyelonephritis and in prediction of renal scarring." J Nucl Med 43:27-32.

Herz D, Merguerian P, McQuiston L, Danielson C, Gheen M, Brenflerk L. (2010). "5-year prospective results of Dimercapto-Succinic Acid Imaging in children with febrile urinary tract infection: Proof that the top-down approach works." J Urol 184:1703-1709.

Houle AM, Vernet O, Jednak VR, Pippi Salle JL. (1998). "Bladder function before and after selective dorsal rhiztomy in children with cerebral palsy." J Urol 160:1088-1091.

Hsu LY, Tan TY, Tam VH, Kwa A, Fisher DA, Koh TH. (2010). "Surveillance and correlation of antibiotic prescription and resistance of Gram-negative bacteria in singaporean hospitals." Antimicrobiol Agents & Chemotherapy 54:3:1173-1178.

Hedin CR, Mullard M, Sharratt E, Jansen C, Sanderson JD, Shirlaw P. et al. (2010). "Probiotic and prebiotic use in patients with inflammatory bowel disease: a case-control study." Inflammatory Bowel Disease16(12):2099-2108.

Johnson JR. (1991). "'Virulence factors in Escherichia coli urinary tract infection." Clin Microbiol Rev 4:1:80-128.

Karoly E, Fekete A, Banki NF, Szebeni B, Vannay A, Szabo AJ. et al. (2007). " Heat shock protein 72 (HSPA1B) gene polymorphism and toll-like receptor (TLR) 4 mutation are associated with increased risk of urinary tract infection in children." Pediatr Res 61:371-374. .

Kavanagh E. Ryan S. Awan A.McCourbrey S, O'Connor R, Donoghue V. (2005). "Can MRI replace DMSA in the detection of renal parenchymal defect in children with urinary tract infection?" Pediatr Radiol 35:275-281.

Klar A, Hurvitz H, Berkuny, Nadjari M, Blinder G, Israeli T. (1996). "Focal bacterial nephritis in children." J Pediatr 128:6:850-853.

Kennedy KM, Glynn LG, Dineen B.(2010)." A survey of the management of urinary tract infection in children in primary care and comparision with the NICE guidelines." BMC Family Practice 11:6:

Kundson MJ, Austin JC, McMilan ZM, Hawtrey CE, Cooperes CS. (2007). "Predictive factors of early spontaneous resolution in children with primary vesicoureteral reflux." J Uro 178:1684-1688.

Levitchenko EN, Lahy C, Lévy J, Ham HR, Piepsz A. (2001). "Role of Tc-99m DMSA scintigraphy in the diagnosis of culture negative pyelonephritis." Pediatr Nephrol 16:503-506.

Lonergan GJ, Pennington DJ, Morrison JC, Haw RM, Grimley MS, Kao TC. (1998). "Childhood pyelonephritis: comparison of gadolinium enhanced MR imaging and renal cortical scintigraphy for diagnosis." Radiology 207:377-384.

Langley JM, Hanakowski M, Le Blanc JC. (2001). "Unique epidemiology of nosocomial urinary tract infection in children." Am J Infect Control 29:94-98.

Lakshmanan Y, and Fung LC. (2000). "Laparoscopic extravesicular ureteral reimplantation for vesicoureteral reflux: recent technical advances." J Endourol 14:7:589-593.

Loening-Baucke V. (1997). "Urinary incontinence and urinary tract infection and their resolution with treatment of chronic constipation of childhood." Pediatr 100:2:228-232.

Lim IS, Lee HS, Kim WY. (2009). "The effect of latic acid bacteria isolates on the urinary tract pathogens to infants in vitro." J Korean Medical Science 24:557-562.

Matsuoka H, Nakashima Y, Oshima K. (2006). "Prognostic significance of the number of renal glomeruli in reflux nephropathy." BJU International 98:172-176.

Naber K, Bergman B, Bishop MC, et al. (2001). "Guidelines on urinary and male genital tract infections." Amhem. The Netherlands: European Association of Urology.

Nicolau DP. (2011). "Current challenges in the management of the infected patient." Curr Opin Infect Dis. 24:1:S1-10.

Nikfar R, Khotaee G, Ataee N, Shams S. (2010)." Usefullness of procalcitonin rapid test for the diagnosis of acute pyelonephritis in children in the emergency department". Pediatr International 52:2:196-198.

Olianti C. Imperiale A, Materassi M, Seracini D, Ienuso R, Pupi A, La Cava G, Tommasi M. (2004). "Urinary endothelin-1 excretion according to morpho-functional damage lateralization in reflux nephropathy." Nephrol Dial Transplant 19:1774-1778.

Orrett F, Brooks P, Richardson E, Mohammed S. (1999). "Pediatric nosocomial urinary tract infection at a regional hospital." Int Urol Nephrol 31:173-179.

Őborn H and Herthelius M. (2010). "Lower urinary tract symptoms in children and adolescents with chronic renal failure." J Urol 183:312-316.

Parrex P, Willi JP, Kossovsky MP, Girardin E. (2008). "Longitudinal analyses of renal lesions due to acute pyelonephritis in children and their impact on renal growth." J Urol 180:6:2602-2606.

Piepsz A, Colarinha P, Gordon I, Hahn K, Olivier P, Roca I.et al. (2001). Paediatric Committee of the European Association of Nuclear Medicine. "Guidelines for 99 mTc-DMSA scintigraphy in children." Eur J Nucl Med 28:3:37-41.

Preda I, Jodal U, Sixt R, Stokland E, Hansson S. (2011). "Imaging strategy for infants with urinary tract infection: a new algorithm." J Urol 185:1046-1052.

Prelog M, Schieficker D, Fille M, Brunner A, Zimmerhackl LB. (2007). "Acute nosocomial urinary tract infection in children." Infect Control Hosp Epidemiol 28:1019-1023.

Rathore NH, Barton LL, Luisiri A. (1991). "Acute lobar nephronia: a review." Pediatrics 87:728-734.

Routh JC, Inman BA, Reinberg Y. (2010). "Dextranomer/hyaluronic acid for pediatric vesicoureteral reflux: systemic review." Pediatrics 125:5:1010-1019.

Rendeli C, Ausili E, Tabacco F, Focarelli B, Massimi L, Caldarelli M. et al. (2007). "Urodynamic evaluation in children with lipomeningocele: Timing for neurosurgery, spinal cord tethering and follow-up." J Urol 177:2319-2324.

Rosenberg HK, Eggli KD, Zerin JM, Ortega W, Wallach MT, Kolberg,et al. (1994). "Begnin cystitis in children mimicking rhadomyosarcoma. J Ultrasound in medicine." 13:2:921-932.

Routh JC, Huang L, Retik AB, Nelson CP. (2010). "Contemporary epidemiology and characterization of newborn males with prune belly syndrome." Urology 76(1): 44-48.

Riccabona M, and Fotter R. (2009). "Urinary tract imaging in infants." Pediatr Radiol 39:3:436-445.

Sureshkumar P, Jones M, Cumming R G and Craig JC. (2009). "Risk factors for urinary tract infection in children: a population-based study of 2856 children." J of Paediatrics and Child Health 45:87-97.

Smellie JM, Normand ICS, Katz G. (1981). "Children with urinary infection: a comparison of those with and those without vesicoureteral reflux." Kidney Int 20:6:717-722.

Sillén U, Bradström P, Jodal U. Holmdahl G, Sandin A, Sjöberg Z, Hansson S. (2010). "The Swedish reflux trial in chilfen:v. Bladder dysfunction" J Urol 184:298-230.

Silveri M, Capitanucci ML, Capozza N, Mosiello G. Silvano A, De Gennaro M. (1997). "Occult spinal dysraphism: neurogenic voiding dysfunction and long-term urologic follow-up." Pediatr Surg Int 12:148-150.

Siomou E, Girapros V, Fotopoulos A, Aasioti M, Papadopoulou F, Serbis A.et al. (2009). "Implications of 99mTc-DMSA scintigraphy performed during urinary tract infection in neonates." Pediatrics 124:3:881-887.

Thomas MAJ, Wiswell MC, John LTC, Roscelli MC. (1986)." Corolorative evidence for the decreased incidence of urinary tract infections in circumcised male infants". Pediatr 78:1:96-99.

Uehling DT, Hahnfeld LE, Scanlan KA. (2000). "Urinary tract abnormalities in children with acute focal bacterial nephritis." BJU International 85:885-888.

Wheeler D, Vimalachandra D, Hodson EM, Roy LP, Smith G, Craig JC. (2003). "Antibiotics and surgery for vesicoureteral reflux: a meta-analysis of randomized controlled trials." Arch Dis Child 88:688-694.

Weber J. Sheridan R, Pasternack M, Tompkins R. (1997). "Nosocomial infections in patients with burns." AJIC Am J Infect Control 25:195-201.

Whelan CM, and McKenna PH. (2004). "Dysfunctional voiding as a co-factor of recurrent UTI." Contemp Urol. 16:58-73.

Yabel Y, Berdeli A, Mir S. (2007)." Association of TLR2 gene Arg753Gln polymorphism with urinary tract infection in children." International J Immunogenetics 34:399-405.

Youssif M, Dawood W, Shabaan S, Mokhless Z, Hanno A. (2009). "Early valve ablation can decrease the incidence of bladder dysfunction in boys with posterior urethral valves." J Urol 182(4):1765-1768.

Zamir G, Sakran W, Horowitz Y, Koren A, Miron D. (2004). "Urinary tract infection: is there a need for routine renal ultrasonography?" Arch D's Child 89:466-468.

Zaontz MR, Pahira JJ, Wolfman M, Gargurevich AJ, Zeman RK. (1985). "Acute focal bacterial nephritis: a systemic approach to diagnosis and treatment." J Urol 133: 752-757.